ON THE STANDARD NOMENCLATURE OF TRADITIONAL CHINESE MEDICINE

by Prof. Xie Zhufan

Foreign Languages Press   Beijing

First Edition   2003

Home Page:
http://www.flp.com.cn
E-mail Addresses:
info@flp.com.cn
sales@flp.com.cn

ISBN 7-119-03339-5

© Foreign Languages Press, Beijing, 2003

Published by Foreign Languages Press
24 Baiwanzhuang Road, Beijing 100037, China

Distributed by China International Book Trading Corporation
35 Chegongzhuang Xilu, Beijing 100044, China
P.O. Box 399, Beijing, China

Printed in the People's Republic of China

CONTENTS

FOREWORD

Any scientific discipline should have its special terminology. Traditional Chinese medicine (TCM) is no exception. The nomenclature of TCM was first established in the *Canon of Medicine* or even in earlier writings that are no longer extant. Over many centuries, TCM's technical vocabulary has been increased, and is familiar to Chinese medical circles. An integral system of TCM nomenclature in Chinese has existed for many years.

In recent decades, TCM has been introduced to the Western world and aroused extensive interest because of its holistic and natural approaches to healing. However, owing to the cultural gap and language barriers between the East and the West, the rendering of the technical terms of TCM into English is still in an unsettled state. One Chinese medical term often has several or even many different renderings, while the same English term may refer to different Chinese concepts. This certainly greatly hampers normal international exchanges. Both the writers (or translators) and the readers are anxious to have the international TCM terms standardized.

The author of this book, Prof. Xie Zhu-fan, has been engaged in the translation of TCM terms and writing TCM books in English for more than 20 years. To solve the above-mentioned problem, he collected a considerable amount of recently published TCM books written in English, including almost all the influential textbooks, monographs and Chinese-English TCM dictionaries, made a comparative study of the different renderings of each commonly used term in these books, and selected the most appropriate expression as the proposed standard. The comparative study was performed from various angles. First of all, the English expression had to accurately and precisely reflect the Chinese original. Secondly, the available terms were studied and compared from the grammatical, philological and etymological perspectives. Thirdly, among the qualified equivalents selection was made according to the frequency of use. The term used by more authors was considered preferable. Lastly, the expressions proposed as the standard were carefully examined from the viewpoint of Western medicine, so as to avoid either using the same wording for different concepts in Chinese and Western medicine or offering different expressions for the same phenomenon in the two systems of medicine. Furthermore, the proposed standard terminology had to meet the basic requirements of scientific nomenclature.

The rhetorical components in Chinese terms with no substantial significance have been omitted from the proposed standard. So, such a comparative study was a complex work; it needed a wide and sound knowledge of Chinese medicine, Western medicine, the English language, the classical Chinese language and Chinese history.

In his discussions, Prof. Xie gives the necessary explanations for the appropriate English equivalents to facilitate their general acceptance as the proposed standard, and makes comments on the inappropriate expressions to prevent their further use and their further causing of misunderstanding. Since the majority of the terms selected as the proposed standard are based not only on accuracy and preciseness, but also on the frequency of use (the number of users), they are likely to be generally accepted. The comments made on inappropriate expressions play an even more important role in the proposed standardization. From these comments readers can learn much about Chinese medicine, the Chinese language, and sometimes Western medicine as well. Through his discussions, Prof. Xie makes great efforts to promote cultural exchanges between the East and the West, to clear up misunderstandings resulting from seemingly literal translation without a real understanding of the Chinese medical terms (including a proper understanding of the related Chinese characters). Therefore, the scope of this book is not confined to the proposal of standard TCM nomenclature; it is actually a collection of discussions on the unique and difficult points of TCM. I believe that this book will make important contributions to the formulation of a formally recognized standard international nomenclature of TCM. In addition, readers will acquire a lot of interesting knowledge that is not easily found, or is even neglected, in standard TCM books.

Prof. Han Qide
Academician of the Chinese Academy of Sciences;
President of the Peking University Health Science Center;
Executive Vice-President of Peking University; and
Vice-Chairman of the Standing Committee of the National
People's Congress, P.R. China

July, 2003

INTRODUCTION

Since the introduction of acupuncture to the American and European countries in the 1970s, the interest in traditional Chinese medicine (TCM) has been growing rapidly all over the world. As English is a generally recognized international language, dozens of TCM textbooks have been published in English, hundreds of seminars and conferences on TCM have been held with English as the formal language, and thousands of papers, pamphlets and popular readings written in English have come into being. Most of the technical terms used in these publications and verbal communications are translations of Chinese terms. Owing to the archaic Chinese language used in traditional medicine, as well as the abstruse ancient philosophical thinking and the unique cultural background, translation of traditional Chinese medical terms is an extremely difficult task, and the majority of the terms are translated in several or many different ways by different authors. The confusion of terms greatly hampers the correct understanding of TCM by Westerners, and so the need for TCM nomenclature to be internationalized and standardized is pressing. Such uniformity will greatly facilitate teaching, practice, research and information exchange.

In order to formulate an internationalized and standardized TCM nomenclature, it is neither necessary nor reasonable to initiate or create a new series of English translations, for many forerunners have already made great efforts and significant contributions in this field. It is possible to formulate standard TCM nomenclature on the basis of the terms now available. The major task at present is to do a comparative study of the various renderings appearing in the recent English TCM publications and select the appropriate terminology as the standard. Since most of the terms thus selected have been used by the majority of authors, these terms are apt to be generally accepted. On the other hand, some individual authors have made brilliant suggestions on certain terms. Careful analysis and comparison with other expressions may further expose the advantages of making these suggestions more acceptable.

BRIEF HISTORICAL REVIEW OF TCM TERMINOLOGY

A historical review made by Paul U. Unschuld showed that translation of Chinese medical works into Western languages can be dated back more than three hundred years.[1] In 1682, Andreas Cleyer published, in Frankfurt, a Latin version of the Mai Jue (脈訣), a treatise on pulse diagnosis. Thereafter, a number of Chinese medical works, such as Nan Jing (難經, *Classic of Difficult Issues*)，Bin Hu Mai Xue (瀕湖脈學, *Binhu's Sphygmology*), Yin Hai Jing Wei (銀海精微, *Essentials of Ophthalmology*) and Zhen Jiu Jia Yi Jing (針灸甲乙經, *Systematic Classic of Acupuncture and Moxibustion*) were translated into German or French. Ben Cao Gang Mu (本草綱目，*Compendium of Materia Medica*) was partly translated into English, German, French and Latin. In the early twentieth century, William R. Morse, dean of the Medical School and head of the Department of Anatomy and associate in surgery, West China Union University, translated part of the Yi Zong Jin Jian (醫宗金鑒, *the Golden Mirror of Medicine*, 1742, the official textbook in the Qing Dynasty) into English[2]. The Huang Di Nei Jing (黃帝內經, *The Yellow Emperor's Internal Classic* or *Canon of Medicine*), the greatest medical classic extant in China, was partly translated into English by Ilza Veith and published in 1949, and a revised edition was published in 1966.[3, 4] Needless to say, all these works involved a lot of problems concerning the translation of Chinese medical terms, and every author had to make efforts to solve these problems. Besides the translation of classical TCM works, books written in English introducing Chinese medicine also appeared many years ago. For example, William R. Morse wrote a book titled *Chinese Medicine*, and published in 1934.

In the last two decades more efforts were made in this respect. More than a dozen Chinese-English TCM dictionaries have been compiled and published. In these dictionaries, each TCM term is taken as an entry, annotated and rendered into English. Most of the dictionaries include at least 5,000 entries, covering all the commonly used terms. Besides the compilation and publication of Chinese-English TCM dictionaries, quite a few classical TCM works have been rendered into English, including the Nan Jing (難經, *Classic of Difficult Issues*, 1986), Jin Gui Yao Lue Fang Lun (金匱要略方論, *Synopsis of Prescriptions of the Golden Chamber*, 1987),

Shang Han Lun (傷寒論, *Treatise on Febrile Diseases Caused by Cold*, 1993), Ling Shu (靈樞 *the Spiritual Pivot*, 1993), Pi Wei Lun (脾胃論 *Treatise on the Spleen and Stomach*, 1993) and the full text of the Huang Di Nei Jing (*Yellow Emperor's Canon of Internal Medicine*, 1997). Meanwhile, special symposia or conferences on TCM terminologies were conducted. For example, in 1986 an international symposium on translation methodologies and terminologies was conducted in Munich under the auspices of the International Association for the Study of Traditional Asian Medicine. This symposium brought together, for the first time, Asian, European and American scholars working on the translation, editing, and analysis of ancient Chinese medical texts into contemporary languages. The participants presented many brilliant views and illustrative examples associated with terminological choices and basic translation methodologies, helpful for reaching a common understanding. However, the symposium was chiefly an exchange of experiences, and no concrete conclusions were reached.

The most fruitful meetings were organized by the World Health Organization (WHO). The WHO's initiative to stipulate standard acupuncture nomenclature began in 1980. Three working groups and one consultation meeting on the standardization of acupuncture nomenclature were organized by the WHO Regional Office for the Western Pacific in 1982, 1984, 1985 and 1987, respectively. Afterwards, a WHO scientific group meeting was held in Geneva in 1989 and *A Proposed Standard International Acupuncture Nomenclature* was published in 1991 as the report of the scientific group. In the same year, the WHO Regional Office for the Western Pacific published *Standard Acupuncture Nomenclature (Revised Edition)*. Although the standard nomenclature is confined to a limited number of acupuncture terms and the related names of internal organs, it indicates that a consensus on the standardization of English TCM terminology can be reached after exchanges of views and careful discussion

GENERAL CONSIDERATIONS

From the above discussion we can see that there is already a sound base on which an international standard nomenclature of TCM can be preliminarily established. However, it is by no means an easy task to formulate a generally accepted standard nomenclature. The difficulty chiefly lies in the different cultural backgrounds of the East and West, and of ancient China and the modern Western world. Language barrier is one of the major reflections of different cultural backgrounds. Philosophical disparity plays a more important role. It makes the knowledge of TCM hardly be understandable from the Western perspective. Historical development has also had an impact on medical terminology. All these factors result in diversified renderings of TCM terms into English. Before starting a comparative study on the existing renderings, discussion of the following issues may be helpful. First of all, we must differentiate standard nomenclature in English from standardized translation. Although standard nomenclature of Chinese medicine should be based on the translation of the Chinese terms, they are two different affairs, and some difficulties in translation can be avoided in the nomenclature. Secondly, we have to distinguish professional technical terms from non-professional common terms. Not every word, phrase or sentence frequently encountered in the ancient and modern Chinese medical literature can be regarded as a technical term. Thirdly, standardization of the terms in Chinese is prerequisite for the standard nomenclature in English. The Chinese government and medical circles have made great efforts to standardize or unify the Chinese terminology of traditional medicine. Now, we are able to select the clinical terms from those approved by the Chinese government and the basic theoretical terms from the national Chinese textbooks. Fourthly, we should pay attention to the impact of the ancient Chinese type of writing on the medical terms. The standard nomenclature should fully reflect the unique features of Chinese medicine, but should get rid of purely linguistic influences, particularly the rhetoric influences that diversify the medical terms without academic or technical significance. Lastly, the most important issue is to define the basic requirements for the selection of standard nomenclature from the present terminologies appearing in recent publications. The standard nomenclature can only be established, provided that the terminologies precisely reflect the concept of Chinese medicine and at the same time are widely accepted through common practice.

DIFFERENCE BETWEEN STANDARDIZED TRANSLATION AND STANDARD NOMENCLATURE

Standardized translation and standard nomenclature of Chinese medicine in English differ in the source of terms and quantity of glossary.

Translation involves all the terms used in ancient and modern literature. Even the alternative names and euphemisms should also be considered. For example, lip is also called "flying door" (飛門 [féi mén]); head is also called "confluence of all yang meridians" (諸陽之會 [zhū yáng zhī huì]), and has a euphemistic name: "house of intelligence" (精明之府 [jīng míng zhī fǔ]). In the translation of Chinese medical literature, all these terms should be rendered into English differently from the basic terms "lip" and "head", but for the formulation of standard international nomenclature only "lip" and "head" are enough; it is unnecessary to take notice of the rest. This is because the standard nomenclature is prepared for those who wish to write papers and books by themselves. The writers should keep the terminology consistent throughout in order to avoid confusion.

More examples may further clarify this issue. The term 四診 [sì zhěn] is translated by different authors as "four diagnostics", "four techniques of diagnosis", "four diagnostic methods", "four methods of diagnosis", "four examinations", "four methods of examination", "four physical examinations", and "four methods of physical examination". In a word, the character 四 [sì] is translated as "four". No one can say that the translation is wrong, but the subsequent description will be baffling, for there are five examinations, namely, examinations through looking, listening, smelling, asking and touching. The Chinese character 聞 [wén] means realization either through listening or through smelling. There is neither such a concept nor such a word in the Western world. This is one of the cultural disparities between the East and West. In translation, we should not avoid the disparity, but in formulating the standard terminology, we are not at all obliged to solve this kind of problem, for it is not related to the medicine itself; it is purely a linguistic issue. There is no doubt that the correct translation is "four examinations", and what the translator can do is to explain why five categories of examination are called four examinations in an attached annotation. In the standard nomenclature, the problem can be easily solved: Delete the word "four" and simply call it "examinations".

In the translation of Chinese medical terms, some scholars have made great efforts to search for English equivalents of some polysemous characters that reflect ancient Chinese culture. For example, 青 [qīng] is a character that means the color of the east, i.e., spring. Since spring is the season when plants and trees (wood) start to grow, the color of seedlings and young leaves is designated 青 [qīng]. The normal color of the east is believed to be blue, but the young leaves and grass are green in color. In Chinese, the blue sky is called 青天 [qīng tiān], and green grass, 青草 [qīng cǎo], both attributed to 青 [qīng]. This puzzles many Westerners. According to the theory of the five elements, wood checks earth, and the color of earth is yellow. The seedling breaks through the soil in spring, so its color is intermingled with yellow, and becomes green[*]. That is why both blue and green are designated by the same character, 青 [qīng]. In addition, any color associated with blue can be called 青 [qīng]. In painting there are three basic colors: blue, yellow and red. Blue mixed with red is violet, and so violet belongs to 青 [qīng]. This is also true in English because another word for violet is bluish-purple. A mixture of all the three basic colors is black. and so 青 [qīng] may also refer to black, e.g., 青布 [qīng bù] "black cloth", and 青魚 [qīng yú] "black carp".

For the Chinese, there is no difficulty differentiating the meaning of the character 青 [qīng] in these commonly used words, but for the translators, it is impossible to find an English word exactly equivalent to such a polysemous character, even as far as only "blue" and "green" are concerned. To solve this problem, Nigel Wiseman and Paul Zmiewski proposed a rarely used or archaic English word that can be pressed into service and suggested the word cyan[5]. Unfortunately, this suggestion has not been widely accepted. English-speaking people are not familiar with this word, and from the dictionaries one can only find blue or dark blue (but not green) as its meaning. This kind of puzzling issue comes from the ancient cultural background, which exerted an impact on the development of Chinese medicine but no longer plays an important role in the present practice of Chinese medicine. For translation, it may cause difficulty, but for the formulation of standard nomenclature, it is unnecessary to consider such a puzzling way of wording.

DIFFERENCE BETWEEN MEDICAL TERMS AND COMMON WORDS

A medical term is a word or phrase used to designate some definite thing or phenomenon in medicine. Chinese medical literature first appeared two thousand years ago. At that time, owing to limitation of

---

[*]"青，東方色也。凡青之屬皆從青。" "五行之理，有相生者，有相尅者，相生爲正色，相尅爲間色。…綠者青黃之雜，以木尅土故也。"（說文解字義證）

material prerequisites (e.g., bamboo slips were used for writing), conciseness was highly advocated in writing. In such a style of writing, the sentences were usually short, often composed of 3 or 4 characters. Since these sentences have been repeatedly cited in later generations, many medical professionals may regard them as medical terms. For example, "腎主骨 [shèn zhǔ gǔ]" and "腎爲水臟 [shèn wéi shuǐ zàng]" are collected in the dictionaries as entries. They are actually two complete sentences. The first sentence is composed of a subject 腎 [shèn] (kidney), a transitive verb 主 [zhǔ] and an object 骨 [gǔ] (bone), and the second sentence, a subject 腎 [shèn] (kidney), a linking verb 爲 [wéi] and a predicate 水臟 [shuǐ zàng] (water viscus). The verb 主 [zhǔ] is a common word that is rendered by different authors as "govern", "manage", "control", "direct", "be in charge of", "take charge of", etc. No word is more common than 爲 [wéi], which is equivalent to the English verb "be". Among the various renderings of these two examples it is impractical and impossible to determine which rendering can be taken as a standard term, because none of them is really a medical term.

The following two examples may give a further illustration. 壯水之主，以制陽光 [zhuàng shuǐ zhī zhǔ, yǐ zhì yáng guāng] ("strengthen the mains of water to obstruct the bright sunshine") and 益火之源，以消陰翳 [yì huǒ zhī yuán, yǐ xiāo yīn yì] ("supplement the source of fire to remove the cloudy shades") are a pair of sentences that have been repeatedly cited in the Chinese medical literature because of the flowery language and matching words. They are two lines of exquisite verse, but neither the whole lines nor any of the component parts can be taken as medical terms. Even 水 [shuǐ], 火 [huǒ], 陰 [yīn], and 陽 [yáng] are used as words with double meanings. They express the principle of treating exuberant yang by replenishing yin and treating excessive yin by reinforcing yang in a lively, metaphorical way.

In conclusion, when we try to formulate a standard TCM nomenclature in English, we have to select the technical terms and exclude the common words and expressions.

DIFFERENTIATION OF CULTURE-SPECIFIC TERMS FROM GENERIC TERMS

At the International Symposium on Translation Methodologies and

Terminologies, 1986, Paul U. Unschuld made an impressive exposition on the translation of generic terms encountered in editing a commentated Nan-Ching (*Classic of Difficult Issues*, ca the first century A.D.). He proposed as a rule that generic terms should be rendered as generics. He gave examples to illustrate that many terms refer to generic phenomena, and are not culture-specific. It is perfectly justifiable to render the Chinese term 血 [xuè] into English as "blood", because both refer to the same substance. There is difference in conceptual interpretation between 血 [xuè] and blood, but "the conceptual interpretation of reality cannot be part of the translation of the generic term employed to designate this reality; otherwise, a translation would become unfeasible, if not impossible. Generic terms remain identical through the centuries and millennia, but the conceptual associations accompanying them may vary significantly in the course of time." If the reality should be designated differently to conform to different conceptual interpretations, Western physicians could not use the term "blood", as their concept of blood differs greatly from that of ordinary laymen.

Unschuld applied the same argument to all instances in which designations of real anatomical facts have to be rendered into English, and showed ample evidence that the organs lungs, heart, spleen, liver and kidneys were known as real, tangible entities. He further expounded that the *Canon of Medicine* and the *Classic of Difficult Issues* appear to have differed in their respective uses of the term 腎 [shèn]. "If we insist on interpretational rendering reflecting the different meanings of 腎 [shèn] in these two texts, we will find two different target terms for our translation."[6]

In fact, we can extend this argument to other generic phenomena. The terms designating symptoms are usually not culture-specific. Except for some metaphorical expressions, for most of these terms English equivalents can be found. The major problem is whether the equivalents are standard terms. In this connection, the recent edition of the WHO's *International Classification of Diseases*, 1998, (ICD-10) can be taken as the guide to standardization. For example, 納呆 [nà dāi] is rendered as "anorexia", "want of appetite", "poor appetite", "loss of appetite", and "torpid intake" by different authors. All these expressions can reflect the concept of the Chinese medical term. According to the frequency of usage, particularly according to ICD-10, "anorexia" (R63.0 in ICD-10) is selected. Anorexia is loss of appetite, and 納呆 [nà dāi] is also loss of appetite. We do not think there is difference between the Chinese loss of appetite and the Western loss of appetite. Dispute can thus be avoided, as the words and terms used in ICD are generally recognized as standardized.

Similarly, the above-mentioned argument can be applied to most disease names. In fact, Chinese medical professionals have already realized the disadvantages of the terminological gap in the respect of disease names between traditional Chinese medicine and modern Western medicine. Traditional Chinese orthopedists pioneering the modernization of disease names have replaced all the orthopedic disease names with the terms used in modern Western medicine. In other branches of clinical medicine, although traditional disease names are partially retained, the corresponding names used in modern Western medicine are clearly labeled in Chinese textbooks. For example, "丹痧 [dān shā] ('red rash') is also called 喉痧 [hóu shā] ('throat rash'), 疫痧 [yì shā] ('epidemic rash'), and 爛喉丹痧 [làn hóu dān shā] ('red rash with putrefying throat'). This disease is called 猩紅熱 [xīng hóng rè] ("scarlet fever" or "scarlatina") in Western medicine."* Apparently, it is unnecessary to use any literal translation of the traditional terms as the standard nomenclature. As for the selection between "scarlet fever" and "scarlatina", the latter is a better choice because it tallies with ICD-10 (A38); in addition, it also fits well the original Chinese term 丹痧 [dān shā] literally.

STANDARDIZATION OF TCM NOMENCLATURE IN CHINESE

In the Chinese medical literature it is not rare to encounter one thing designated with multiple names. For example, 水瀉 [shuǐ xiè] (watery diarrhea) is also called 水泄 [shuǐ xiè] (watery discharge), 注泄 [zhù xiè] (pouring discharge), 泄注 [xiè zhù] (discharging-pouring), 注下 [zhù xià] (pouring downward). Even such a simple term for a common symptom has so many designations, and each designation can be rendered into English in its own way of wording. This will certainly cause a lot of difficulties in the standardization of English nomenclature.

---

*"丹痧又称喉痧、疫痧、爛喉丹痧。本病西醫學稱猩紅熱。" cited from Zhong Yi Er Ke Xue (*Traditional Chinese Pediatrics*) (in Chinese), the Textbooks Series for Programmed Courses of the TCM Universities and Colleges, Shanghai Science and Technology Press, 1997, p.126.

In the past decade the Chinese government has paid great attention to the standardization of Chinese TCM terminology, not only for academic needs but also for practical use. In 1994, the State Administration of Traditional Chinese Medicine of the P.R. China promulgated *Criteria of Diagnosis and Therapeutic Effect of Diseases and Syndromes in Traditional Chinese Medicine* (in Chinese, with English translation of disease names attached to the text) as a professional TCM standard work. In this document, 400 standardized disease names are collected, and many irregular disease names are discarded.

In 1997, the State Technology Supervision Bureau of the P.R.C. issued a series called *Clinical Terminology of Traditional Chinese Medical Diagnosis and Treatment*. The series is in three parts: syndromes (800 entries); diseases (930 entries); and therapeutic methods (1050 entries). They are written in Chinese with no English equivalents. These documents cover all of the common clinical terms of TCM.

As for the basic theoretical terms of TCM, the normal terms (if not formally standardized) can be found in the recent editions of national Chinese textbooks. Since 1992, a series of textbooks for programmed courses of higher TCM education has been compiled and published. In these textbooks special attention is paid to the terminology. For example, in one of the serial textbooks, *Diagnostics of Traditional Chinese Medicine* (in Chinese), 1998, a special section discusses the concept of the terms 病 [bìng] (disease), 症 [zhèng] (symptom) and 證 [zhèng] (syndrome or pattern), as well as the classification and nomenclature of diseases. In *Fundamental Theories of Traditional Chinese Medicine* (in Chinese), 1995, the terms used are carefully selected, and in many sections the text starts by defining the related terms.

In short, we now have adequate sources for the selection of standard TCM terms in Chinese.

THE IMPACT OF ANCIENT WRITINGS ON TCM TERMINOLOGY IN CHINESE

The creation of Chinese medical terms was greatly influenced by the style of writing prevalent in different historical periods. Most terms associated with the fundamental theories were formed at the very beginning, when the theoretical system of Chinese medicine was first established, i.e., during the period when the *Internal Classic* (also called the *Canon of Medicine*) was compiled in the 3rd–5th centuries B.C. In that period, the written Chinese language was characterized by primitive simplicity. This was closely related to the level of technology. Since paper had not been invented, and bamboo slips were used, there was great limitation on writing and a piece of writing had to be as short as possible. Thus, medical terms formed during and before that time were mostly single-charactered.

Owing to the limitation of pictographic characters, the measures adopted to meet the increasing needs for representing concepts were chiefly extension of the meaning and phonetic loan. Both made the characters polysemous, with big changes of meaning at different historical periods. That is why annotations and commentaries are usually necessary for classical works, and different commentators may have different opinions on the same character or medical term. For example, the character 後 [hòu] has the following meanings in common language: (1) posterior (in opposition to anterior – 前 [qián]), (2) late (in opposition to early – 先 [xiān]), (3) descendant, (4) behind, and (5) an interjection. When this character is used in Chinese medicine, its meaning is further extended, including (1) defecation[*], (2) anus[**] and (3) absence of response[***]. Some of the meanings fell out of use later, but some are still in use at present, such as 裏急後重 [lǐ jí hòu zhòng], in which 後 [hòu] refers to the anus. Because of the polysemy of the characters, single-charactered terms often caused confusion and were gradually replaced by double-charactered terms. For example, the character 飲 [yǐn] is commonly encountered in Chinese medicine either as a noun or as a verb. As a noun, it is used in medicine with several specific meanings: (1) a collective term for food and drink, (2) decoction taken cold, and (3) a morbid condition characterized by retention of fluid. Use of the single character 飲 [yǐn] not only causes confusion with its ordinary meaning (drinking or beverage) in

---

[*]"得後與氣則快然如衰。" (素問·脈解篇) "The patient will feel very comfortable when loosening the bowels and breaking wind." (*Plain Questions*: Chapter 49)

[**]"裏急後重" (難經·五十七難) means "abdominal urgency and anal heaviness", i.e., tenesmus. (*Classic of Difficult Issues*: Item 57)

[***]"一候後則病, 二候後則病甚, 三候後則病危。" (素問·三部九候論) "If one subdivision (of pulse taking) has no response, it is a symptom of disease; when two subdivisions are not responding, the disease is serious, when three subdivisions are not responding, the patient is in danger." (*Plain Questions*: Chapter 20)

common language, but it is also difficult to determine its specific meaning as a medical term. Therefore, the single-charactered term 飲 [yǐn] in the first sense has been replaced by 飲食 [yǐn shí] (food and drink, or diet), the term in the second sense by 飲子 [yǐn zi] (cold decoction), and the term in the third sense by 飲證 [yǐn zhèng] (retained-fluid syndrome). However, the ancient terms are still well kept in modern literature, and the statements in the classics using the ancient terms are often cited. In translation, this will lead to a lot of difficulties, for the translator has to determine the exact meaning of a single-charactered term, usually from the context. For the formulation of a standard English term, this problem can be easily solved by avoiding polysemous Chinese words.

In contrast to simplicity, the use of excessive modifiers in the terms is also a puzzle. In the second and third centuries, along with the invention of paper, the prevalent writing style in China underwent great changes. There emerged rhythmical prose characterized by parallelism and ornaments with sentences composed of four and six characters in alternation, which became more and more popular in later centuries. This certainly had a strong impact on the style of medical writings and the word building of medical terminologies. No more single-charactered terms were created, and few terms consisting of odd-numbered characters. If we make a comparison between the following two terms indicating mechanism of disease – 寒邪傷肺 [hán xié shāng fèi] ("pathogenic cold damaging the lungs") and 寒滯肝脈 [hán zhì gān mài] ("cold stagnating in liver vessel"), we can clearly see that the addition or subtraction of the character 邪 [xié] simply depends on the total number of characters in the term. In the first term, if we simply say 寒傷肺 [hán shāng fèi] ("cold damaging the lungs") with deletion of the word 邪 [xié] ("pathogenic"), it is clear enough, as cold that damages the lungs must be pathogenic. In the second term, if we say 寒邪滯肝脈 [hán xié zhì gān mài] ("pathogenic cold stagnating in the liver vessel"), we do not make any mistake because the cold that stagnates is bound to be pathogenic. Neither 寒傷肺 [hán shāng fèi] nor 寒邪滯肝脈 [hán xié zhì gān mài] can be accepted as Chinese medical terms, simply because it goes against the customs of writing. To date, such an influence still exists. In the *State Standard of P.R. China: Clinical Terminology of Traditional Chinese Medical Diagnosis and Treatment* (in Chinese), 1997, 寒邪犯胃 [hán xié fàn wèi] ("pathogenic cold invading the stomach") and 寒滯胃脘 [hán zhì wèi wǎn] ("cold stagnating in the stomach cavity") are listed as synonyms. In the two terms, there is practically no difference between 寒邪 [hán xié] and 寒 [hán], and between 胃 [wèi] and 胃脘 [wèi wǎn]. The only difference is the number of characters[*]. Whether all the characters should be expressed in English is an issue of translation, but in the formulation of standard English nomenclature it is not at all necessary to follow the modifications made according to the rules of Chinese prose writing. The important factors for the word building of technical terms used in medicine are their academic and scientific qualities as well as correctness, accuracy and succinctness. If any rhetorical modification is needed, it should follow English usage, and not Chinese usage, particularly not the rules of Chinese rhythmical prose.

Another problem related to writing style is the omission of the so-called "function word" (roughly equivalent to preposition or conjunction in English). This is particularly common in the terminologies of treatment principles or therapeutic methods. The basic terms in this category are usually composed of a transitive verb and its object, such as 清熱 [qīng rè] ("clear heat"), 化痰 [huà tán] ("resolve phlegm"), 活血 [huó xuè] ("activate blood"), 調經 [tiáo jīng] ("regulate menstruation"), 止血 [zhǐ xuè] ("stop bleeding"), and 定痛 [dìng tòng] ("relieve pain"). In most instances, complex phrases are used, each consisting of two basic terms, and in order to meet the requirements of rhythmical prose, the function word (character), as a rule, is omitted, for example, 清熱化痰 [qīng rè huà tán], 活血調經 [huó xuè tiáo jīng], and 止血定痛 [zhǐ xuè dìng tòng]. But without the function word it is difficult to determine the relationship between the two basic terms contained in the complex term, so that the latter may be defined in diverse ways by different authors. In fact, the relationships between the basic terms can be classified into three patterns. Pattern 1: The two basic terms are placed side by side. Pattern 2: The former is the means, and the latter the end. Pattern 3: The former is principal, and the latter subordinate. According to the explanation given in *The State Standard of P.R. China: Clinical Terminology of Traditional Chinese Medical Diagnosis and Treatment* (in Chinese) 1997,

---

[*]One may argue that 胃 and 胃脘 are not exactly the same. The former means "stomach" and the latter means "stomach cavity". It should be stressed that the entire system of Chinese medicine is not founded on a strictly anatomical basis. Both 寒邪犯胃 and 寒滯胃脘 can be abbreviated as 胃寒, but never abbreviated as 胃脘寒 to indicate the precise anatomical location. So, even making an abbreviation is still guided by the rules of writing.

the term 清熱化痰 [qīng rè huà tán] is defined as "treatment by using heat-clearing and phlegm-resolving drugs"*, and so it belongs to pattern 1, and its proper translation is "clear heat and resolve phlegm"; the term 活血調經 [huó xuè tiáo jīng] is defined as "regulation of the menstruation by means of activating blood and *qi* flow"**, so it belongs to pattern 2, and its proper translation is "activate blood to regulate menstruation"; the term 止血定痛 [zhǐ xuè dìng tòng] is defined as "hemostatic treatment as the principal and sedation and analgesia as the subordinate"***, so it belongs to pattern 3, and its proper translation is "stop bleeding as well as relieve pain". The above discussion is based on the definition given by the State Standard. No matter how authoritative the State Standard is, different opinions still exist because the wordings themselves are logically imperfect. Undoubtedly, if one administers blood-activating agents together with menstruation-regulating agents to treat a menstrual disorder, the treatment should also be called 活血調經 [huó xuè tiáo jīng]. In fact, the above expressions can easily be clarified by adding the function words 與 [yǔ] (and), 以 [yǐ] (to), and 及 [jí] (as well) to patterns 1, 2 and 3, respectively. Since the customary style of TCM writing rejects the insertion of function words between basic terms, the best way is to standardize the basic terms and leave their various combinations to be determined by the users. Many authors have already made translations in this way, for example, they translate 活血調經 [huó xuè tiáo jīng] as "activate blood, regulate menstruation" with no indication about the relationship between the two basic terms.

BASIC REQUIREMENTS FOR STANDARD NOMENCLATURE

We can make a long list of requirements for standardized TCM nomenclature, but in the final analysis any standard terminology must meet

---

*"清熱藥與祛痰藥並用" cited from 中華人民共和國國家標準·中醫臨床診斷術語－治法部分 (*The State Standard of P.R. China: Clinical Terminology of Traditional Chinese Medical Diagnosis and Treatment — Therapeutic Methods*) (in Chinese), 1997, p.32.

**"通過活血理氣以達調理月經目的" ditto, p.15.

***"以止血爲主，並兼鎮定止痛" ditto, p.15.

the following two basic requirements, i.e., correct reflection of the original Chinese concept and proper expression as medical terms in English.

No one will wonder that correct reflection of the original TCM concept is a prerequisite for standard terminology in English. However, many existing terms in English do not express the real concept of TCM, chiefly due to misunderstanding of the ancient Chinese language. Two trends of misunderstanding may occur. One is negligence of the real meaning of the character when the related medical term was initiated. The other is to take it for granted that the primary meaning of a character is always suitable for the rendering. These two trends are often closely related. Following are some examples.

Many authors render 苗竅 [miáo qiào] as "sprout and orifice". Literally, 苗 [miáo] means "a young plant, seedling or sprout", and 竅 [qiào], "an opening or orifice". The key question is the grammatical structure of the term. Unfortunately, many Chinese texts only give an explanation of each character, seldom indicating the grammar. This double-charactered term may have two possible constructions: one is coordinative, and the other subordinative. In TCM, the two characters 苗 [miáo] and 竅 [qiào] can be used separately, each showing a similar meaning. For example, 舌爲心之苗 [shé wéi xīn zhī miáo] (The tongue shows symptoms of the heart.) and 心開竅於舌 [xīn kāi qiào yū shé] (The heart opens into the tongue.) are practically the same. This may create a false impression that the term 苗竅 [miáo qiào] is composed of two synonyms in coordination.

This can be rejected by *reductio ad absurdum*. In TCM there are various designations containing the character 竅 [qiào] such as 心竅 [xīn qiào] (orifice of the heart), 肺竅 [fèi qiào] (orifice of the lung), 清竅 [qīng qiào] ("sense organs on the head" or "brain"), 精窍 [jīng qiào] ("orifice of the male urethra"), none of which is a coordinative compound. If 苗竅 [miáo qiào] were a coordinative compound, there would be a contradiction. 苗 [miáo] refers to the five sense organs while 竅 [qiào] refers to the five sense organs plus the external genitalia and anus. It is obviously illogical to put them together as coordinates.

Grammatically, 苗 [miáo] is an attributive of 竅 [qiào], and the two characters in combination form a compound noun, which means the orifice (or sense organ) that gives the symptom of a trend or suggests what is going to happen in the internal organs. Here, 苗 [miáo] more or less corresponds to the word 苗頭 [miáo tóu] (symptom of a trend).

Therefore, among the available renderings, "signal" is more appropriate than "sprout".

The character 真 [zhēn] is used in many TCM terms, but its meaning may vary. Because it means "true" in modern Chinese, many authors render it into English as "true". In the terms 真寒假熱 [zhēn hán jiǎ rè] ("true cold with false heat") and 真虛假實 [zhēn xū jiǎ shí] ("true deficiency with false excess"), 真 [zhēn] does mean "true". But these terms were initiated by Zhang Jing-yue and first appeared in Jing-Yue Quan Shu (*Jing-yue's Complete Works*, 1624). This character is a pictograph, resembling a vehicle. It was first created to signify the vehicle that bears the immortal being to heaven.* So, in the *Canon of Medicine* (written in the 3rd—5th centuries B.C.), the character 真 [zhēn] was used in a sense other than "true". For example, 真人 [zhēn rén] refers to one who has a full knowledge about the law of nature and behaves accordingly to enjoy longevity. 真氣 [zhēn qì] and 元氣 [yuán qì] are synonyms, both of which can be rendered as "original *qi*". 真氣 [zhēn qì] is the *qi* that exists from the beginning of one's life and may have some other categories of *qi* as its derivatives, but there is no "false *qi*" as its opposite.

The term 募穴 [mó xué] may serve as another example. In modern Chinese, the character 募 [mù] means "collect", for example, 募款 [mù kuǎn] means "to collect money", 募捐 [mù juān] means "to collect donations". Therefore, some authors translate 募穴 [mó xué] as "collecting points". The character 募 can also be written as 幕, which means "curtain", and so other authors render the term as "curtain points". But both renderings are hard to understand. As these points are the sites where the *qi* of *zang-fu* organs accumulates, some authors prefer the term "accumulation point". Again, this is not widely accepted, because there are many other points that should be regarded as the sites where the *qi* of *zang-fu* organs accumulates. Because of the difficulty in translation, many Chinese authors resort to *pinyin*, and suggest "*mu* points", but the *pinyin* name is not accepted by Westerners, for "mu" gives no information other than a sound. In addition, whether this character 募 should be pronounced as "mu" is open to question. According to the Ci Yuan (*Word Sources*), the most authoritative dictionary of classical Chinese, 1979, 募 in the term

---

*真，僊人變形而登天也。從匕從目從乚八，所乘載也。（說文解字）The character 真 [zhēn] refers to an immortal being changing its physical shape and going to heaven. In this character, the vehicle carrying the immortal to heaven is sketched. (*Analytical Dictionary of Characters*, 100 B.C.)

募穴 is in common with 膜 [mó], and both should be pronounced as "mó". Etymological study also shows that in TCM 募 is actually an alternative for the character 膜 [mó]. 膜原 [mó yuán] is also written as 募原 [mó yuán].

Besides literal translation, there are other approaches to achieving an equivalent in the target language. If an English word or phrase expresses the characteristic features of the Chinese term, it may also be an appropriate equivalent, even with no literal coincidence. 募穴 [mù [mó] xué] is a collective term for a group of points, each of which is situated close to a *zang* or *fu* organ, showing tenderness or other hypersensitive responses when the corresponding organ is diseased. Thus, some authors initiated a new name for these group points, viz "alarm points". This name is becoming more and more popular. Whether it can be taken as a standard translation is open to discussion, for some translators stick to the principle that a good translation must first of all accurately reflect the Chinese original literally, so that the terms in the source language and target language can be easily interchangeable. However, so far as the standard English terminology is concerned, the term "alarm points" is selected, for it provides more acceptable information than the others.

In this context, an important issue open to discussion is whether the English equivalents should always be word-to-word or word-to-character translation. It should be stressed that both the rendering of Chinese medical terms into English and the formulation of standard TCM terminology in English are scientific issues. The wording of Chinese TCM terms reflects Chinese culture, particularly ancient Chinese culture, including customs, social institutions, literature, etc., in addition to medicine. The appropriateness of TCM terms in English should be determined from the medical perspective, and not from the literary or other perspectives.

Of course, literal translation should also be considered. In this respect, etymological study of Chinese medical terms may be helpful. The basic characters are pictographic or ideographic. They often serve as the elements to form other categories of characters, such as associative compounds and pictophonetic characters. Associative compounds are formed by combining two or more elements, each with a meaning of its own, to create a new meaning. Pictophonetic characters are formed by combining two elements, with one element indicating meaning and the other sound. Incorrect etymological understanding of a character may lead to inappropriate translation of that character. For example, many characters with 疒 (which means disease or illness) as a basic structural element are sound-forming characters such as 疝 [shàn] and 痧 [shā]. In some recent publications they are translated as "mounting" and "sand" respectively. Apparently, they are mistaken as characters with a compound association of meanings，with the element 山 [shān] ("mount") and 沙 [shā] ("sand"). In fact, they are sound-forming characters, with 山 [shān] and 沙 [shā] providing the sound but not the meaning. According to the Shuo Wen Jie Zi (*Analytical Dictionary of Characters*, 100 B.C.), the earliest and most authoritative book on Chinese philology, 疝 [shàn], signifying "abdominal pain", is a pictophonetic character with the sound of 山 [shān]*. The translation of 痧 as "sand" is more inconceivable, because this character refers to an acute morbid condition characterized by vomiting and diarrhea accompanied by abdominal pain. As a popular name 痧 may refer to measles, still with nothing to do with sand.

PINYIN AND ROMANIZED CHINESE

One of the measures to solve the problems encountered in translating Chinese medical terms into English is the use of *pinyin*. It should be noted that *pinyin* is not translation, and in many instances nor is it transliteration. It just renders the pictographic Chinese into the Latin alphabet, i.e., Romanized Chinese. Strictly speaking, *pinyin* is not a language or a form of language; it is a phonetic transcription. The *pinyin* system was promulgated by the Chinese government in 1958 for the purpose of standardizing the pronunciation of Chinese characters and popularizing the common Chinese language. *Pinyin* can only be used for the pronunciation of the Chinese characters. Usually, it is only used together with Chinese characters as a phonetic attachment. In order to distinguish it from the alphabet used in some Western languages (including English) the printing model and typeface used for *pinyin* should be different. For example, the first vowel should be printed as "ɑ" but not "a", and the letter "ɡ" should not be printed as "g". The *pinyin* alphabet includes ê and ü. The pronunciation of the letters in the *pinyin* alphabet is also different from those used in English.

---

* "疝, 腹痛也。從疒, 山聲。" （說文解字） "疝" [shàn] is abdominal pain. It pertains to 疒 (illness) and is pronounced 山 [shān] (*Analytical Dictionary of Characters*)

Strictly speaking, the use of *pinyin* cannot be regarded as transliteration. To transliterate means "to represent, as a word, by the alphabetic characters of another language having the same sound"[*] In many instances, by *pinyin* one cannot achieve such a goal. Some Western authors put an attachment "(pronounced as chee)" or "(ch'i)" when they use the word *qi*, for instance.

Another problem is the presence of homonyms in TCM terms. Many Chinese medical terms difficult to render into English are monosyllabic words. Some of them are pronounced alike, for example, 正 [zhèng], 症 [zhèng], 證 [zhèng], and 癥 [zhēng]. In written language there is no difficulty in making the differentiation for they are printed in different shapes. But when they are printed in *pinyin*, no such differentiation can be made; even with the addition of tone symbols, the majority of them are still indistinguishable. Nevertheless, all the above four terms are commonly used in TCM and it is difficult to find an exact English equivalent for any of them. In 1995, the State Administration of Technical Supervision, P.R. China, issued a document entitled *Classification and Codes of Diseases and ZHENG of Traditional Chinese Medicine*, but two years later, in 1997, they changed the word ZHENG into Syndrome in the standard clinical terminology of TCM.

In recent TCM publications in English, *pinyin* is used in two categories of conditions: one is to deal with abstract or conceptual objects or ideas that cannot be satisfactorily expressed by corresponding English words or phrases, and the other is to deal with terms indicating actual things or events but with multiple inclusions, to which no single English word or phrase is equivalent. Yin, yang and *qi* belong to the first category. Since yin and yang have already been collected in the Oxford and Webster's English dictionaries, they can be taken as English words without hesitation. Divergence exists about the word "qi", but the majority of authors have accepted it. Beside "qi", *pinyin* is used as proposed standard terms only for proper nouns, weights and measures.

As for the terms of the second category, none of *pinyin* names are adopted in this scheme. Any terms designating actual things or events should have corresponding English equivalents unless they have never been known to or encountered by Westerners. Take disease names as an example. If a *pinyin* name is used to designate a disease, it makes an impression that that disease has never been known to Westerners, because

---

[*]Cited from *the New International Webster's Comprehensive Dictionary of English Language*, 2000, p.1334.

pinyin gives no information other than a sound that is entirely meaningless to Westerners who have no knowledge of the Chinese language.

ADOPTION OF THE WHO'S STANDARD ACUPUNCTURE NOMENCLATURE

Although the WHO's Standard Acupuncture Nomenclature, 1991, only contains the nomenclature of the 14 meridians, 361 classical acupuncture points, 8 extra meridians, 48 extra points, scalp acupuncture lines and a few related terms about needles, it took ten years and a considerable amount of funds to accomplish this work. Since its publication, it has been well received by many traditional (complementary or alternative) medical circles, particularly by the researchers, teachers and practitioners of acupuncture, and has made important contributions to teaching, research and clinical practice, as well as international exchanges of information on this subject. On the other hand, it proves the stipulation of English-language standard terms for international communication of TCM to be both necessary and possible.

In addition, the WHO's Standard Acupuncture Nomenclature has solved a knotty problem, i.e., the standardization of the names of the *zang-fu* organs. This problem has been discussed for many years with no definite conclusion. Because of the differences in knowledge about the functional activities of individual internal organs between traditional Chinese and modern Western medicine, how to designate these organs in English was an outstanding question. Manfred Porkert even initiated a set of Latin terms[7], but his estimable efforts were of no effect. Most English-speaking people have not been trained in Latin. To become familiar with such words as *orbes horreales* and *orbes aulici* is not easier than to learn the Chinese 臟 [zàng] and 腑 [fǔ]. More important, that rendering the Chinese terms into Latin gives no help for closing the cultural gap between the east and the west. The designation of the twelve regular meridians with ordinary English "heart", "lung", "spleen", etc., in the WHO's standard nomenclature naturally solved this problem, for the meridian names must indicate the corresponding internal organs. In the past two decades almost all authors have used these ordinary English words in their writings. Except for 三焦 [sān jiāo]*, the other eleven terms have been generally

---

*Some authors insist on using the term "triple burner" instead of "triple energizer".

accepted. This is a great achievement, for these terms are the very basic elements upon which rendering of hundreds of TCM terms covering all fields of Chinese medicine becomes feasible.

In this scheme of proposed standard nomenclature, the WHO's Standard Acupuncture Nomenclature will be strictly followed, even though some minor revisions are suggested.

USE OF WESTERN MEDICAL TERMS

Traditional Chinese medicine has many unique points conceptually different from modern Western medicine. For expressing this uniqueness, technical terms are indispensable, but merely by creating new terms we can hardly accomplish the task. In this respect, exposition is much more important. China's experience in introducing Western medicine may have some reference use. More than a century ago, when modern Western medicine was first introduced to China, Western missionaries tried to create many new Chinese characters, but none of them were accepted by the Chinese. By using the available characters, a number of Western medical terms were formulated in Chinese. Even ordinary Chinese people with a minimal medical knowledge find no difficulty in differentiating 肝炎 [gān yán] (hepatitis) of Western medicine from 肝火 [gān huǒ] (liver fire) or 肝火上炎 [gān huǒ shàng yán] (up-flaming of liver fire) of Chinese medicine, though the same character 肝 [gān] is used in the two terms. Chinese people also appreciate that 神經 [shēn jīng] refers to "nerve" but not "mentality" or "meridian".

In recent decades the trend of development of TCM in China is to get onto the common track with modern science. TCM is not an antique whose value relies on retaining all the old traditional features. It is a practical discipline of medicine that is useful for the health service at present. Both medical circles and the administrative institutions have devoted much attention to the modernization of TCM in order to meet the requirements of the modern health service. This certainly has had a great impact on terminology. For example, many diseases, though designated with traditional names, have been redefined with modern diagnostic cri-

---

The insistence is probably based on defective knowledge of Chinese philology. This term will be discussed in the next chapter.

teria and specified with the corresponding diagnosis in modern Western medicine. Under such conditions, it is impractical to stick to such traditional terms as "wasting-thirst" (消渴 [xiāo kě]) and "sudden turmoil" (霍亂 [huò luàn]) in this scheme, for determination of fasting blood sugar and glucose tolerance test have already been listed as the diagnostic criteria for the former, and the presence of *vibrio cholera* in the excreta for the latter.

Another important point that should be emphasized is the difference between the English-Chinese glossary and Chinese-English glossary. In the former, English terms are the primary entries, while the attached Chinese terms serve as the predicative, but in the latter the English terms are predicative. Generally speaking, the Chinese terms usually have wider connotations than the corresponding English terms. For example, 肌痹 [jī bì] is traditionally defined as obstruction of *qi*-blood flow in muscles, manifested by muscle pain associated with muscular weakness and wasting. According to modern Chinese standards, electromyographic changes such as low amplitude, shorter duration and polyphasic action potentials, fasciculation and persistent insertional activity are added to confirm the diagnosis of 肌痹 [jī bì][*]. Therefore, it might not be perfectly correct if we say 肌痹 [jī bì] is called polymyositis in Western medicine, as this conclusion excludes other possible diseases, but we ensure that polymyositis is called 肌痹 [jī bì] in TCM.

In short, the proper use of Western medical terms is necessary and may facilitate the correct understanding of TCM. Insisting on intentionally keeping TCM terminology apart from Western medical terms in every respect will make a false impression that TCM is an esoteric system of medicine

SUMMARY

As stated at the very beginning of this chapter, TCM terminology has been studied by many authors in their translation and writing of TCM textbooks and monographs. In addition, more than a dozen Chinese- English TCM dictionaries have come into being (some of which are also

---

[*]Professional TCM Standard of P.R. China: *Criteria of Diagnosis and Therapeutic Effect of Diseases and Syndromes in Traditional Chinese Medicine* (in Chinese), issued by the State Administration of Traditional Chinese Medicine, 1994, p.31.

English-Chinese TCM dictionaries). The key issue is how to unify the diversified opinions to achieve the standard nomenclature. The practical way is to collect the various expressions and select the most appropriate one through comparative study.

In 2000, we were sponsored by the State Administration of Traditional Chinese Medicine to do research on the the standard English translation of TCM terms. In the course of that research, we collected various translations of commonly used terms from recent publications. Among all the source literature, we paid more attention to dictionaries and books, because their authors and compilers usually gave comprehensive consideration to the terminological issue. Except for some distinguishing ideas on terminology, the terms used in English TCM journals published either in the East or in the West are generally not collected because the terms often vary in the same journal.

In 2002, the World Health Organization also asked us to contribute to the standard TCM nomenclature for international use. We further expanded the source references and re-examined the comparative studies. The final list of the source references is attached at the end of this book. We do not think that the proposed standard nomenclature in the scheme is ideal, but since most of the entries are in common with majority opinion, we hope this scheme can become the basis on which a formal standard nomenclature is established after revision. We also did our best to analyze the improper renderings that distort the original Chinese concepts, and hope that these expressions will no longer appear in publications.

REFERENCES

[1] Paul U. Unschuld (ed.) *Approaches to Traditional Chinese Literature*. Kluwer Academic Publishers, 1989; pp. ix–xix.

[2] William R. Morse. *Chinese Medicine*. Paul B Hoeber, Inc., New York, 1934, pp. xiii-xiv.

[3] Huang Ti Nei Ching Su Wen – *The Yellow Emperor's Classic of Internal Medicine,* translated by Ilza Veith. The Williams & Wilkins Company, 1949.

[4] Huang Ti Nei Ching Su Wen – *The Yellow Emperor's Classic of Internal Medicine*, translated by Ilza Veith. University of California Press, Berkeley and Los Angeles, 1966.

[5] Nigel Wiseman and Paul Zmiewski. Rectifying the names: Suggestions for Standardizing Chinese Medical Terminology. *Approaches to*

Traditional Chinese Literature. Kluwer Academic Publishers, 1989; pp. 55-66.

[6] Paul U. Unschuld. Terminological Problems Encountered and Experiences Gained in the Process of Editing a Commentated Nan-Ching Edition. *Approaches to Traditional Chinese Literature*. Kluwer Academic Publishers, 1989; pp. 100-102.

[7] Manfred Porkert. *Chinese Medicine*. William Morrow & Co., Inc. New York and Seattle, 1988.

FUNDAMENTAL THEORIES

PHILOSOPHICAL TERMS

Since traditional Chinese medicine was established and developed in the light of ancient Chinese natural philosophy, a number of philosophical terms are used for the exposition of basic medical theories. The related philosophical terms can be classified into three categories: theory of (essential) *qi*, theory of yin-yang, and theory of the five elements.

THEORY OF (ESSENTIAL) QI

This theory is an ancient Chinese philosophical concept, which explains the formation of the universe including all things, living and non-living, by an invisible substance called *qi*. The movement and transformation of *qi* causes all kinds of changes and the essential part of *qi* gives rise to life. The terms involved in this theory are mainly "essence", "*qi*", "vitality", "spirit", and "essential *qi*". The former three are collectively called the "three treasures". In addition, two more terms are closely related to this theory. They are "movement of *qi*" and "transformation of *qi*".

Proposed Standard Nomenclature

theory of essential *qi* 精氣學說 [jīng qì xué shuō][1]

theory of *qi* 氣論 [qì lùn][1]

qi 氣 [qì][3]

essence 精 [jīng][2]

essential *qi* 精氣 [jīng qì][5]

vitality 神 [shén][4]

ascending, descending, exiting, and entering 升降出入 [shēng jiàng chū rù][8]

spirit 精神 [jīng shén][6]

qi movement 氣機 [qì jī][7]

qi transformation 氣化 [qì huà][9]

Discussion

1. This theory is developed from the philosophical concept of *qi*, and the word "*qi*" alone is enough to express the whole picture of the theory. Probably there are two reasons to explain why this concept is called essential *qi* (精氣 [jīng qì]) instead of *qi*. In ancient China, Guan Zhong, a famous philosopher, discoursed on *qi* in terms of essence. According to his proposition, "so-called essence is the essential part of *qi*", and this part of *qi,* capable of moving and changing, is the fundamental substance that forms the universe and human beings. Traditional Chinese medicine did adopt this concept as one of the basic theories, but in the *Canon of Medicine (Internal Classic)* the term "essential *qi*" is only used in its narrow sense, referring to reproductive essence and nutritive essence, while the single character 氣 [qì] is used to represent the fundamental substance which forms the universe and human beings. In addition, the movement and change of this fundamental substance is called "transformation of *qi*" (氣化 [qì huà]) but not "transformation of essential *qi*" (精氣化 [jīng qì huà]).

It should be noticed that 精氣學說 [jīng qì xué shuō] is a modern term. The development of Chinese medical terms must follow the rules of the Chinese language. Most TCM terms in Chinese are customarily composed of even-numbered characters in order to avoid monosyllabic words that are not so kind to the ears and easily cause confusion. There is no problem in pronouncing "theory of *qi*" in English, but it will be difficult to pronounce and hear 氣學說 [qì xué shuō] in Chinese. In the Chinese national TCM textbooks, when theory of *qi* is talked about, the wording is changed to 氣論 [qì lùn]*. The latter is apparently not so smooth-reading as 精氣學說 [jīng qì xué shuō], but better than 氣學說 [qì xué shuō] in enunciation.

In conclusion, as a translation of the Chinese term, "theory of essential *qi*" is accurate, for it includes all the characters with no omission, but as an international standard term, "theory of *qi*" may be better, for it reflects a full view. In fact, English-speaking authors (but not translators) would rather use the term "theory of *qi*" than "theory of essential *qi*".

2. The term 精 [jīng] has a dual meaning: in the broad sense it refers

---

*Wu DX (chief editor). Zhong Yi Xue Ji Chu Li Lun, *Fundamental Theories of Traditional Chinese Medicine* (in Chinese), The Textbook Series for Programmed Courses of the TCM Universities and Colleges, Shanghai Science and Technology Press, 1995, p.38.

to the fundamental substance that constitutes the human body and maintains human life, and in the narrow sense it refers to the reproductive essence, particularly of the male (namely, semen). In the theory of *qi*, the word 精 [jīng] is used in its broad sense, and most authors take essence as its equivalent, while a few authors render it as "essence of life" or "vital essence".

3. *Qi* (氣 [qì]) is one of the most important concepts in Chinese medicine. It is a unique concept both philosophically and medically. How to express this important concept in English or other Western languages is an issue of dispute that has lasted for many years. Paul Unschuld made a historical review about the translation of this concept. In 1682, Andreas Cleyer used the Latin word *spiritus*, which was defined as subtle matter and immaterial substance, very close to the concept of *qi*. Afterwards, Western mainstream medicine turned its interest away from "vital spirit" to physical and chemical processes as the foundation of life, and the idea of *spiritus* soon became obsolete[*]. In this context, Unschuld emphasized the importance of terminology. Along with the discarding of the notion of *spiritus*, Cleyer's introduction of Chinese medicine as a system of ideas centered around a *spiritus* soon became an obsolete presentation, followed by lack of interest in Europe in this Asian health care system.

In recent decades, energy or vital energy has been used to represent the concept of *qi*, but it cannot cover all the major fields of the concept, particularly when the word *qi* refers to substance. Since *qi* is such an important concept in TCM and in Oriental culture as a whole, the use of romanized characters is generally agreed. Most authors use the *pinyin* scheme, but this scheme causes difficulty in pronunciation, because in English *q* is always followed by *u* and pronounced *kw*. Even in some foreign names such as Qishm, *qi* is pronounced as *ki*. Therefore, some authors express this term as *qi* (pronounced *chee* or *ch'i*). In the present scheme, *qi* (*ch'i*) is suggested when it first appears in writing, and then *qi* when it appears afterwards.

It should be noted that the character 氣 [qì] as a medical term is polysemous. The proposed standard term *qi* is only an equivalent (or a symbol) of the word in its philosophical sense. In 氣促 [qì cù] and 氣短 [qì duǎn], for example, the character 氣 [qì] is better rendered as "breathing" or "breath".

---

[*]Paul U. Unschuld (ed.) *Approaches to Traditional Chinese Literature*, Kluwer Academic Publishers, 1989; pp. ix–xix.

4. One of the three major components that form the theory of essential *qi* is the concept of 神 [shén]. The translation of 神 [shén] has aroused a lot of controversy. The word 精 [jīng] refers to the essential substance which produces life activities, and is therefore often rendered "vital essence" or simply "essence", while 神 [shén] is the manifestation or activity of the essence. As the essence has multifarious manifestations and activities, 神 [shén] may refer to (1) that which governs all life activities, either physiological or psychological, (2) the outer manifestation of all the vital energy, and (3) all kinds of mental activities including consciousness, thinking, feelings, etc. Therefore, different authors have suggested different equivalents, such as "spirit", "mind", "vitality", and "divinity". It is difficult to determine the standard translation of 神 [shén], but the problem can be solved in the reverse way: it is feasible to determine the Chinese equivalent of the English terms. Although all of them can be rendered as 神 [shén], their difference in meaning can be easily shown by using a compound word derived from this character: vitality – 神 [shén] in its most general sense, spirit – 神 [shén] as an abbreviation of 精神 [jīng shén], mind – 神 [shén] as an abbreviation of 心神 [xīn shén], mentality – 神 [shén] as an abbreviation of 神明 [shén míng], consciousness – 神 [shén] as an abbreviation of 神志 [shén zhì]. Giovanni Maciocia made a brilliant exposition on the translation of 神 [shén]. He strongly opposed the translation into "spirit" by many Occidental authors. "The translation of *Shen* simply as 'Spirit' (as opposed to the material body) was influenced by Western Christian missionaries in China during the second half of the 19th century. A Christian philosophical outlook would use the word *Shen* indicating the 'Spirit' (or even 'God') as opposed to the 'body', reflecting a typical Western dualistic attitude to matter and Spirit which is totally alien to Chinese Philosophy."[*]

5. About the term 精氣 [jīng qì], the divergence in its English equivalents comes from the ambiguous grammatical structure of the Chinese. Grammatically, the term may be regarded as a simple combination of two juxtaposed nouns 精 [jīng] and 氣 [qì], and thus translated as "essence and *qi*" and the like (including "essence *qi*", "essence-*qi*"). But this is probably not the case, and the first character 精 [jīng] can be an adjective describing the character 氣 [qì]. In this case the translation is

---

[*]Giovanni Maciocia. *The Foundations of Chinese Medicine*. Churchill Livingstone, 1989, p.75-76.

"essential *qi*". Even if 精 [jīng] remains a noun, it can be used in the possessive case, and the translation becomes "*qi* of essence." The national Chinese textbook of TCM clearly defines 精氣 [jīng qì] as 氣中之精粹 (the essential part of qi), and then the translation is "essence of qi". When translating the Chinese into English, one can find that any of the above four forms of expression might be useful in different contexts. As a basic TCM term in English, "essence of qi" fits in with the definition. However, as "essential qi" is actually synonymous with "essence of qi" and is more succinct, it is therefore proposed as the standard term.

6. Both medical professionals and laypersons use the word 精神[jīng shén]. In layman's language, it is a polysemant, referring to "spirit", "vigor" and "liveliness". As a medical term, it refers to the combination of essence and its outward manifestations. The English expressions suggested by various authors include "spirit", "vitality", "vital spirit", "essence-spirit", "mind", "mentality", and "mental power". The expression that can be widely accepted by both laymen and professionals is "spirit".

7. The Chinese term 氣機 [qì jī] is rendered in various ways in recent publications. They include "functional activities of qi", "function of qi", "activity of *qi* (or *qi* activity)", "movement of *qi* (or *qi* movement)", "mechanism of *qi* (or *qi* mechanism)", and "*qi* dynamic". The national textbook of traditional Chinese medicine in Chinese gives this term a clear-cut definition. "The movement of *qi* is called 氣機 [qì jī]"[*]. So, "*qi* movement" is the best choice.

8. *Qi* movement usually takes the form of ascending, descending, exiting and entering, corresponding to 升 [shēng], 降 [jiàng], 出 [chū], and 入 [rù] respectively. It should be noted that these terms come from intransitive verbs, expressing the movement of *qi* itself. But sometimes 升 [shēng] and 降 [jiàng] are used in the transitive form with a direct object; in other words, they may bear the meaning of causing something to move upwards or downwards. In this instance the equivalents will be discussed elsewhere.

9. Different authors have suggested multifarious ways to express the Chinese concept 氣化 [qì huà]: "*qi* transformation", "transformation of

---

[*]"氣的運動稱爲氣機。" — cited from Wu DX (chief editor), *Fundamental Theories of Traditional Chinese Medicine* (in Chinese), The Textbook Series for Programmed Courses of the TCM Universities and Colleges, Shanghai Science and Technology Press, 1995, p.40.

qi", "transformation by *qi*", "transformative action of *qi*", "functional activity of *qi*", "activity of *qi*", "*qi* activity", "*qi* functional activity", "functional activity of *qi*". These expressions can be classified into two groups — one associated with the word "transformation", and the other with "activity". "Transformation" is better than "activity" to express the concept of 化 [huà], and so "transformation of *qi*" or "*qi* transformation" is selected. In addition, "transformation" has a dual meaning of transforming and being transformed. This tallies with the Chinese original, which refers to transforming something by *qi*, and also to the transformation of *qi* itself. The word "activity" merely means being active, excluding the change of *qi* itself.

THEORY OF YIN AND YANG

This is an ancient Chinese philosophical concept of naive dialectics, expressing the law of the unity of opposites. According to this theory, everything in the universe can be classified into two fundamental principles, properties or aspects, i.e., yin and yang, which are ever opposing and complementing each other. This concept introduced into Chinese medicine is widely applied to indicate various antitheses in anatomy, physiology, pathology, diagnosis and treatment and explaining health and various disease processes. The terms used in the theory of yin-yang mainly include those describing the relationship between yin and yang, such as opposition, interdependence, waxing and waning, transformation, intercourse, harmony, balance, disharmony, and alternative preponderance, as well as the terms derived from these relationships, such as yin within yin, yin within yang, yang within yin and yang within yang.

Proposed Standard Nomenclature

theory of yin and yang 陰陽學說 [yīn yáng xué shuō][1]

yin and yang 陰陽 [yīn yáng][2]

opposition of yin and yang 陰陽對立 [yīn yáng duì lì][3]

interdependence of yin and yang 陰陽互根 [yīn yáng hù gēn][4]

waxing and waning of yin and yang 陰陽消長 [yīn yáng xiāo zhǎng][5]

inter-transformation of yin and yang 陰陽轉化 [yīn yáng zhuǎn huà][6]

intercourse of yin and yang 陰陽交感 [yīn yáng jiāo gǎn][7]

harmony of yin and yang 陰陽調和 [yīn yáng tiáo hé][8]

balance of yin and yang 陰陽平衡

disharmony of yin and yang 陰陽失調 [yīn yáng shī tiáo][10]

yin within yin 陰中之陰 [yīn zhōng zhī yīn][12]

yin within yang 陽中之陰 [yáng zhōng zhī yīn][12]

yang within yang 陽中之陽 [yáng zhōng zhī yáng][12]

[yīn yáng píng héng][9]

alternative preponderance of yin and yang 陰陽勝復 [yīn yáng shèng fù][11]

yang within yin 陰中之陽 [yīn zhōng zhī yáng][12]

Discussion

1. There is no much dispute about this term. The word "theory" is used much oftener than "doctrine" or "hypothesis". A more succinct form, i.e., "yin-yang theory" is frequently encountered.

2. Since the words yin and yang have already been included in English dictionaries (e.g., Webster's Dictionary and the Oxford Dictionary) as a pair of terms used in Chinese philosophy, there is no more argument about the English equivalents of 陰 [yīn] and 陽 [yáng]

3. Most authors, Occidental and Oriental, use the word "opposition" for 對立 [duì lì], but some others prefer "antagonism". The latter has no advantage, as it implies active opposition with hostility. "Opposition" is more appropriate, for it means either the state or the action of opposing.

4. Most authors, Occidental and Oriental, use the word "interdependence" for 互根 [hù gēn] but some others prefer "mutual rooting", probably because the word "rooting" is an exact equivalent for the character 根 [gēn]. Indeed, the primary meaning of this character is root, but there are other meanings, such as "base", "source", "origin", "foundation", and so on. It is difficult to understand that yin and yang are mutually rooting. In the opposition of yin and yang, one's position depends upon the contrary position of the other.

5. For the phrase 消長 [xiāo zhǎng], different authors use different English expressions: "wax and wane" (or "waxing and waning", "wane and wax"), "growth and decline", "ebb and flow", "natural flux", "mutual consumption", "mutual growth and reduction" etc. Among these expressions, the phrase "wax and wane" (or "waxing and waning") seems to be the most appropriate because it is often used to describe the gradual periodic change of the area of brightness of the moon, and is very close to the Chinese concept of this term related to ancient astronomy. "Waxing and waning" may be better than "wax and wane" for showing a process rather than a state. Another issue is about the word order. In Chinese, it is cus-

tomarily to put 消 [xiāo] which means "wane" before 長 [zhǎng] which means "wax", but in English the two words are usually used in reverse order, i.e., "wax and wane". From the medical point of view, there is no difference between the two word orders. In addition, "ebb and flow" may be equally appropriate, but "waxing and waning" has already been used by many authors.

6. Most authors express this concept as "transformation of yin and yang" (or "yin-yang transformation"), "transformation between yin and yang", "inter-transformation of yin and yang", or "mutual transformation of yin and yang". Here, the transformation is that either from yin into yang, or from yang into yin. Therefore, it is appropriate to call it inter-transformation or mutual transformation. The word "inter-transformation" is thus selected, and the whole term can be rendered as "inter-transformation of yin and yang" or "yin-yang inter-transformation". Some author suggests the word "conversion". "Yin-yang conversion" may be equally good or even better. However, since most authors use the word transformation or inter-transformation, the word conversion is left for further discussion.

7. This is a new term developed from the Yi Jing (*The Book of Changes*). The original statement is: Interaction of the heaven (yang) and earth (yin) leads to transformation and generation of myriad of things ("天地感而萬物化生"). It not only refers to sexual intercourse that gives birth to a new human life, but also refers to the generation of all kinds of things in the world.

8. "Balance between yin and yang" and "harmony between yin and yang" are often used as synonyms, but the latter seems to be more commendatory and determinant of a healthy state while "balance between yin and yang" may have a neutral sense including balance at an abnormal level.

9. Either "balance" or "equilibrium" can be used as an equivalent of 平衡 [píng héng]. Since "balance" is not only a noun, but also a verb, and can be easily turned into an adjective ("balanced"), while "equilibrium" is always a noun, the former word is more frequently used. Strictly speaking, this term is somewhat modernized. According to the ancient Chinese texts, the state of yin and yang in a healthy individual should be 陰平陽秘 [yīn píng yáng mì] which may be literally translated as "Yin is even (or steady) and yang is sound (or firm)." However, quite a few authors also translate this term as "balance between yin and yang" or "yin-yang balance." The translation is somewhat modernized, not identical with the original Chinese text.

10. The term 失調 [shī tiáo] is modernized. It is the antonym of harmony (調和 [tiáo hé]), and hence disharmony. The antonym of balance is imbalance (失衡 [shī héng]). There is no difference between yin-yang disharmony and yin-yang imbalance, both being abnormal.

11. The concept 勝復 [shèng fù] is expressed by different authors in various ways: "alternation of excessiveness and deficiency between yin and yang"; "alternation of overabundance and deficiency between yin and yang"; "preponderance between yin and yang"; "alternative predominance between yin and yang"; "alternate excesses and deficiencies of yin and yang"; "alternate excess of yin and yang"; "yin-yang retaliation". Some of them are actually explanations and cannot be taken as medical terms. "Yin-yang retaliation" is the most concise one, but the word "retaliation" is usually used in a bitter sense, referring to repaying an injury or insult, or repaying evil with evil. The relation between yin and yang is not so hostile.

12. Different English expressions exist for these terms. Taking "yang within yin" as an example, other expressions include "yang aspect of yin", "aspect of yang within yin", or "component part of yang within yin". All these are less succinct.

THEORY OF THE FIVE ELEMENTS

The terms used in this theory mainly include the name of the theory itself and the relationships among the five elements. About the name of the elements, viz, wood, fire, earth, metal and water, there has never been any big argument in English publications. The medical terms formed in the light of this theory such as "wood restricting earth" (木克土 [mù kè tǔ]), "fire failing to generate earth" (火不生土 [huǒ bù shēng tǔ]) are derived from the sentences "Wood restricts earth" and "Fire fails to generate earth". Their standardization depends chiefly upon the proper selection of the equivalents for the verbs 生 [shēng], 克 [kè], 乘 [chéng], 侮 [wǔ].

Proposed Standard Nomenclature

theory of the five elements 五行學說 [wǔ xíng xué shuō][1]
generation [promotion] in the five

the five elements 五行 [wǔ xíng][1]
the five (circuit) phases 五運 [wǔ yùn][2]

elements 五行相生 [wǔ xíng xiāng shēng][3]

restriction and generation in the five elements 五行制化 [wǔ xíng zhì huà][5]

reverse restriction in the five elements 五行相侮 [wǔ xíng xiāng wǔ])[7]

qi of "mother" (organ) 母氣 [mǔ qì][9]

restriction [control] in the five elements 五行相克 [wǔ xíng xiāng kè][4]

subjugation in the five elements 五行相乘 [wǔ xíng xiāng chéng][6]

"mother-child" involvement in the five elements 五行母子相及 [wǔ xíng mǔ zǐ xiāng jí][8]

qi of "child" (organ) 子氣 [zǐ qì][9]

Discussion

1. There are two basic forms to express the character 行 [xíng] in this term: Considering that the five 行 [xíng] refer to wood, fire, earth, metal and water, many authors use the term "five elements" or the "five elementals". However, 行 [xíng] does not mean "element"; it means "movement". Wood, fire, earth, metal and water are called five 行 [xíng] because they are characterized by constant movement and change. Therefore, some other authors use the phrase "five transformation phases", "five evolutive phases", or simply "five phases". The problem of the latter translations lies in that classification of things into the five phases may cause difficulty. For instance, the liver pertains to wood, the spleen to earth, and hyperactivity of the liver impairing the spleen function is often expressed as "wood restricting earth". In this case, it may cause confusion if wood (the liver) and earth (the spleen) are taken as two phases. In the Chinese national textbook, 五行 [wǔ xíng] is defined as "five sorts of substances, namely wood, fire, earth, metal and water, as well as their movements and changes."* According to this definition, the term "five elements", though not complete, is better than the terms mentioning merely the movements and changes with omission of the substances. In addition, the translation "five elements" has a longer history and more advocates than any of the other expressions.

2. This term is somewhat different from the "five elements". It emphasizes the movements and changes of the five elements rather than the elements themselves. The English expressions include the "five circuit

---

* "五行，即木、火、土、金、水五種物質及其運動變化。" — cited from Wu DX (chief editor). *Fundamental Theories of Traditional Chinese Medicine*. (in Chinese), The Textbook Series for the Programmed Courses of the TCM Universities and Colleges, Shanghai Science and Technology Press, 1995, p.23.

phases", "five movements", "five motions", "five evolutive phases", "condition of the energies of the five elements", etc. The term "five circuit phases" is selected because it better reflects the original concept and can be abbreviated as "five phases".

3. The character 相 [xiāng] does not necessarily mean "mutual" or "each other". In many instances, it only stresses an action on somebody or something else. Even the modern Chinese language continues this kind of usage. For example, 實不相瞞. [shí bù xiāng mán] means "tell you the truth" (瞞. [mán] means "hide the truth from"), but it does not at all mean that you and I should not hide the truth from each other; 有事相告 [yǒu shì xiāng gào] means "I have something to tell you", but not "we have something to tell each other." Many authors translate 相生 [xiāng shēng] into "mutual generation", "mutual promotion", "mutual production", "inter-generation", or "inter-promotion". All these expressions may cause misunderstanding that A generates (promotes or produces) B, and at the same time B also generates (promotes or produces) A. This is certainly not correct. According to the five-element theory, wood generates fire, but fire does not generate wood.

One may argue that in the five elements there is always a cyclic movement. When A generates B, B may indirectly generate A through the sequential generating action, i.e., B generating C, C generating D, D generating E, and finally E generating A. Of course, this is purely hypothetical. Even so, the word "mutual" is still misleading. Some authors would rather express it as "generating sequence".

About the translation of the character 生 [shēng], various words have been used: "generating" ("generation"), "promoting" ("promotion"), "producing" ("production"), "engendering", and "creating". It is difficult to say which one is the best. According to rough statistics, generation and promotion are the words most frequently used In comparison with "promotion", the word "generation" is closer to the meaning of the original character, but the word promotion has its own advantage when it is used in contrast with 克 [kè] (restriction).

4. About the character 相 [xiāng], please see above (the note on "generation in the five elements"). One might argue that in this case the action can be directly reversed; for example, wood restricts earth, and earth may restrict wood. But in the latter case, the reverse restriction is called 侮 [wǔ]. It should be noted that, generally speaking, 克 [kè] (restriction) refers to the relationship in a normal condition, while 侮 [wǔ]

(reverse restriction) refers to an abnormal condition. That is to say, the two opposite actions can never manifest themselves in the same person at the same time, and so the word "mutual" is still not acceptable.

Regarding 克 [kè], the following words are frequently taken as its equivalents: "restriction", "control", "controlling", "conquest", "checking", "counteracting", "overacting", "overpowering", "subjugation", "restraining", etc. According to the frequency of use, restriction and control (controlling) are selected.

5. The Chinese term 制化 [zhì huà] is closely associated with generation and restriction in the five elements. Literally, it is synonymous with 生克 [shēng kè]. The English expressions for this concept found in recent publications are "inhibition and generation", "restriction and generation", and "promoting and checking", also very similar to 生克 [shēng kè].

6. Different authors express the action 乘 [chéng] in different ways: "subjugation", "over-acting", "encroachment", "overwhelming", "invasion", etc. The word "subjugation" is selected because of its frequent use.

7. As the English equivalent of 侮 [wǔ], the following expressions have appeared in recent publications: "insulting", "subjugation", "violation", "rebellion", "reversal of restriction", and "reverse restriction". More authors accept the last one.

8. A newly developed term to summarize pathological changes in the generation sequence of the five elements, including "disorder of a child-organ affecting its mother-organ (子病及母 [zǐ bìng jí mǔ])" and "disorder of the mother-organ affecting the child-organ" (母病及子 [mǔ bìng jí zǐ])

9. It is a metaphoric expression to call the element or organ that generates in the generation sequence of the five elements the "mother", and call the element or organ that is generated the "child". Most authors use quotation marks and an additional word such as organ or element to avoid confusion with similar obstetrical terms, for example, child's *qi* 子氣 [zǐ qì] in Chinese obstetrics refers to gravid edema.

ANATOMICAL TERMS

Any system of medicine must be founded on anatomy. Chinese medicine is no exception. As early as 2,000 years ago, autopsies were performed in China, as described in the *Canon of Medicine*. "A well-developed man can be measured from outside on the skin and flesh, and after death the body can be dissected to examine the firmness of the *zang* organs, the size of the *fu* organs, the volume of food contents, the length of vessels, the turbidity of blood, and the content of *qi*......"* Since the names of organs and tissues used in Chinese medicine and those used in Western medicine refer to the same anatomical entities, they are apparently equivalents. There is no reason to designate the same reality with two different names. Of course, the understanding of the anatomical entities is different in Chinese and Western systems of medicine, but the conceptual interpretation of reality cannot alter the translation, otherwise, in Western medicine these terms should not be kept in use, as the conceptual associations accompanying them have varied significantly since the anatomical names were first established.

ZANG-FU ORGANS

Zang-fu (臟腑 [zàng fǔ]) is the collective name for all internal organs. The *zang* organs are regarded as the core of the structure and functions of the human body, and each *zang* organ is connected with a corresponding *fu* organ by the meridians. The *zang-fu* organs are closely related to other organs and tissues functionally, thus making the human body as an integral entity. The terms involved in this section are chiefly the names of individual internal organs. The terms related to the functions of *zang-fu* organs will be listed as physiological terms.

Proposed Standard Nomenclature

zang-fu organs 臟腑 [zàng fǔ][1]

zang organs 臟 [zàng][1]

yang *zang*-organs 陽臟 [yáng zàng][2]

yin *zang*-organs 陰臟 [yīn zàng][2]

heart 心 [xīn][3]

liver 肝 [gān][3]

lung 肺 [fèi][3]

spleen 脾 [pí][3]

pericardium 心包[絡] [xīn bāo [luò]][3]

kidney 腎 [shèn][3]

---

* "若夫八尺之士，皮肉在此，外可度量切循而得之，其死可解剖而視之，其臟之堅脆，府之大小，穀之多少，脈之長短，血之清濁，氣之多少……" — cited from *Spiritual Pivot, Canon of Medicine*

fu organs 腑 [fǔ][1]

gallbladder 膽 [dǎn][3]

large intestine 大腸 [dà cháng][3]

bladder 膀胱 [páng guāng][3]

upper energizer 上焦 [shàng jiāo][4]

lower energizer 下焦 [xià jiāo][4]

stomach 胃 [wèi][3]

small intestine 小腸 [xiǎo cháng][3]

triple energizer 三焦 [sān jiāo][4]

middle energizer 中焦 [zhōng jiāo][4]

extraordinary organs 奇恒之腑 [qí héng zhī fǔ][5]

Discussion

1. One of the most difficult issues in the translation of Chinese medical terms has been the names of internal organs. Because of the great disparities between the Western and Chinese descriptions of the functions of internal organs, many authors have initiated various ways to express the internal organs in their Chinese medical sense. Manfred Porkert created a set of Latin terms for the internal organs, e.g., *orbis cardialis* for the word heart used in Chinese medicine. Some others insisted on using *pinyin*. This problem has already been solved in the *Standard Acupuncture Nomenclature* recommended by the WHO. No more *pinyin* or Latin names appear in the recent publications, except *sanjiao* (the triple energizer). However, the name for the internal organs in general is still a controversial issue. In Chinese, they are collectively called 臟腑 [zàng fǔ], and either internal organs or viscera may be taken as an appropriate equivalent. But the Chinese term can be separated into 臟 [zàng] and 腑 [fǔ], each possessing its own definition. Internal organs or viscera cannot be treated in a similar way. Various suggestions have appeared in recent publications. The terms "bowels" or "hollow organs" for 腑 [fǔ] and "viscera", and "solid organs" for 臟 [zàng] can not be generally accepted because the word "bowels" only refers to the intestines while "viscera" also includes the intestines; the lung cannot be taken as a solid organ, and the gallbladder is not hollow. The most promising way of expression is to render 臟 [zàng] into yin organs and 腑 [fǔ] into yang organs. This is advocated by many authors, and causes no contradiction in most instances. The only disadvantage is that the nomenclature cannot always follow the principle of relativity of yin and yang, for 臟 [zàng] pertains to yin only when it is contrasted to 腑 [fǔ]. When yin-yang classification is applied to 臟 [zàng], there are yin yin organs (referring to the heart and liver) and yang yin organs (referring to the spleen, lung and kidney). We had better not use such perplexing terms. Since 臟腑 [zàng fǔ], 臟 [zàng] and 腑 [fǔ] are such important concepts and no exact equivalents can be

found in English, use of Romanized Chinese seems to be acceptable.

2. The yin-yang classification of *zang* organs is based on the property but not on the location, so it has more clinical significance. The terms yin *zang*-organs and yang *zang*-organs show the disadvantage of naming yin organs for 臟 [zàng] and yang organs for 腑 [fǔ]. It would be very confusing to say yin yin organs and yang yin organs.

3. Regarding the English names of these organs, there is no more dispute. Owing to the great disparities existing in the concept of the internal organs between Chinese and Western medicine, many authors use capitalization for *zang-fu* organs in Chinese medicine. No such rule is made in this proposal, because it leads to two problems. One is to what extent should capitalization be used. All anatomical terms of Chinese medicine as well as the term indicating substances are conceptionally different from those in Western medicine. For example, in Chinese medicine a tooth is believed to be surplus bone, and is nourished by kidney essence. Should this word also be capitalized? If so many words were capitalized, many sentences would become unsightly. The other problem is the compliance with English grammar, for not all these terms are proper nouns.

4. Although the term triple energizer has been recommended by the WHO since 1991 or even earlier, quite a few authors refuse to use this term. Some of them insist on the use of *sanjiao*, and some others adhere to "triple burner". *Sanjiao* is not such an important concept in Chinese medicine as *qi* and *zang-fu*; on the contrary, even in China there is much dispute about this term, for example, whether the upper energizer includes the upper limbs or not, and whether the liver is an organ of the middle energizer or an organ of the lower energizer. There is really no adequate reason to keep such a *pinyin* name in the standard English nomenclature. The word "burner" is used on the basis of misunderstanding of the character 焦 [jiāo]. As a common word, this character does mean "burnt" or "charred", but as a medical term, it means "passage or space within the body". This definition is well explained in some specialized Chinese dictionaries.[*]

5. Most authors use the word "extraordinary" to express the concept

---

[*] "焦鬲導達，呼吸開利，快然若未始有疾者。"（《藥戒》）"The passage and the diaphragm being free and the breathing unobstructed, the patient feels comfortable as if no illness had ever occurred." (*Medication Taboos*) — cited from Jian Ming Zhong Yi Zi Dian (*Concise Dictionary of Characters in Chinese Medicine*) (in Chinese), Guizhou People's Publishing House, 1985, p.369

奇恒 [qí héng], which seems better than. "curious", "peculiar", or "unusual". Disparity also exists in the expression of 腑 [fǔ]. Owing to the fact that none of extraordinary organs function as *fu* organs, many authors simply call them "extraordinary organs" instead of "extraordinary *fu* (or yang or hollow) organs".

OTHER SPECIAL ANATOMICAL NAMES

Many anatomical names in Chinese medicine have their corresponding English names in Western medicine. Since these terms used in the two systems of medicine refer to the same anatomical entities, we had better not regard them as specific terms for Chinese medicine. So they are not included in this proposal, and the commonly used ones are listed in the attached table. Some anatomical terms, however, are only used in Chinese medicine. Standardization of their English equivalents is necessary.

Proposed Standard Nomenclature

signaling orifices 苗竅 [miáo qiào][1]

thoracic center 膻中 [dàn zhōng][2]

cardio-diaphragmatic interspace 膏肓 [gāo huāng][4]

elixir fields 丹田 [dān tián][3]

interior-exterior interspace 膜原 [mó yuán][5]

dorso-ventral boundary (of the Hand or foot) 赤白肉際 [chì bái ròu jì][6]

house of blood 血府 [xuè fǔ][7]

sea of marrow 髓海 [suǐ hǎi][7]

house of marrow 髓府 [suǐ fǔ][7]

essence chamber 精室 [jīng shì][7]

sea of blood 血海 [xuè hǎi][7]

blood chamber 血室 [xuè shì][7]

life gate 命門 [mìng mén][8]

Discussion

1. Many authors translate 苗竅 [miáo qiào] into "sprout and opening" or "sprout and orifices". They all take the character 苗 [miáo] as an independent noun, and adhere to its original meaning of "sprout" in the common language. From the Chinese medical point of view, such translation is inexplicable. Even as a common word, 苗 [miáo] does not always mean sprout. It may refer to anything (including a phenomenon) that begins to appear or develop. For example, 苗頭 [miáo tóu] means a symptom of a trend or suggestion of a new development. If one interpreted it as "sprout and head" literally in a word-for-word way, one

would make a funny mistake. Interpretation of 苗竅 [miáo qiào] as "sprout and opening" is the same. In this term, the two characters are not placed side by side as A and B. A is an attributive noun, describing the action or quality of B. Some authors use the word "signal", which better shows the real meaning. "Signaling orifices" are thus suggested as a standard term, for some body orifices such as the eyes and the mouth, particularly the tongue, can give signals indicating disease of related internal organs.

2. The term 膻中 [dàn zhōng] refers to central part of the chest, between the two breasts. *Pinyin* is by no means the best choice. Many Chinese scholars make mistake about the pronunciation, and so Jian Ming Zhong Yi Zi Dian (*Concise Dictionary of Characters in Chinese Medicine*) (in Chinese) has a special note on the character 膻 [dàn], that it should not be pronounced dǎn or tǎn, and when it is pronounced shān, it does not mean the "chest" but refers to the "smell of mutton". Even the *Standard Acupuncture Nomenclature* published by the World Health Organization Regional Office for the Western Pacific makes a mistake on this *pinyin* name. Of the two *pinyin* names for 膻中 (CV17) — Tānzhōng and Shànzhōng, neither is correct. Only in the *Proposed Standard International Acupuncture Nomenclature* published by the World Health Organization, Geneva, the correct *pinyin* dànzhōng is given. Since the *pinyin* name of this term is in such a confused condition, there is no reason to ask Westerners to take it as the standard.

3. To translate the Chinese term *dantian* (丹田 [dān tián]) into an anatomical name is difficult because it is a collective name of three different sites of the body. Two ways of expression are often adopted. One is the use of *pinyin*, and the other, literal translation. Both are acceptable. The literal translations frequently encountered: are "cinnabar field" and "elixir field". The character 丹 [dān] does mean "cinnabar", but the word "elixir" more vividly reflects its implication. In medicine, 丹 [dān] usually refers to pellets, and in Taoist practice the process of making refined pellets, particularly the pellet of immortality, is called 煉丹 [liàn dān]. Dantian, the region(s) of the body to which one's mind is focused in *qigong* and other practices, is compared to the place where the agent that makes people live forever is manufactured.

4. In Chinese medicine the term 膏肓 [gāo huāng] refers to the region below the heart and above the diaphragm, situated deeply in the body. It is an anatomical reality. Like the heart has BL15 as its transport

point on the back and the diaphragm has BL17 as its transport point, this anatomical reality also has BL43 as its transport point. If we accept the heart and the diaphragm as the English equivalents of the corresponding Chinese medical terms, we have no reason to resist such an expression as cardio-diaphragmatic interspace. In Chinese medicine, it is believed that diseases of this region cannot be effectively treated with medicines. Probably because the idiom 病入膏肓 [bìng rù gāo huāng] which means "the disease is beyond cure" is a commonly used phrase in the Chinese language, many authors prefer *pinyin* to the anatomical location. However, *pinyin* is no more than a meaningless sound to Westerners who have not learned the Chinese language.

5. The Chinese term 膜原 [mó yuán] is also called 募原 [mù yuán]. Both terms were used in *the Canon of Medicine*. It is difficult to say which one can be taken as the standard Chinese, and hence which *pinyin* name should be the standard equivalent. This term refers either to the pleurodiaphragmatic interspace or to the interior-exterior interspace. The former is somewhat obsolete, but the latter is still useful, particularly in the field of epidemic febrile diseases, for example, a pathogen in the interior-exterior interspace usually gives rise to a half-exterior half-interior syndrome.

6. Several expressions have been suggested by different authors, such as "boundary between the whitish and pinkish skin", "junction of the red and white skin", "border of the red and white flesh", "red-white border", "border separating the light-colored skin from the darker-colored skin", "border of the light and dark skin", and "dorso-ventral boundary (of the hand or foot)". The last one is the most succinct and fully reflects the meaning of the Chinese original.

7. The terms house of blood (血府 [xuè fǔ]), house of marrow (髓府 [suǐ fǔ]), sea of blood (血海 [xuè hǎi]), sea of marrow (髓海 [suǐ hǎi]), blood chamber (血室 [xuè shì]), and essence chamber (精室 [jīng shì]) are alternative names for blood vessel, bone, liver (or conception vessel), brain, uterus (or conception vessel), and life gate respectively. There is not much dispute about these English equivalents.

8. For this term most authors agree that literal translation is better than *pinyin* and suggest the following equivalents: "gate of life", "life gate", "vital gate", "gate of vitality", and "vital portal". Most authors prefer the word "life" for 命 [mìng] and "gate" for 門 [mén], and hence the succinct term "life gate" is selected.

Anatomical Names Common to both Chinese and Western Medicine

brain 腦 [nǎo]

bone 骨 [gǔ]

uterus 女子胞 [nǚ zǐ bāo]

afterbirth 胞衣 [bāo yī]

nostril 鼻孔 [bí kǒng]

nasal septum 鼻柱 [bí zhù]

apex nasi 鼻准 [bí zhǔn]

dorsum nasi 鼻梁 [bí liáng]

mouth 口 [kǒu]

tooth 齒 [chǐ]

tongue 舌 [shé]

retropharynx 咽底 [yān dǐ]

uvula 蒂丁 [dì dīng]

epiglottis 會厭 [huì yàn]

pylorus 幽門 [yōu mén]

anus 肛門 [gāng mén]

skin 皮 [pí]

down 毫毛 [háo máo]

muscle 肌 [jī]

tendon 筋 [jīn]

cranium 頭顱骨 [tóu lù gǔ]

vertex 巔 [diān]

hairline 髮際 [fà jì]

ophryon 闕中 [què zhōng]

temporal 顳顬 [niè rú]

supra-orbital ridge 眉棱骨 [méi léng gǔ]

orbit 目眶 [mù kuàng]

palpebra 胞瞼 [bāo jiǎn]

lower eyelid 目下胞 [mù xià bāo]

canthus 目眥 [mù zì]

outer canthus 外眦 [wài zì]

palpebral conjunctiva 瞼內 [jiǎn nèi]

auricle 耳廓 [ěr kuò]

earlobe 耳垂 [ěr chuí]

eardrum 耳膜 [ěr mó]

tragus 耳門 [ěr mén]

marrow 髓 [suǐ]

blood vessel 脈 [mài]

placenta 人胞 [rén bāo]

nose 鼻 [bí]

nasal orifice 鼻竅 [bí qiào]

ala nasi 鼻翼 [bí yì]

radix nasi 鼻根 [bí gēn]

vibrissa 鼻毛 [bí māo]

lip 唇 [chún]

gum 齦 [yín]

pharynx 咽 [yān]

laryngopharynx 咽喉 [yān hóu]

tonsil 喉核 [hóu hé]

cardia 賁門 [bēn mén]

ileocecal conjunction 闌門 [lán mén]

hair 毛 [máo]

sweat pore 玄府 [xuán fǔ]

flesh 肉 [ròu]

diaphragm 鬲 [gé]

vertex cranii 巔頂 [diān dǐng]

fontanel 囟 [xìn]

mid-frons 天庭 [tiān tíng]

forehead 額 [é]

sideburns 銳髮 [ruì fà]

eyebrow 眉 [méi]

eye 目 [mù]

lacrimal punctum 淚竅 [lèi qiào]

upper eyelid 目上胞 [mù shàng bāo]

inner canthus 內眥 [nèi zì]

eyelash 睫 [jié]

iris 黃仁 [huáng rén]

ear 耳 [ěr]

helix 耳輪 [ěr lún]

external auditory meatus 耳道 [ěr dào]

malar eminence 顴 [quán]

philtrum 人中 [rén zhōng]

mandibular arch 曲頰 [qū jiá]

mandible 頜 [hé]

neck 頸 [jǐng]

laryngeal prominence 結喉 [jié hóu]

shoulder 肩 [jiān]

arm 臂 [bì]

elbow 肘 [zhǒu]

supraclavicular fossa 缺盆 [quē pén]

xiphoid process 鳩尾 [jiū wěi]

costal region 脅 [xié]

abdomen 腹 [fù]

lower abdomen 小腹 [xiǎo fù]

umbilicus 臍 [qí]

pubic symphysis 曲骨 [qū gǔ]

pubic margin 毛際 [máo jì]

scrotum 陰囊 [yīn náng]

penis 陰莖 [yīn jīng]

knee 膝 [xī]

popliteal fossa 膕 [guó]

calf 腨 [chuǎi]

lateral malleolus 外踝 [wài huái]

skeleton 骸 [hái]

lumbus 腰 [yāo]

tibia 骭骨 [gàn gǔ]

trochanter 髀樞 [bì shū]

sacral region 尻 [kāo]

fibula 外輔骨 [wài fǔ gǔ]

chin 頷 [hàn]

cervical vertebra 頸骨 [jǐng gǔ]

occipital bone 枕骨 [zhěn gǔ]

nape 項 [xiàng]

scapula 肩胛 [jiān jiǎ]

upper arm 肱 [gōng]

humerus 臑骨 [nào gǔ]

suprasternal notch 上橫骨 [shàng héng gǔ]

pectoral muscle 膺 [yīng]

hypochondriac region 季肋 [jì lèi]

upper abdomen 大腹 [dà fù]

inguinal region 少腹 [shào fù]

pubic bone 橫骨 [héng gǔ]

perineum 會陰 [huì yīn]

vaginal orifice 陰戶 [yīn hù]

testis 睾 [gāo]

thigh 股 [gǔ]

patella 膝臏 [xī bìn]

shin 脛 [jìng]

medial malleolus 內踝 [nèi huái]

heel 踵 [zhǒng]

spine 脊 [jǐ]

lumbar vertebra 腰骨 [yāo gǔ]

femur 髀骨 [bì gǔ]

coccyx 尾閭 [wěi lú]

sacrum 尻骨 [kāo gǔ]

PHYSIOLOGICAL TERMS

In traditional Chinese medicine the knowledge of physiology was obtained chiefly through observation of human beings in the light of natural philosophy and by analogy with natural nomenclature, daily life and even government administration at that time. This makes the Chinese physiological terms unique if they are reviewed from the perspective of modern physiology.

The Chinese physiological terms can be classified into two main categories: the names of the basic substances involved in physiological activities, and the names of the physiological activities. Traditional Chinese medicine holds that the visceral organs, particularly the five *zang* organs, form the core of the human body. They control all kinds of life activities, and through their outer manifestations their physiological functions as well as pathological changes can be detected. Therefore, Chinese physiology is included in the theory of organ manifestation.

BASIC PHYSIOLOGICAL SUBSTANCES

The basic physiological substances comprise *qi*, essence, blood, body fluids, and nutrients. They are further classified according to the organ or tissue to which they are supplied, for example, spleen *qi*, kidney essence, liver blood, stomach fluid, heart nutrient, and so forth. It should be noted that, although these substances are distributed all over the body, special names are only given to those with clinical significance. For example, when we talk about the blood, "heart blood" and "liver blood" have special significance and hence are so named, but no special names are designated for the blood of other organs.

Proposed Standard Nomenclature

innate (or inborn) 先天 [xiān tiān][1]

acquired 後天 [hòu tiān][1]

health (or normal) *qi* 正氣[zhèng qì][2]

genuine *qi* 真氣 [zhēn qì][3]

pectoral *qi* 宗氣 [zōng qì][5]

original *qi* 原[元]氣 [yuán qì][4]

nutritive *qi* 營氣 [yíng qì][7]

defensive *qi* 衛氣 [wèi qì][6]

organ *qi* 臟腑之氣[zàng fǔ zhī qì][9]

meridian *qi* 經氣 [jīng qì][8]

fu organ *qi* 腑氣 [fǔ qì][9]

zang organ *qi* 臟氣 [zàng qì][9]

liver *qi* 肝氣 [gān qì][10]

heart *qi* 心氣 [xīn qì][10]

lung *qi* 肺氣 [fèi qì][10]

spleen *qi* 脾氣 [pí qì][10]

kidney *qi* 腎氣 [shèn qì][10]

stomach *qi* 胃氣 [wèi qì][10]

kidney essenc 腎精 [shèn jīng][11]

essence 精 [jīng][11]

heart blood 心血 [xīn xuè][12]

blood 血 [xuè][12]

nutrient 營 [yíng][13]

liver blood 肝血 [gān xuè][12]

nutrient-yin 營陰 [yíng yīn][13]

nutrient-blood 營血 [yíng xuè][13]

lung fluid 肺津 [fèi jīn][14]

body fluids 津液 [jīn yè][14]

yin 陰 [yīn][15]

stomach fluid 胃津 [wèi jīn][14]

liver yin 肝陰 [gān yīn][15]

heart yin 心陰 [xīn yīn][15]

lung yin 肺陰 [fèi yīn][15]   spleen yin 脾陰 [pí yīn][15]
stomach yin 胃陰 [wèi yīn][15]   kidney yin 腎陰 [shèn yīn][15]
heart yang 心陽 [xīn yáng][15]   yang 陽 [yáng][15]
spleen yang 脾陽 [pí yáng][15]   liver yang 肝陽 [gān yáng][15]
kidney yang 腎陽 [shèn yáng][15]   lung yang 肺陽 [fèi yáng][15]
stomach yang 胃陽 [wèi yáng][15]

Discussion

1. The meanings of 先天 [xiān tiān] and 後天 [hòu tiān] are quite clear. They refer to "before birth" and "after birth" respectively. It is not difficult to find English equivalents of the two terms, but a number of authors adhere to the literal translation and render them as pre-heaven (or before heaven, earlier heaven) and post-heaven (or after heaven, later heaven). Such literal translations may cause misunderstanding. The English word "heaven" is the place believed to be the home of good people after death. So the term post-heaven may be misunderstood as "after death". As a matter of fact, such an expression for death also exists in Chinese language. For example, 歸天 [guī tiān] literally means "return to heaven", which is a euphemism for "die".

Besides "pre-heaven", "post-heaven" and the like, the following words are often used for 先天 [xiān tiān]: "congenital", "prenatal", "innate", and "inborn", and for 後天 [hòu tiān]: "acquired", and "postnatal". "Congenital" is not so good a word for describing *qi* and essence, because it is often used in Western medicine with special application to defects, anomalies or diseases, while in Chinese medicine the *qi* and essence endowed before birth are normal, physiological and vitally important. "Prenatal" vs. "postnatal" does not totally conform to the Chinese original. The word "prenatal" means "existing or occurring before birth", with reference to the fetus, and "postnatal" means "existing or occurring after birth", with reference to the newborn. The exact meaning of "postnatal" can be easily understood from its related word "postpartum", which means "occurring after childbirth", with reference to the mother. So, "prenatal" and "postnatal" are only related to the fetus before birth and the infant after birth. But the original Chinese concept, no matter whether it is concerned with *qi* or essence, refers to that which exists in the human body lifelong. Therefore, "inborn (or innate)" is selected for 先天 [xiān tiān], and "acquired" for 後天 [hòu tiān]

2. Many words have been used by different authors for expressing

the character 正 [zhèng] in 正氣 [zhèng qì]. They include "health(y)", "normal", "upright", "right", "vital", "genuine", "orthopathic", "antipathogenic", etc. Some of them are literal translations, and some are free translations. Each has its own grounds and advocates, and it is difficult to make a selection merely according to the frequency of use. Probably we had better make the selection with reference to its opposite. In Chinese medicine, 正 [zhèng] is most frequently used in opposition to 邪 (xié). If the latter is expressed by "pathogenic", the most appropriate expression for the former is "health(y)" or "antipathogenic". The word "normal" might also be considered, but the opposite of normal *qi* is abnormal *qi*, which often refers to *qi* in abnormality, e.g., sunken *qi*, which is pathological but not pathogenic. The word "right" refers to what is just and honorable, and "upright" means strictly honest or honorable. They are good translations of the character 正 [zhèng] in 正氣 [zhèng qì] when the latter refers to noble moral quality. "Song of Uprightness" (正氣歌 [zhèng qì gē]) is a famous poem to show the loyalty written by a patriotic Chinese general who chose death rather than surrender to the enemy. Here, the word 正氣 [zhèng qì] has a different connotation from the same word used in medicine.

3. Many translators render 真氣 [zhēn qì] as "true *qi*". Literally, it seems to be right, but the character 真 [zhēn] has other meanings than "true". It means "original" in some instances, for example, in the Chinese idiom 歸真返璞 (return to original purity and simplicity), the title 真人 [zhēn rén] (well-practised Taoist), and the common word 天真 [tiān zhēn] (innocent or naive). That is why Chinese medicine holds that 真氣 [zhēn qì] is the same as 元氣 [yuán qì] (original *qi*). Since this term is in frequent use, it had better be kept in the standard nomenclature with an appropriate equivalent. "Genuine *qi*" is the choice.

4. The term 原氣 [yuán qì] and 元氣 [yuán qì] are regarded as one term. As its equivalent, several expressions have appeared in recent publications. They are "original *qi*", "original vital *qi*", "primordial *qi*", "source *qi*", and "renal *qi*". Among these expressions, "primordial *qi*" seems to be the most specific and scientific, but it does not suit the Chinese concept. The word "primordial" has a specific meaning in modern biology. It refers to the first in order of appearance in the growth of an organism, but the primordial one (e.g., primordial cell) no longer exists in the later development. This is not the case for 原[元]氣 [yuán qì]; the latter exists in the human body lifelong. "Renal *qi*" only partly reflects the

concept of this term, and is confused with "kidney *qi*". "Source qi" is not recommendable either, because the word "source" is a literal translation of the character 源 [yuán] but not 原[yuán]. The meanings of the two characters may have some overlap, but they are not exactly the same. In conclusion, "original *qi*" is the best choice.

5. It is extremely difficult to find an appropriate equivalent of the term 宗氣 [zōng qì]. The English equivalents suggested by different authors can be classified into two groups: literal translations and explanatory expressions. The former include "ancestral *qi*", "genetic *qi*", and "initial *qi*", which may cause confusion with "inborn qi". The latter include "gathering qi", "chest qi" (or "qi of the chest"), "pectoral qi" and "thoracic qi", which are derived from the concept that 宗氣 [zōng qì] is the qi that gathers in the chest, formed by the combination of fresh air inhaled into the lungs and the qi absorbed from food. "Gathering qi" and "pectoral qi" are the two words most often used by different authors. Comparatively speaking, the word gathering seems to be less promising, for it does not exclude the qi gathering in other parts of the body. Therefore, "pectoral qi" is selected, and in fact it is most frequently used.

6. Most authors use "defensive" (or defense) qi" and "protective qi" to express the concept of 衛氣 [wèi qì]. There is not much dispute so far as the character 衛 [wèi] is concerned. So far as the frequency of use is concerned, "defensive" is preponderant.

7. Nigel Wiseman takes 營氣 [yíng qì] as an example to illustrate that even those who favor literal translation do not necessarily choose the same renderings[*]. 營氣 [yíng qì] is rendered by some as "nutritive qi" or "nourishing qi", and by others as "construction qi" or "constructive qi". Nourishment and construction do have some relation, but they are not the same thing. The character 營 [yíng] is polysemantic. It means "manage" in the word 經營 [jīng yíng], "construct" in the word 營造 [yíng zào], and "camp" in the word 營地 [yíng dì]. However, in medicine it has its proper meaning. In the ancient Chinese language 營 [yíng] is written 榮 [róng]. The *Canon of Medicine* states that 榮 [róng] is the essential qi derived from food.[**] In the Japanese language 榮養 [róng yǎng] is the equivalent of the Chinese word 營養 [yíng yǎng], both signifying nutri-

---

[*]Nigel Wiseman. English-Chinese Chinese-English Dictionary of Chinese Medicine. Hunan Press of Science and Techonology, 1996, p.39.

[**] "榮者，水穀之精氣也。"（素問・痹論）— cited from *Spiritual Pivot, Canon of Medicine*

tion. Furthermore, in the latest edition of the Chinese national TCM text-book, the term 營氣 [yíng qì] is clearly defined as "the qi that runs within the vessels and has a nutritive action."[*] From this example, we can see that, although many characters are polysemants, most of them still have a specific meaning when they are used in medicine. Rendering them into English, we should, first of all, carefully differentiate the specific meaning from their other non-medical meanings.

8. Meridian *qi* (經氣 [jīng qì]) is an abbreviation of "*qi* of meridians and collaterals" (經絡之氣 [jīng luò zhī qì]). For simplicity, the meridians and collaterals can be expressed as meridian system, and the latter when used as an attributive noun can be further shortened to meridian. The main problem for this term is the choice of meridian or channel. This has already been discussed elsewhere.

9. With reference to the *zang* and *fu* organs, we had better say "*zang-fu* organs" instead of "internal organs", "visceral organs", or simply "viscera". But if we are talking about the internal organs with no reference to *zang* or *fu* organ, it seems too wordy to say *zang-fu* organs all the time. So, "visceral *qi*" or "organ *qi*" is good enough to express the concept of 臟腑之氣 [zàng fǔ zhī qì]. More authors prefer "organ *qi*".

10. For the *qi* of each individual organ, a rule of nomenclature can be set according to the cooresponding expressions used by most authors, i.e., the name of the organ + *qi*. Here, it needs stressing that only the original noun form of the organ name is used as the attributive of the word *qi*. Use of the adjective form of the organ names (i.e., cardiac, hepatic, splenic, pulmonary, renal, etc.) should be avoided in order to minimize the confusion of the Chinese and Western concepts.

11. Most authors employ the word "essence" to express the concept of 精 [jīng] in its broad sense. (精 [jīng] in its narrow sense. refers to semen or sperm.) Some authors modify it to "vital essence" or "essence of life" in order to distinguish 精 [jīng] used in medicine from that used in common language, but this seems unnecessary, because traditional Chinese medicine holds that the essence of the human is integrated with that of heaven and earth (i.e., the universe), and life arises only after the intercourse of yin and yang. In addition, if we adopt this expression, a

---

* "營氣，是行於脈中、具有營養作用之氣。" — cited from Wu DX (chief editor). *Fundamental Theories of Traditional Chinese Medicine.* (in Chinese) The Textbook Series for Programmed Courses of the TCM Universities and Colleges, Shanghai Science and Technology Press, 1995, p.45.

number of problems emerge, for example, .腎精 [shèn jīng] would be "kidney essence of life" instead of "kidney essence", 水穀之精 [shuǐ gǔ zhī jīng] would be "vital essence of food" but not simply "food essence".

12. Regarding the word "blood", some authors insist on using *xue* or *hsüeh* to express the Chinese concept of the red fluid circulating in the blood vessels, because the concept of 血 [xuè] in Chinese medicine is different from that in Western medicine. Paul Unschuld made an incisive comment on this issue. He classified Chinese medical terms into generic and metaphoric, and set a rule "to render generic terms as generic." (cf. p.7) He totally disagreed with DeWoskin's suggestion of rendering 血 [xuè] as "vital fluid" "If we were to follow recent suggestions to render the Chinese 血 [xuè] not as 'blood' but as 'vital blood' because the connotations associated with the term 血 [xuè] in traditional Chinese medicine differ from the understanding of blood in modern science, ……a Western physician or scientist should no longer use the term 'blood' because his scientific conception of 'blood' differs from that of ordinary laymen, who employ the word 'blood' as part of their vernacular".*

13. The English expression of the character 營 [yíng] has already been discussed in the term 營氣 [yíng qì]. Here, this character is used as a noun, and so "nutrient" is the best term. There is some argument about "nutrient" and "nutrition". Since 營 [yíng] is taken as a kind of physiological substance in this context, "nutrient" is naturally more appropriate. This can also be shown in the term nutrient-blood (營血 [yíng xuè]), which means nutrients and blood, and in the term nutrient-yin (營陰 [yíng yīn]), which means nutrients and other substances.

14. The term "body fluids" is equivalent to 津液 [jīn yè] in Chinese medicine. Strictly speaking, 津 [jīn] and 液 [yè] are different. The former refers to thin fluid that permeates the skin and muscles, and the latter is thick fluid that moistens the joints and the brain and marrow.** Now, this differentiation seems unnecessary. It is no more stressed in the latest edition of the Chinese national TCM textbook, and, except in occasional instances, the two Chinese characters are almost always used in

---

*Unschuld PU. Terminological Problems Encountered and Experiences Gained in the Process of Editing a Commentated Nan-Ching Edition, in *Approaches to Traditional Chinese Medical Literature*, Kluwer Academic Publishers,1989, pp. 100-101.

** "腠理發泄，汗出溱溱，是謂津。……穀入氣滿，淖澤注於骨，骨屬屈伸，泄澤，補益腦髓，皮膚潤澤，是爲液"。(靈樞・決氣) — cited from Chapter 30, *Spiritual Pivot, Canon of Medicine*

combination as one single term.* Even in the exceptional cases, i.e., 傷津 [shāng jīn] and 脫液 [tuō yè], both 津 [jīn] and 液 [yè] can be rendered as "fluid". Therefore, there is no need to differentiate between thin and thick fluid in the standard nomenclature, and it is rational to designate the fluid that moistens the lung as lung fluid (肺津 [fèi jīn]) and the fluid produced by the stomach as stomach fluid (胃津 [wèi jīn]).

15. Besides their philosophical concepts, yin and yang in medicine also refer to concrete realities. In this context, yin represents the structural or material aspect while yang represents the active or functional aspect. They can further be classified in accordance with the *zang-fu* organs. Nomination of the organ yin or yang should follow the rule for organ *qi*, i.e., the name of the organ + yin or yang, and only the original noun form of the organ name should be used as the attributive of the word yin or yang. No adjective forms of the organ names (such as cardiac, hepatic, splenic, pulmonary, renal, and gastric) should be adopted in order to avoid confusion with the Western concepts.

ORGAN MANIFESTATIONS

Kwnoledge of organ manifestation is obtained by observation of life activities both in healthy persons and patients, but the conclusions chiefly deal with physiology. For example, edema manifested in the upper portion of the body is often associated with respiratory symptoms and can be relieved by administering herbal medicines for treating respiratory diseases, such as *Herba Ephedrae*. This treatment is metaphorically called "easy pouring of the pot by taking off the lid". The conclusion thus derived is physiological, namely, "the lung regulates water passages".

Regarding physiological terminology, a general issue should be discussed first. In traditional Chinese medicine, organ manifestations are usually expressed in simple sentences, and the verb most frequently used as the predicate is the character 主 [zhǔ]; for example, 肺主氣 [fèi zhǔ qì] (the lung governs qi), and 脾主升清 [pí zhǔ shēng qīng] (the spleen is in charge of sending the clear upward). It is apparently irrational to take

---

* "津液常並稱，一般不予嚴格區別。" — cited from Wu DX (chief editor). *Fundamental Theories of Traditional Chinese Medicine.* (in Chinese) The Textbook Series for Programmed Courses of the TCM University and Colleges, Shanghai Science and Technology Press, 1995, p.50.

the whole sentence as a technical term, but in many TCM dictionaries the above sentences and many others are listed in the entries. "Term" is ordinarily defined as a word or phrase used to designate some definite thing. If a sentence could be taken as a term, there would be confusion between exposition and terminology. The real problem is the difficulty in the demarcation of terms. In the above examples, it is easy to determine that the subject of the sentence can be excluded from the term, but it is hard to determine whether the predicate verb 主 [zhǔ] can be excluded. In the first example, 主氣 [zhǔ qì] (governing qi) is a term of physiological function, but in the second example, 升清 [shēng qīng] (sending the clear upward) is such a term without 主 [zhǔ]. An effective way to determine whether the character 主 [zhǔ] is a part of the term is to delete it from the sentence first. If the sentence with and without this character has basically the same meaning, it should not be included in the term, but if the sentence without this character no more represents the original meaning, it should be a part of the term. Thus, according to the exposition of organ manifestation, the physiological functions of *zang-fu* organs expressed by using the character 主 [zhǔ] can be divided into two groups as shown in the following table.

English	Chinese	English	Chinese
govern the blood	(心) 主血	govern the vessels	(心) 主脈
govern the blood vessels	(心) 主血脈	govern the mentality	(心主) 神明
rise and grow	(肝主) 升發	smooth the qi flow	(肝主) 疏泄
govern the tendons	(肝) 主筋	transport and transform	(脾主) 運化
send the clear upward	(脾主) 升清	control the blood	(脾主) 統血
govern the muscles	(脾) 主肌肉	govern the limbs	(脾) 主四肢
Move the water	(肺主) 行水	regulate water passage	(肺主) 通調水道
govern *qi*	(肺) 主氣	disperse	(肺主) 宣散
govern the voice	(肺) 主聲	purify and send downward	(肺主) 肅降
govern the skin and hair	(肺) 主皮毛	receive *qi*	(腎主) 納氣

store essence	(腎主) 藏精	govern water	(腎) 主水
govern the bones	(腎) 主骨		

From the above-listed visceral manifestations, some terms are specifically defined with traditional Chinese features, and so the related nomenclature should be standardized. Since all the terms are associated with certain physiological activities, it is better to render them in verb forms, which can be changed in nouns whenever necessary.

Proposed Standard Nomenclature

rise and grow; rising and growth 升發 [shēng fā][1]

move water; movement of water 行水 [xíng shuǐ][3]

send the clear up; up-sending of the clear 升清 [shēng qīng][5]

regulate water passages; regulation of water passages 通調水道 [tōng tiáo shuǐ dào][6]

purify and send downward; purification and down-sending 肅降 [sù jiàng][8]

smooth the qi flow; smoothing of *qi* flow 疏泄 [shū xiè][2]

transport and transform; transportation and transformation 運化 [yùn huà][4]

disperse; dispersion 宣發；宣散 [xuān fā][7]

receive qi; reception of qi 納氣 [nà qì][9]

control the blood; control of blood 統血 [tǒng xuè][10]

Discussion

1. 升發 [shēng fā] is a word group consisting of two verbs with no objects. It is rendered as "rising", "rising and growth" "flourishing growth", "ascending of qi", "upbearing and effusion", or "upward dispersion" by different authors.

2. The English equivalents of 疏泄 [shū xiè] found in recent publications are extremely diversified, including "smoothing and regulating the flow of qi", "smoothing and regulating the flow of qi and blood", "ensure the smooth flow of qi", "control the smooth flow of qi", "regulation of the flow of qi", "free flow of qi", "free coursing", "flowing and spreading", "dispersing and discharging functions", "dispersive effect", etc. The major problem comes from the absence of an object. In Chinese, particularly in Chinese medical literature, the object is self-evident. But as a standard physiological term in English, a direct literal translation of the Chinese can hardly be accepted. According to Zhong Yi Da Ci Dian (*Grand Dic-*

tionary of Traditional Chinese Medicine, 1995), the most authoritative TCM dictionary at present, 疏泄 [shū xiè] is explained as "to free or smooth the movement of qi throughout the body"* Another problem is the differrence between 疏 [shū] and 泄 [xiè]. The verb 疏 [shū] means "to dredge" or "to unblock". Although 泄 [xiè] generally means "to discharge" or "to let out", it is actually synonymous with 疏 [shū].** Rendering the whole term into English, the use of one verb is enough. Therefore, "smooth the qi flow" of "smoothing of qi flow" is proposed on the basis of the above-mentioned expressions.

3. The term 行水 [xíng shuǐ] basically has renderings: "movement of water" and "water metabolism". The latter is not only too westernized, but also inexact.

4. Most authors use "transport and transform" or "transportation and transformation" to express the concept of 運化 [yùn huà], one of the most important activities of the spleen. In order to make the term clearer, some authors add an object, e.g., "transportation and transformation of nutrients". This seems unnecessary, for the transporting and transforming function of the spleen is not confined to nutrients. Some authors prefer "digestion" to "transformation". This is not selected also because this function of the spleen not only refers to the change of food into nutrients, but also deals with water metabolism. The sequence of the words may be reversed in some authors' writings. Corresponding to the Chinese original, "transportation and transformation" is the regular sequence, but if we say "transformation and transportation", it is also logical. It should be noted that vagueness to some degree is allowed in Chinese medicine. No one can definitely say whether transportation precedes transformation, or transformation precedes transportation, or they occur simulataneously.

5. The character 升 [shēng] is a common word, but it is extremely difficult to find an English equivalent. In Chinese, it is used both as an intransitive verb and a transitive verb. There are some English words that are equivalent to the character in its intransitive sense, and some other English words equivalent to the character in its transitive sense,

---

*"舒暢全身氣機" –cited from Zhong Yi Da Ci Dian (*Grand Dictionary of Traditional Chinese Medicne*, ed. by Li JW et al., People's Publishng House of Health, 1998, p.788.

** "泄：宣通，疏利。" – cited from Jian Ming Zhong Yi Zi Dian, *Concise Dictionary of Characters in Traditional Chinese Medicine* (in Chinese), Guizhou People's Publishing House, 1985, p.150.

but no single English word can fit both. For standardization of English expressions two words may be used as equivalents, one reflecting the intrasitive 升 [shēng], and the other reflecting the transitive 升 [shēng]. The following expressions are used in this instance: "send up essential substance", "sending clarity upward", "sending the nutrients upward", "transporting nutrients upwards", and "upbearing of the clear". The word "upbear" (apparently derived from "bear" and "up") may not be appropriate, particularly when we say "The spleen upbears the clear." The word "bear" means carry, particularly while moving. The spleen has a lifting effect, and sends the clear upward. But it is hard to imagine how the spleen carries the clear while the latter is moving up to the upper portion of the body. The word "transport" is too specific in this instance. So, more authors use the common word "send", which means "cause to go without going oneself". As for the object, the word "the clear" seems the best, other words such as "nutrients" and "essential substance" can not include all what the Chinese medicine calls 清 [qīng].

6. The term 通調水道 [tōng tiáo shuǐ dào] is also a physiological term of category I, but the verb is a two-charactered compound and the object is also composed of two characters. About 水道 [shuǐ dào], most of the authors render it as "water passages", while some individual authors use the word "waterways" or "water course". As for the word 通調 [tōng tiáo], there are various expressions: "regulate", "clear and regulate", "dredge", and "open up and regulate". To make the selection, we should again pay attention to the rule of Chinese wording. In this term, if only one character were used as the verb, either 通水道 [tōng shuǐ dào] or 調水道 [tiáo shuǐ dào] would be unacceptable. The two characters, though somewhat different in meaning, are closely related. The character 通 [tōng] (open up) makes the term clearer that the regulation (調 [tiáo]) is aimed at opening. In reality, it is needless to say that physiologically the water passages should be open but not closed. So the addition of the character 通 [tōng] is chiefly for the purpose of making the term readable with two-character words. There are no such requirements in English, and so "regulate water passages" or "regulation of water passages" is regarded as the standard terminology.

7. The terms 宣發 [xuān fā] and 宣散 [xuān sàn] are synonyms. In fact, the characters 宣 [xuān] 發 [fā] and 散 [sàn] are very close in meaning. In the Chinese language many characters have multiple meanings. A common way to prescribe the proper meaning of a polysemant is

to add another character with a similar meaning. The character 宣 [xuān], when used as a verb, has at least two meanings: (1) to declare or announce, and (2) to lead off. 告 [gào] is similar to the first meaning, and 發 [fā] and 散 are similar to the second meaning. Therefore, 宣告 [xuān] means "to declare" or "to announce", and 宣發 [xuān fā] or 宣散 [xuān sàn] means "to lead off". It should be noted that both 宣發 [xuān fā] and 宣散 [xuān sàn] can be abbreviated as 宣 [xuān], but not as 發 [fā] or 散 [sàn]. The English equivalents that have appeared in recent publications include "dispersion", "diffusion", "perfusion", "dissemination", and "spreading". Literally, all these expressions are basically in keeping with the original Chinese, but considering the function of the lungs, "perfusion" may not be appropriate, for it is usually used with reference to a liquid. The words "dissemination" and "spreading" seem to be too general, and correspond more to 散 [sàn] than 宣 [xuān]. Between "dispersion" and "diffusion", more authors use the former, probably because it indicates an active process rather than a passive one.

8. The term 肅降 [sù jiàng] includes two functions: 肅 [sù] is an abbreviated of 清肅 [qīng sù], which means to purijy, and 降 [jiàng] has a dual meaning, to descend and also to make something descend. Many authors render this term as "purifying and descending", "purification and descendance" and "purity and secending". All these cannot exactly reflect the Chinese original. Some authors create "downbear" for 降 [jiàng]. It is better than "descend", but still cannot conform with the real Chinese meaning. The lungs are believed to have such an action to cause qi or water descend. This does not mean the lungs bear it downward. The word "send" might be better, for the lungs themselves do not move downward while the qi or water goes down..

9. The term 納氣 [nà qì] is rendered as "receive qi", "reception of qi", "qi absorption", "absorbing gases" and "promoting inspiration" by different authors. The words "inspiration" and "absorption" are somewhat too Westernized, and the function indicated by this term may have a wider sense. For example, it may involve the entire respiratory process and even other related functions. Therefore, most authors prefer the literal translation "reception of qi"

10. The spleen keeps the blood flowing within the vessels. This function is called 統血 [tǒng xuè]. Rendered into English, it is expressed as "regulate the blood", "be in charge of the blood", "govern the blood" and "control the blood". The last one is accepted by more authors.

ETIOLOGICAL TERMS

In traditional Chinese medicine the main factors that cause disease can be classified into three groups: (1) pathogenic factors from without, including the "six excesses" and other various infectious factors; (2) emotional disturbance and unhealthy life style; and (3) other miscellaneous pathogenic factors such as trauma.

A very important point that should be emphasized is the intimate relationship between causal factors and clinical manifestations. The Chinese knowledge of etiology was chiefly derived from the observation of clinical manifestations. This is called "seek the cause from syndromes" (審證求因 [shěn zhèng qiú yīn]). Sometimes there may be a circular argument. Take wind as an example. "Wind syndrome" is defined as a group of clinical manifestations that resemble the meteorological phenomena caused by natural wind. Deduced by analogue, "wind" is considered as the cause of "wind syndromes", and also so defined. Here, the so-called "wind" may or may not be related to the air moving as a result of natural forces. The quintessence of Chinese etiology is that it is not only associated with clinical manifestation and diagnosis, but also with the treatment. The therapeutic methods, formulas and drugs that are effective for wind syndromes are designated as "wind-dispelling therapy", "wind-dispelling formulas" and "wind-dispelling drugs". A patient with wind syndrome can often be effectively treated with a wind-dispelling therapy or formula, or drugs. From the terminological perspective, all the terms related to the same etiological term should have consistent wording.

EXTERNAL CONTRACTIONS

The processes by which external pathogenic factors, after attacking the human body, result in illness are collectively called "external contractions". The main pathogens are the six excesses (i.e., wind, cold, summer heat, dampness, dryness and fire) and various infectious or pestilential factors.

Proposed Standard Nomenclature

cause of disease 病因 [bìng yīn][1]   etiology 病因學 [bìng yīn xué][1]
pathogenic *qi* 邪氣 [xié qì][2]   pathogenic factor 邪 [xié][2]

pathogen 邪 [xié][2]

external contraction 外感 [wài gǎn][3]

external pathogen 外邪 [wài xié][4]

yin pathogen 陰邪 [yīn xié][5]

yang pathogen 陽邪 [yáng xié][5]

seasonal pathogen 時邪 [shí xié][6]

pestilential *qi* [pathogen] 癘氣 [lì qì][7]

six excesses 六淫 [liù yín][8]

wind 風 [fēng][9]

pathogenic wind 風邪 [fēng xié][9]

external wind 外風 [wài fēng][11]

endogenous wind 內風 [nèi fēng][12]

cold 寒 [hán][9]

pathogenic cold 寒邪 [hán xié][9]

external cold 外寒 [wài hán][11]

endogenous cold 內寒 [nèi hán][11]

summer heat 暑 [shǔ][10]

summer pathogen 暑邪 [shǔ xié][10]

summer heat 暑熱 [shǔ rè][10]

summer damp 暑濕 [shǔ shī][10]

dampness 濕 [shī][9]

pathogenic damp 濕邪 [shī xié][8]

external damp 外濕 [wài shī][11]

endogenous damp 內濕 [nèi shī][11]

dryness 燥 [zào][9]

pathogenic dryness 燥邪 [zào xié][8]

external dryness 外燥 [wài zào][11]

fire 火 [huǒ][9, 12]

endogenous dryness 內燥 [nèi zào][11]

pathogenic fire 火邪 [huǒ xié][9, 12]

pathogenic heat 熱邪 [rè xié][13]

heat 熱 [rè][13]

toxin 毒 [dú][15]

warm pathogen 溫邪 [wēn xié][14]

fire toxin 火毒 [huǒ dú][15]

heat toxin 熱毒 [rè dú][15]

endogenous toxin 內毒 [nèi dú][15]

damp toxin 濕毒 [shī dú][15]

intruding pathogen 客邪 [kè xié][16]

poison 毒 [dú][15]

wind-cold 風寒 [fēng hán][17]

combined pathogen 合邪 [hé xié][17]

wind-heat 風熱 [fēng rè][17]

cold-damp 寒濕 [hán shī][17]

wind-damp 風濕 [fēng shī][17]

damp-heat 濕熱 [shī rè][17]

wind-cold-damp 風寒濕 [fēng hán shī][17]

wind-dryness 風燥 [fēng zào][17]

dryness heat 燥熱 [zào rè][18]

dryness-heat 燥熱 [zào rè][18]

dryness fire 燥火 [zào huǒ][18]

dryness-fire 燥火 [zào huǒ][18]

Discussion

1. Most authors use "cause of disease" to express the concept of 病因 [bìng yīn] in Chinese medicine. Others render it as "pathogenic factor" or "etiological factor", or more freely as "origin of disharmony". "Pathogenic factor" usually refers to individual fact(s) that produce(s) a certain disease, corresponding to the Chinese concept of 病邪 [bìng xié]. The word "etiology" can certainly be used in Chinese medicine, but it is not an equivalent for 病因 [bìng yīn]. It comes from the Greek *aitia* cause and *logos* study, and so corresponds to 病因學 [bìng yīn xué] in Chinese.

2. The Chinese character 邪 [xié] is an adjective, but can also be used as a noun. In recent publications on Chinese medicine there are two ways to express this character in English: one is "evil" (as an adjective and also as a noun), and the other "pathogenic" or "pathogen". "Evil" is a literal translation of 邪 [xié]. In common Chinese language, 邪 [xié] means "morally bad" or "wickedness", but in medicine it is an abbreviation of 病邪 [bìng xié], referring to any material or influence that causes disease. Therefore, "pathogenic" or "pathogen" conforms more exactly to 邪 [xié]. There is no problem when pathogenic is used to reflect the adjective 邪 [xié], but the word "pathogen" might be controversial. In modern Western medicine a "pathogen" is often defined as a disease-producing micro-organism. However, this should not be regarded as absolute. In *Merriam-Webster's Medical Desk Dictionary*, 1996, "pathogen" is defined as "a specific causative agent (as a bacterium or virus) of disease, that is to say, agents other than micro-organisms are not excluded. In the earlier edition of *Dorland's Illustrated Medical Dictionary*, the definition of "pathogen" is "any disease-producing micro-organism or material". In other words, "pathogen" is not confined to micro-organism. In addition, etymologically the word pathogen is formed from the Greek elements *pathos* (disease) and *gennaō* (to produce), without any element referring to a micro-organism. On the other hand, in traditional Chinese medicine micro-organisms are not excluded from the disease-producing agents. Particularly in modern texts of traditional Chinese medicine, micro-organisms are stressed as the etiological factors, for example, in the *Criteria of Diagnosis and Therapeutic Effect of Diseases and Syndromes in Traditional Chinese Medicine* promulgated in 1995 by the State Administration of Traditional Chinese Medicine, People's Republic of China, the diagnostic criteria for dysentery include "growth of dysentery bacilli in stool culture or discovery of trophozoites or cysts in the fresh stool". Based on the above discussion, the word "pathogen" can be taken as the appropriate equivalent of 邪 [xié] where externally contracted diseases are concerned. In reality, the word "pathogen" has already been satisfactorily used in writing English books on Chinese medicine by quite a few Occidental authors. On the other hand, for internal injuries the term 病邪 [bìng xié] is seldom used. If there is any need for the use of this term, it can be replaced by "pathogenic factor" or "pathogenic *qi*".

3. Many authors use the word affection to express the character 感

[gǎn], but Nigel Wiseman suggests the word "contraction". The word "affection" may signify an affliction or disease, which is equivalent to the Chinese term, but the primary meaning of "affection" usually refers to a state of emotion or feeling. Since the emotional change is highly emphasized in Chinese medicine, it is better to avoid any confusion of an externally contracted disease with a disorder that relates to emotion.

4. There are several ways to express the Chinese concept of 内 [nèi] versus 外 [wài] in the causes of disease. As two adjectives, they can be rendered as internal versus external, endogenous versus exogenous, and endopathic versus exopathic. Each term has many advocates. According to *Webster's Comprehensive Dictionary* (1996), the English word endopathic means "pertaining to those diseases originating from within the organism", and exopathic means "of or resulting from causes external to the organism." In *Dorland's Illustrated Medical Dictionary*, there is only the word exopathic, with the meaning described similarly as above. There is no problem if we say exopathic disease, but it is redundant if we say exopathic pathogen or exopathic pathogenic factor (both –pathic and patho- come from the Greek *pathos*). In fact, the authors who agree with the word exopathic usually combine it with the word evil. Some authors further develop it into exopathic factor. The word "exogenous" means "originating outside the organism" (*Webster's Comprehensive Dictionary*, 1996). Some authors prefer this word, probably because they use the word "endogenous" for the pathogenic factors originating inside the body. However, most authors use the word "external" which simply means "outside the body". This is logical and reasonable, because external pathogenic factors naturally originate outside the body. They are different from internal pathogenic factors which may either originate inside the body, or originate outside and then go into the body.

5. The yin-yang classification is applicable to pathogenic factors. Pathogenic factors that tend to impede and injure yang are classified as yin pathogens, and those that tend to take the form of heat and injure yin are classified as yang pathogens. Generally speaking, cold and dampness pertain to yin, and wind, summer heat, dryness and fire pertain to yang. But there are different opinions. In addition, in some texts yin pathogen and yang pathogen also refer to the pathogenic factors that attack the yin meridians and yang meridians respectively. In the present proposed standard so defined terms are not included because the definition is too sweeping.

6. Most authors use the word "seasonal" to express the concept of 時

[shí] in the term 時邪 [shí xié]. The diversity lies in the expression of 邪 [xié] as "pathogens", "pathogenic factors", "evil", "evil factors", or simply "factors". The word pathogen is particularly suitable in this case.

7. Generally there are two main expressions for the Chinese concept 癘氣 [lì qì]: one is "epidemic pathogen" or "epidemic pathogenic *qi*", and the other, "pestilential *qi*" or "pestilential pathogen". The second one is used by more authors for its conformity with the original Chinese concept.

8. 六淫 [liù yín], the six excessive or untimely climatic influences, is a very commonly used term collectively denoting a group of pathogenic factors in Chinese medicine. Since these pathogenic factors are originally associated with climatic changes, and the Chinese character 淫 [yín] means excessive rain, which is also related to meteorological phenomena, many authors use such expressions as the "six climatic excesses", "six abnormal climatic factors", "six climatic pathogens", "six climatic conditions in excess", and "six climates excessively victorious". However, the pathogenic factors included in this term, except summer-heat, are also used for naming the pathogenic factors that are produced within the human body, and the meaning of 淫 [yín] as "excessive" is not necessarily confined to rain. Some other English terms have been initiated such as the "six pathogenic factors", "six evils", "six factors", and "six pernicious influences". All these expressions, though not erroneous, do not exactly reflect the original Chinese concept. Bensky D, Maciocia G, O'Connor J, Sivin N, Unschuld PU, and Wiseman N render this term as the "six excesses", which is now widely accepted.

9. The six excesses are individually called "wind" (風 [fēng]), "cold" (寒 [hán]), "summer heat" (暑 [shǔ]). "dampness" (濕 [shī]), "dryness" (燥 [zào]), and "fire" (火 [huǒ]). For "wind", "cold", "dryness" and "fire", there are practically no different views on their English equivalents. Divergence exists in the expression of 濕 [shī]: "damp(ness)", "moist", "wetness", or "humor". "Humor" is a Latin word, and so it is not widely accepted. The words "moist (moistness)", "damp (dampness)" and "wet (wetness)" have similar meanings but are different in degree. "Moist" is slightly wet, and the moist air may not be harmful to the health, but on the other hand it often makes one feel pleasant. "Damp" means not as dry as (something) should be, or slightly wetter than one would like[*]. So it refers

---

[*]Tom McArthur, *Longman Lexicon of Contemporary English*. Longman Group Ltd. 1981, p.560

to an abnormal condition, and for English-speaking people "damp in the air" is also believed to be harmful. "Wet" means containing or covered in liquid, and signifies rainy when referring to the weather. It is certainly harmful, but seems too severe a condition of 濕 [shī]. Most authors prefer damp(ness).

In Chinese when any of the six excesses is used singly, the character 邪 [xié] is often added. This is only partially for the purpose of differentiating the pathogen from the syndrome bearing the same name, e.g., differentiating pathogenic cold from cold syndrome. The major purpose, however, is the avoidance of mono-charactered words or the formation of a phrase with an even number of characters. For example, if we compare the term 風邪犯肺 [fēng xié fàn fèi] (pathogenic wind invading the lung) with 風熱犯肺 [fēng rè fàn fèi] (wind-heat invading the lung) we can see that both "wind" and "wind-heat" are pathogens, but the character 邪 is only used in the former case but not in the latter. It sounds awkward if we say 風犯肺 [fēng fàn fèi] or 風熱邪犯肺 [fēng rè xié fàn fèi], though there is no mistake at all in either expression. The difference in wording is purely a rhetorical matter of the Chinese language, and has nothing to do with Chinese medicine. Therefore, the proposed standard nomenclature should follow the English idiom and the scientific wording.

10. The character 暑 [shǔ] has two meanings: heat (or hot weather) and summer. Almost all authors use summer heat to express the Chinese concept of 暑 [shǔ]. The only difference is the use of a hyphen or the union of the two words. Thus, there are three types of expression: summer heat, summer-heat, and summerheat. In the present scheme, "summer heat" is taken as the equivalent of both 暑 [shǔ] and 暑熱 [shǔ rè], because 暑 [shǔ] when used singly as a medical term is usually an abbreviation of 暑熱 [shǔ rè]. In the terms 暑邪 [shǔ xié] and 暑濕 [shǔ shī], however, the character 暑 [shǔ] refers to the hot season or summer, and the equivalents are "summer pathogen" and "summer damp" respectively. In the latter two terms it is better not to render the character 暑 [shǔ] as summer-heat. "Summer pathogen" (暑邪 [shǔ xié]) includes summer heat and summer damp, while "summer-heat pathogen" excludes summer damp. Many authors render 暑濕 [shǔ shī] as "summer-heat and damp(ness)". Since the word summer already has the meaning of "the hottest season", the word "heat" is redundant.

11. Most authors render the character 外 as external, and so "external

wind" for 外風 [wài fēng], "external cold" for 外寒 [wài hán], "external dampness" for 外濕 [wài shī], and "external dryness" for 外燥 [wài zào]. The word "external" means "situated on the outside" and "coming from the outside". Translation of 外邪 as external pathogen is appropriate, and there is no need for such expressions as "exogenous" and "exopathic" to give special emphasis to the origination, as all external pathogenic factors must originate outside the body. In Chinese terminology, there is only 外邪 [wài xié], but no 內邪 [nèi xié]. If someone uses the latter term, it is merely an abbreviation of 內生之邪 [nèi shēng zhī xié] (pathogen originating from inside the body). The word "internal" only means "of the inside of the body", and does not signify origination from the inside. Therefore, it is reasonable to render 內風 [nèi fēng] as "endogenous wind", 內寒 [nèi hán] as "endogenous cold", 內濕 [nèi shī] as "endogenous dampness", and 內燥 [nèi zào] as "endogenous dryness", when they are regarded as pathogenic factors.

12. All authors render 火 [huǒ] as "fire". As a pathogenic factor, it is an abbreviation for "pathogenic fire" 火邪 [huǒ xié]. It should be noted that "fire" is not always a pathogenic factor. Sometimes it refers to a pathological change, and sometimes it refers to a physiological action. Generally, its real implication can be easily distinguished from the context. If it causes any confusion, the better way is to use "pathogenic fire", "pathological fire", and "physiological fire" instead of the single word "fire". In addition, "fire" may also be an abbreviation of fire syndrome, a syndrome caused by pathogenic fire. However, it is better to call it "fire syndrome" than simply "fire".

13. There is no disagreement about the term "heat" (熱 [rè]) as an abbreviation for pathogenic heat (熱邪 [rè xié]). Similarly to the term "fire", the abbreviated term "heat" also has multiple implications and applications. It may refer to a pathogenic factor, a pathological process or a syndrome. Whenever confusion may arise, it is better to employ the unabbreviated form.

14. In Chinese medicine, acute febrile diseases with seasonal prevalence are collectively called "warm disease" (溫病 [wēn bìng]), and any pathogenic factor that causes warm disease is called "warm pathogen" (溫邪 [wēn xié]. Most authors use the word "warm" to express the Chinese concept of 溫 [wēn]. Some authors suggest the word "warmth", but it is not widely accepted. There is not much divergence in rendering 溫 [wēn] as "warm". Divergence exists in the selection of "pathogen" or "evil" as

the equivalent of 邪 [xié].

15. 毒 [dú] in Chinese medicine has multiple meanings. As its equivalent, various expressions have appeared in recent publications, such as "poison", "toxin", "venom", "toxic substance", and "poisonous substance". In addition, it also refers to ulcers in external diseases. "Toxin" and "poison" are selected as the proposed standard terminology, for both are frequently used. Venom is a poisonous fluid of certain snakes, scorpions, etc. injected by a bite or sting, and so it is only used in snake-bite and insect-sting. The terms toxic substance and poisonous substance are not succinct enough. In external diseases yin ulcer and yang ulcer are equivalents of 陰毒 [yīn dú] and 陽毒 [yáng dú], but they are not pathogenic factors.

The concept of 毒 [dú] may be clear-cut, referring to some concrete substances, but may also be vague, representing the virulence of any of the external pathogens, particularly if the pathogen has been accumulated and retained. For example, retained pathogenic damp may become toxic, giving rise to an intractable lesion with profuse exudation. In Chinese medicine, the pathogenic factor is believed to be damp toxin (濕毒 [shī dú]) instead of simple damp pathogen (濕邪 [shī xié]). Most authors render 濕毒 [shī dú] as "damp toxin". Other expressions such as "noxious dampness", "toxic material produced by wetness-evil", "toxin produced by damp" are not widely accepted. Similarly, the toxin derived from retained pathogenic heat is called "heat toxin" 熱毒 [rè dú] which often gives rise to abscesses and sores. For this term, various equivalents have been proposed: "noxious heat", "pyretic toxicity", "toxic heat", "virulent heat", "toxin heat", and "heat toxin". Among them, "heat toxin" seems to be most consistent with the original Chinese concept. Selection of the proper equivalent of 火毒 [huǒ dú] is even more complicated, for the term itself has dual implications. On the one hand, it refers to the toxin that originates from stagnation of pathogenic fire, mostly occurring in inflammations accompanying external diseases; on the other hand, it can also mean the toxin that causes infection in cases of burns. Therefore, this term is translated in various ways, such as "noxious fire", "virulent fire", "burn infection", "burn complicated by infection", and "infection caused by fire", but most authors prefer "fire toxin". In this scheme, "fire toxin" is selected with one single definition, excluding the issue of burns.

The term 內毒 [nèi dú] refers to heat toxins arising inside the body instead of coming from without. For this concept, "endogenous toxin" is more appropriate than "internal toxin", for the latter may come from without. Some author even renders it "endotoxin", but this seems to be amiss, for "endotoxin" is specifically defined in Western medicine as the toxin present in bacteria but separable from the cell body only on its integration.

16. Any pathogenic factor from without that has entered the body is called "intruding pathogen" (客邪 [kè xié]). Although the Chinese character 客 [kè] means "guest", it also has several other meanings. One of them is "intrude from outside"* Translations such as "visiting pathogen" and "guest pathogen" are not recommendable.

17. "Combined pathogen" (合邪 [hé xié]) is a combination of two or more pathogenic factors invading the human body simultaneously. Most authors recommend inserting a hyphen (or hyphens) between the pathogens when they are regarded as a combined pathogen, but for a compound name of two pathogens with the transformation of one from the other, no hyphenation is used. Thus, most authors prefer "wind-cold" (風寒 [fēng hán]), "wind-heat" (風熱 [fēng rè]), "wind-dryness" (風燥 [fēng zào]) "wind-damp" (風濕 [fēng shī]), "cold-damp" (寒濕 [hán shī]), damp-heat (濕熱 [shī rè]), etc. Only a few authors add the word "pathogen" to distinguish a term from the related syndrome, e.g., "wind-cold pathogen" as a pathogenic factor and "wind-cold syndrome" as a syndrome name.

It should be noted that in Chinese 風寒 [fēng hán] (wind-cold) and 風濕 [fēng shī] (wind-damp) are common terms, but for a combination of 風 [fēng], 寒 [hán] and 濕 [shī] the terminology is usually 風寒濕邪 [fēng hán shī xié] (wind-cold-damp). This does not at all mean that wind-cold and wind-damp are not pathogenic, or wind-cold-damp is particularly pathogenic. The Chinese seldom say 風寒邪 [fēng hán xié] and 風濕邪 [fēng shī xié] simply because these terminologies are against "the law of even-numbered characters" in writing and speaking. If they really want to say so, they have to add a functional character 之 [zhī], which has no substantial meaning but makes the characters of the term even-numbered. It is certainly unnecessary to coin the standard English nomenclature in the traditional mold of Chinese characters.

---

* cf. Ci Hai (辭海), 1979, p. 1021, and Jian Ming Zhong Yi Zi Dian, *Concise Dictionary of Characters in Chinese Medicine* (簡明中醫字典) (in Chinese), Guizhou People's Publishing House, 1985, p. 196

Usually, the name of a combined pathogen is also used as the name of the syndrome caused by that pathogen. For example, "wind-damp" is a combined pathogen, and the syndrome caused by wind-damp is also called "wind-damp". Actually, the former is an abbreviation of "pathogenic wind-damp" or "wind-damp pathogen", and the latter, an abbreviation of "wind-damp syndrome". Whenever there is any possible confusion, use of the full name is preferred.

18. In the cases of dryness and heat and the cases of dryness and fire, the condition may be different. There may be pathogenic heat or fire transformed from dryness, and there also may be a simple combination of dryness and heat or dryness and fire. That is why different authors often give diversified English expressions, for example, "dry heat", "dry-heat", "dryness and heat", "dryness- and-heat", and "dryness-heat" for 燥熱 [zào rè]. As mentioned above, in this scheme "dryness heat" and "dryness fire" indicate pathogenic heat or fire transformed from dryness. "Dryness-heat" and dryness-fire" indicate a simple combination of two pathogenic factors.

INTERNAL INJURIES

The causal factors of internal injuries are chiefly emotions and various kinds of improper life style.

Proposed Standard Nomenclature

internal injury 內傷 [nèi shāng][1]	emotions 情志 [qíng zhì][2]
joy 喜 [xǐ][3]	anger 怒 [nù][4]
worry 憂 [yōu][5]	grief 憂 [yōu][5]
anxiety 思 [sī][6]	sadness 悲 [bēi][7]
fear 恐 [kǒng][8]	fright 驚 [jīng][9]
Life-style 生活方式 [shēng huó fāng shì][10]	diet 飲食 [yǐn shí][10]
	fatigue 勞倦 [láo juàn][10]

Discussion

1. In traditional Chinese medicine 內傷 [nèi shāng] means injury to the internal organs, resulting from emotional disturbance or unhealthy life style. In recent publications, several expressions can be encountered for reflecting this concept: "internal damage", "internal disturbance",

"internal impairment", and "internal injury". The majority of authors prefer "injury", probably because it is a general word including damage, impairment, etc.

2. Regarding 情志 [qíng zhì], two collective terms often used in traditional Chinese medicine, are 七情 [qī qíng] (the seven emotions) and 五志 [wǔ zhì] (the five emotions). In these terms either 情 [qíng] or 志 [zhì] is an abbreviation of the word 情志 [qíng zhì], and so 情 [qíng], 志 [zhì] and 情志 [qíng zhì] bear the same implication. As the equivalent, different authors have suggested quite a few English words, such as "affects", "passions", "sentiments", "emotional factors", "modes of emotions". All of these expressions have their own grounds, but each is only used by a few authors. Most authors prefer the term "emotions". In fact, the word emotion that means strong feeling of any kind is more appropriate than the other words.

3. As the equivalent for 喜 [xǐ], most authors prefer the word "joy". Some suggest "pleasure", "elation", "happiness", etc., but these expressions are not widely accepted. Some use "overjoy" or "excessive joy" to show that ordinarily joy is not harmful to the health. As terminology, simply the word "joy" is an exact equivalent of the original Chinese. For overjoy or excessive joy, the Chinese equivalent is 過喜 [guò xǐ].

4. Almost all authors use the word anger for 怒 [nù]. The word rage recommended by some other authors may be used in writing to stress a severe attack of anger or avoid redundancy, but it should not be regarded as the standard nomenclature because it is not an exact equivalent of 怒 [nù]. Rage means violent anger, equivalent to 盛怒 [shèng nù], another commonly used word in classical Chinese medical literature.

5. As a common Chinese character, 憂 [yōu] has two meanings. It means grief as used in the word 憂傷 [yōu shāng], and means worry as used in the word 擔憂 [dān yōu]. In Chinese medicine, both meanings of this character are valid. When 憂 [yōu] injures the lung, it means grief, and when, in combination with 思 [sī], it injures the spleen, it means worry. Therefore, both "worry" and "grief" can be regarded as the appropriate translation, and are advocated by many authors. In English, no corresponding word with such a dual meanings can be found. Two entries are thus collected in this scheme for the same term. There are a number of other translations: "melancholy", "anxiety", "sorrow", and "sadness". Among these words, "melancholy" may lead to confusion with the disease name used in Western medicine, referring to severe forms of major de-

pressive disorder. The word "anxiety" is more appropriate for translating 思 [sī], an emotion close to but different from 憂 [yōu]. "Sorrow" and "sadness" are more suitable for 悲 [bēi].

6. Many authors use the word pensiveness to express 思 [sī]. A number of words such as "reflection", "meditation", "thought", and "thinking" appearing in recent TCM publications, though conforming to the Chinese character 思 [sī] in its common sense, are not related to emotions. Two words are more frequently used: pensiveness and anxiety. Both are of emotional coloring, particularly the latter. Because the Chinese characters denoting the emotions that may cause disease are usually very popular words, the word anxiety is thus selected.

7. Three words are frequently used to express 悲 [bēi]. They are "sadness", "sorrow" and "grief". Each has adequate advocates. Since many authors render 憂 [yōu] as "grief", we had better not use "grief", in order to avoid confusion. Sadness is selected, for more American and British authors prefer this word.

8. The translations made by various authors include fear, fright, terror, shock, panic and apprehension. Most authors use the word fear or fright, and in comparison more authors prefer the word fear to fright.

9. The words most frequently used by various authors to express the Chinese character 驚 [jīng] are "fright" and "terror". Some individual authors recommend the words "shock", "fear", and "apprehension". By comparison with "terror", the word "fright" may be more appropriate, as the Chinese character 驚 [jīng] signifies a feeling of sudden unpleasant fear.

10. Life style is a collective term including diet, work, rest, sexual activities, etc. Various diseases may be caused by improper way of life such as dietary irregularities, physical or mental overstrain, excessive fatigue, over-indulgence in sex, etc. In Chinese medicine the above factors are often discussed separately, but all these and other related factors can be summed up under the heading of life style. Many writers (but not translators) prefer this term to separate headings.

OTHER PATHOGENIC FACTORS

In Chinese medicine, pathological products that cause complications or further development of a disease are often regarded as pathogenic factors. Of them, the common ones are water, damp, phlegm, retained fluid, and stagnant blood. Here, the damp, water, phlegm and retained fluid are all endogenous, and mostly the products of visceral dysfunction, particularly of spleen insufficiency. Stagnant blood is also a pathological product, due to *qi* deficiency, *qi* depression, cold congealing, and heat accumulation. In addition, some other causal factors frequently described in Chinese medicine are also listed in this section.

Proposed Standard Nomenclature

stagnant blood 瘀血 [yū xuè][1]

phlegm 痰 [tán][2]

phlegm-fluid 痰飲 [tán yǐn][2]

trauma 外傷 [wài shāng][3]

water-damp 水濕 [shuǐ shī][2]

retained fluid 飲 [yǐn][2]

non-acclimatization 水土不服 [shuǐ tǔ bù fú][4]

Discussion

1. 瘀血 [yū xuè] is a pathological product of blood stagnation, including extravasated blood and the blood moving sluggishly in circulation or congested in a viscus. Its English terms include two groups of terms: (1) stagnant blood, stagnated blood and congealed blood, (2) stasis of blood, and blood stasis. Group 2 refers to a morbid condition, while group 1 refers to the pathogenic factor. So, blood stasis is usually used for 血瘀 [xuè yū], and stagnant blood for 瘀血 [yū xuè]. Since "stagnate" is an intransitive verb, "stagnant" is more frequently used than "stagnated" as an attributive. The word "congealed" used by some authors is too serious, for congealed blood usually refers to blood in coagulation or blood clots. Of course, congealed blood is stagnant, but stagnant blood is not always congealed.

2. The pathological products of water metabolism are water (水 [shuǐ]), damp (濕 [shī]), phlegm (痰 [tán]) and retained fluid (飲 [yǐn]). Accumulation of damp produces "water", retention of water forms "retained fluid", and condensed fluid becomes phlegm. In other words, "phlegm" is thick, "retained fluid" is thin, "water" is clear, and "damp" is diffused. As for the English expression, most of the authors use "water", and "damp" as the equivalents of 水 [shuǐ], and 濕 [shī], but for the terms 痰 [tán] and 飲 [yǐn] there are diversified expressions.

In modern Chinese the character 痰 [tán] refers only to "sputum", but in traditional Chinese medicine this character is used in a much broader sense. It is a pathological product of diseased internal organs (especially the spleen), sticky and slimy, which, in turn, may cause various troubles, e.g., profuse expectoration when it is accumulated in the lungs, nausea and vomiting when the stomach is affected; dizziness and heavy-headedness when the head is involved, palpitations, impairment of consciousness or even mania when the heart is invaded, and scrofula when accumulating subcutaneously. It is a unique concept of Chinese medicine, referring to such a pathogenic factor that may impair the lungs, the spleen and stomach, the heart (mind) and even the subcutaneous tissue, giving rise to various serious symptoms. There is a saying in Chinese medicine: "Strange diseases are mostly caused by 痰 [tán]". The word "phlegm" is now generally accepted as its equivalent in English. Some authors use "mucus" and "sputum", both of which are too limited in sense, for mucus is the secretion of the mucous membrane and sputum is confined to the mucus coughed up from the respiratory tract. The word "phlegm", though also referring to the thick mucus secreted by the mucosa of the respiratory passages during infections, was used in humoralism as one of the four humors of the body. Of course, the word "phlegm" used in Chinese medicine should not carry its original meaning in humoralism, but at least it reminds us that we should not merely think of the mucus secretion.

As for 飲 [yǐn], "fluid", "fluid retention", "retained fluid", and "rheum" have been proposed. It might be a good suggestion to use "rheum" as the equivalent of 飲 [yǐn], for "rheum" is really a kind of abnormal fluid. Unfortunately, it has already been defined in Western medicine as a catarrhal discharge from the nose and eyes related to a cold. This is certainly not what the term 飲 [yǐn] signifies. In addition, "rheum" comes from the Greek *rheuma* which means a flow, and may refer to any thin watery flux. This is in opposition to 飲 [yǐn] which refers to fluid in retention and stagnation. Since most authors render 津液 [jīn yè] as "body fluids" or "fluids", rendering 飲 [yǐn] as "fluid" may cause confusion. Therefore, "retained fluid" is selected as the proposed standard term, but the addition of attributive "retained" is flexible. If there is no confusion with the concept of normal fluid, e.g., when it is used in combination with phlegm, the word "retained" can be omitted, hence "phlegm-fluid" as the equivalent of 痰飲 [tán yǐn].

3. The term 外傷 [wài shāng] is rendered in the following ways: "external damage", "external injury", "traumatic injury" and "trauma". The

last one seems the best, because it means "an injury to living tissue caused by an extrinsic agent"[*], and any word like "external" is unnecessary. In addition, it conforms with the term "traumatology".

4. Temporary unadaptability of a person to the natural environment of a new dwelling place can be the cause of disease and is called 水土不服 [shuǐ tǔ bù fú]. Since climatic change is often the primary factor, some render it as "climate sickness", which does not exactly tally with the original concept. Quite a few authors use the word "unacclimatization", but it is not a generally recognized English word. More authors prefer the word "non- acclimatization".

PATHOGENETIC TERMS

Pathogenesis is the origination and development of a disease. In traditional Chinese medicine, pathogenesis has the following characteristic features. First of all, the relative forces of the normal *qi* and the pathogenic factors should be sized up, as any disease is considered as a struggling process between the health and evil *qi*. Secondly, disturbances of yin-yang harmony should be reckoned with, as any disease process is a kind of disharmony between yin and yang. Thirdly, the main part of pathogenesis refers to pathological changes upon which disorders of *qi*, blood, fluid, zang-fu organs or meridians develop.

STRUGGLE BETWEEN NORMAL AND PATHOGENIC *QI*

Traditional Chinese medicine defines disease as the struggling process of the body's capacity for maintaining health and normal activities (called "health *qi*" or "normal *qi*") against pathogenic factors. Terms regarding the confrontation between health *qi* and pathogenic *qi* are the very basic terms of pathogenesis in Chinese medicine.

---

[*] *Merriam Webster's Medical Desk Dictionary*, Merriam-Webster, Inc., Massachusetts, U.S.A., 1996, p. 828.

Proposed Standard Nomenclature

pathogenesis 病機 [bìng jī][1]

normal *qi* 正氣 [zhèng qì][2]

health *qi* 正氣 [zhèng qì][2]

exuberance and decline of pathogenic or normal *qi* 邪正盛衰 [xié zhèng shèng shuāi][4]

mechanism of disease 病機 [bìng jī][1]

struggle between normal and pathogenic *qi* 正邪相爭 [zhèng xié xiāng zhēng][3]

Discussion

1. There two trends of rendering the term. 病機 [bìng jī] into English: one is the rendering of 機 [jī] as mechanism, hence "mechanism of disease", "pathomechanism", or "pathological mechanism", and the other is the adoption of the modern term "pathogenesis". Most authors use the latter, but it is somewhat westernized. Both "pathogenesis" and "mechanism of disease" are collected in this scheme for the convenience of writing, for example, using "pathogenesis" to parallel "etiology", and "mechanism of disease" to match "cause of disease".

2. The Chinese word 正氣 [zhèng qì] refers to the body resistance in contrast to pathogenic *qi*, but it cannot be simply nominated as such, because it is a collective term referring to all kinds of functional activities of the human body for the maintenance of a normal life. Various English words have been used to express the character 正 [zhèng] in Chinese medicine, such as "normal", "health", "healthy", "right", "righteous", "upright", "vital", "genuine", "orthopathic", and "anti-pathogenic". The appropriateness of these words can be judged from their antonyms. In Chinese medicine the opposite of 正 [zhèng] is 邪 [xié]. If it is better to render the latter as "pathogenic", as discussed above, then "normal", "health(y)" and "anti-pathogenic" are appropriate. "Right" and "upright" are direct word-for-word translations, their opposites are "wrong (誤 [wù])" and "slanting (斜 [xié])". Quite a few authors recommend the word "upright" or "righteous", probably because it is opposite to "evil (邪 [xié])". They are exact in the case of moral concepts or ethics, but not medicine. The word vital seems too general, and the word genuine comes through a winding course from the saying that 正氣 is also 真氣 (genuine *qi*). Among the words normal, health(y) and anti-pathogenic, the first is selected simply because it is recommended by more authors, and the second is also adopted as a synonym of the first.

3. Besides "struggle", some other words such as "counteraction" and "conflict" have been used to express the concept of 相爭 [xiāng zhēng]. Most authors prefer the word "struggle".

4. The exuberance and decline of pathogenic and health *qi* determines the process and prognosis of a patient, namely, rise of the normal *qi* with decline of the pathogenic *qi* leading to improvement and cure, while exuberance of pathogenic *qi* with decline of normal *qi* resulting in deterioration and even death. The words that have been recommended by different authors for expressing the pathogenetic concept of 盛衰 [shèng shuāi] include "exuberance (exuberant)" or "excess (excessive)" versus "decline (declined)", "deficiency (deficient)", "debilitation (debilitated)" or "exhaustion (exhausted)". For 盛 [shèng], "exuberance" is more appropriate because "excess" is often used to reflect the concept of 實 [shí]. For 衰 [shuāi], "decline" is more appropriate because "deficiency" is often used for 虛 [xū], and "debilitation" and "exhaustion" are too serious.

YIN-YANG DISHARMONY

In Chinese medicine, health is characterized by yin-yang harmony, and all kinds of diseases are regarded by various yin-yang disharmonies. Thus, the words or phrases describing yin-yang disharmony are primary terms of pathogenesis.

Proposed Standard Nomenclature

yin-yang disharmony 陰陽失調 [yīn yáng shī tiáo][1]

yin exuberance 陰盛 [yīn shèng][3]

yang deficiency with yin exuberance 陽虛陰盛 [yáng xū yīn shèng][4]

yin deficiency with yang hyperactivity 陰虛陽亢 [yīn xū yáng kàng][4]

preponderance of yin or yang 陰陽偏盛[勝][yīn yáng piān shèng][5]

yin-yang dual deficiency 陰陽兩虛 [yīn yáng liǎng xū][6]

repelled yin 格陰 [gé yīn][7]

repelled yang 格陽 [gé yáng][7]

yin deficiency 陰虛 [yīn xū][2]

yang deficiency 陽虛 [yáng xū][2]

yang exuberance 陽盛 [yáng shèng][3]

yin exuberance with yang decline 陰盛陽衰 [yīn shèng yáng shuāi][4]

yin deficiency with flaming fire 陰虛火旺 [yīn xū huǒ wàng][4]

decline of yin or yang 陰陽偏衰 [yīn yáng piān shuāi][5]

repelling of yin or yang 陰陽格拒 [yīn yáng gé jù][7]

excessive yin repelling yang 陰盛格陽 [yīn shèng gé yáng][7]

exuberant yang repelling yin 陽盛格陰 [yáng shèng gé yīn][7]

yin collapse 亡陰 [wáng yīn][9]

up-floating of asthenic yang 虛陽上浮 [xū yáng shàng fú][8]

yang collapse 亡陽 [wáng yáng][9]

Discussion

1. The antonym of 失調 [shī tiáo] is 調和 [tiáo hé]. In recent publications quite a few English words are used to express this pair of concepts: "imbalance" vs. "balance", "derangement" vs. "arrangement", "disorder" vs. "order", "incoordination" vs. "coordination", "disharmony" vs. "harmony". The last pair is most acceptable, for they reflect the original concept best and the word "harmonize" fits 調和 [tiáo hé] when the latter is used as a verb.

2. The character 虛 [xū] is a very important word in Chinese medicine. At the International Symposium on Translation Methodologies and Terminologies, 1986, Nigel Wiseman and Paul Zmiewski held a detailed discussion on the rendering of 虛 [xū] and 實 [shí]. They believed that "deficiency" and "excess" were perhaps the most commonly used choices, and were certainly kindest to the ears, but outside the context of eight-principle pattern identification they were rarely suitable equivalents. Their comments were apparently based on the assumption that since the Chinese medical terms in Chinese are composed of characters, the translation should start from searching for a suitable equivalent for each character; until such an equivalent that fits the character in all the meanings of the given character used in medicine is found. This issue will be discussed elsewhere. For the present entry, it should be emphasized that most of the authors do use "deficiency" to express the concept of 虛 [xū] in the statement of pathogenesis.

3. The English equivalent of the Chinese character 盛 [shèng] has been discussed in 邪正盛衰 [xié zhèng shèng shuāi]. The equivalents for 陰盛 [yīn shèng] in recent publications include "excess of yin", "yin excess", "preponderance of yin", "yin predomination"; "excessive yin", "yin sthenia", "exuberant yin", "yin exuberance", "flourishing of yin", "overabundance of yin", etc., and those for 陽盛 [yáng shèng], "excess of yang", "yang excess", "exuberance of yang", "exuberant yang", "yang exuberance", "predominant yang", "preponderance of yang", "hyperactivity of yang", etc. In Chinese, there are several characters synonymous with 盛 [shèng] but different in usage. They are 旺 [wàng], 亢 [kàng],

and 勝 [shèng]. Primarily, 旺 [wàng] is used to describe a blazing fire. By extension, it means "flourishing". 旺盛 [wàng shèng] is often used in combination as one word. The character 盛 [shèng] is composed of two elements. The upper element 成 [chéng] gives the sound, while the lower element 皿 is the pictograph of a utensil. So, the character 盛 (pronounced chéng) means "to fill (a utensil with grains for offering to gods and ancestors)". Since the sacrifice should be abundant, this character is also used to signify "abundant", "plentiful", "prosperous", and "vigorous". The difference between 旺 [wàng] and 盛 [shèng] lies in that the former only refers to actions or activities, but the latter refers to both materials and activities. Another character closely related to 盛 [shèng] is 亢 [kàng], and 亢盛 [kàng shèng] is also often used in combination as one word. The character 亢 usually refers to increase in activity but not to abundance of substance, so we say 陽亢 but we do not say 陰亢. Therefore, the equivalent for 亢 is hyperactivity (hyperactive). The characters 勝 [shèng] and 盛 [shèng] are not only synonyms but also homonyms. Sometimes they can replace each other, for example, 陰陽偏盛 [yīn yáng piān shèng] can be written as 陰陽偏勝 [yīn yáng piān shèng]. Although there is some minor difference between the two characters, both of them are are used in a sense of contrast in this term, and so are often rendered as "preponderance".

For 陰盛 [yīn shèng] and 陽盛 [yáng shèng], various expressions are available, such as "excess of yin (yang)", "yin (yang) excess", "preponderance of yin (yang)", "yin (yang) predomination"; "predominant yin (yang)", "excessive yin (yang)", "yin (yang) sthenia", "exuberant yin (yang)", "yin (yang) exuberance", "flourishing of yin (yang)", "overabundance of yin (yang)", etc. Based on the above discussion, "yin exuberance" and "yang exuberance" are selected.

4. For 陽虛陰盛 [yáng xū yīn shèng], 陰虛陽亢 [yīn xū yáng kàng] and 陰虛火旺 [yīn xū huǒ wàng], each containing two basic terms, the problem lies in the relationship between the basic terms. In the Chinese original the so-called "functional character" joining the two basic terms is omitted for rhetorical reasons. We can try to restore the possible character, such as 與 [yǔ] (and), 並 [bìng] (together with), 伴 [bàn] (accompanied by), 致 [zhì] (resulting in), etc. For the time being, the word "with" is selected.

5. Imbalance of yin and yang may be "preponderance of yin or yang" 陰陽偏勝 [yīn yáng piān shèng] and "decline of yin or yang" 陰陽偏

衰 [yīn yáng piān shuāi]. They are two main categoris of pathological changes with substantial differences. When we say excess of yang, we mean that yang is overabundant while yin is not decreased. But in contrast to the exuberant yang, yin is relatively insufficient. When we say decline of yang, we mean that yang is reduced while yin remains at its regular level, but in contrast to the declined yang, yin is relatively in excess.

6. 兩虛 [liǎng xū] is expressed as "deficiency of both…", "dual deficiency", and "concurrent deficiency" in recent publications. The first two seem more appropriate.

7. 陰陽格拒 [yīn yáng gé jù] is a special form of pathological change in which extremely excessive yin in the interior forces the asthenic yang to spread outward or extremely exuberant yang in the interior keeps the insufficient yin on the outside, forming pseudo-heat or pseudo-cold phenomena. For expressing this concept the characters 格 [gé] and 格拒 [gé jù] have been rendered in English in the following different ways: "repel", "reject", "hinder", "keep out", "screen", "elude", etc. Among these expressions, "hinder" is too vague; "reject" which means refuse to accept, is too weak; "keep out" is too general; "repulse" means drive back by fighting, and is too strong; "screen" and "elude" can only be expressed in the passive voice, but the original term is active; and "repel" means drive back or away, which appears to be the most appropriate word.

陰盛格陽 [yīn shèng gé yáng] is a pathological process in which asthenic yang is forced to float on the body surface while the excessive yin is entrenched in the interior, manifested by intense internal cold with pseudo-heat symptoms. This statement is actually a complete sentence with subject, predicate and object. It can be rendered in English as "Exuberant yin repels yang". As a technical term, the following expressions have appeared in recent publications: "excessive yin rejecting yang", "exuberant yin repelling yang", "excessive yin hindering yang", "yang kept externally by yin-excess in the interior", "interior excess-yin keeping yang out", "excess of yin with elusion of yang", and "predominating yin screened by yang". Among these expressions, "exuberant yin repelling yang" is probably the most appropriate.

In Chinese this term can be abbreviated as 格陽 [gé yáng], and in English the corresponding abbreviation is "repelling of yang" or "repelled yang". As a term indicating pathogenesis, "repelling of yang" seems more suitable.

陽盛格陰 [yáng shèng gé yīn] is a pathological process in which

extremely exuberant yang trapped in the interior keeps the insufficient yin in the exterior, usually referring to high fever with pseudo-cold symptoms. The statement is also a complete sentence, and can be rendered in English as "Exuberant yang repels yin". For similar reasons to those mentioned above, "exuberant yang repelling yin" for this term and "repelling of yin" (格陰 [gé yīn]) as its abbreviation are selected as the proposed standard terms.

8. Since pseudo-heat syndrome is of great clinical significance, besides "exuberant yin repelling yang" there are other statements to express the mechanism. 虛陽上浮 [xū yáng shàng fú] is a commonly used one. The English equivalents available for selection include "vacuous yang floating upward", "upfloating of vacuous yang", "upfloating of asthenic yang", "floating up of asthenic yang", "upward floating of asthenic yang", "floating of weak yang", and "upward floating of yang in deficiency condition". In this case, the word "asthenic" is probably more appropriate than "weak", "vacuous" and "in deficiency condition".

9. An extreme yin-yang disharmony is massive loss of yin or yang. In Chinese medicine it is called 亡陰 [wáng yīn] or 亡陽 [wáng yáng], respectively. In either case, there is sudden and serious functional exhaustion, showing a critical morbid state. According to the description made in the national Chinese textbook of TCM[*], massive loss of either yin or yang is manifested by the following features: (1) functional failure, (2) consumption of *qi*, and (3) profuse sweating. In addition, there is faint, hardly perceivable pulse or very rapid pulse. The availabe expressions seen in recent publications are "yin (yang) exhaustion" or "exhaustion of yin (yang)", "yin (yang) depletion" or "depletion of yin (yang)", and "yin (yang) collapse" or "collapse of yin (yang)". By comparing the three words: exhaustion — a state of extreme mental or physical fatigue, or the state being drained, emptied, consumed or used up, depletion — an exhausted state resulting from excessive loss of blood; and collapse — a state of extreme prostration and depression, with failure of circulation, (cited from *Dorland's Illustrated Medical Dictionary*, 29th edition, 2000), the last word seems the best to fit the Chinese concept.

---

[*] Wu DX (chief ed.) Zhong Yi Xue Ji Chu Li Lun, *Fundamental Theories of Traditional Chinese Medicine* (in Chinese), the Textbook Series for Programmed Courses of the TCM Universities and Colleges, Shanghai Science and Techonology Press, 1997, p. 160-161.

The Chinese term 脫陰 [tuō yīn] or 陰脫 [yīn tuō] is synonymous with 亡陰 [wáng yīn] (yin collapse), and 脫陽 [tuō yáng] or 陽脫 [yáng tuō] is synonymous with 亡陽 [wáng yáng] (yang collapse). Therefore, no special English equivalent other than "collapse" is necessary.

COLD-INDUCED DISEASES, WARM DISEASES AND OTHER EXTERNAL CONTRACTIONS

The pathogenesis of febrile diseases was first systematically described in the book *Treatise on Cold-induced Diseases*, and later under the heading of Warm Diseases. To date, both cold-induced diseases and warm diseases exist in parallel as two schools for studying febrile diseases. Some terms are only used in cold-induced diseases, and some only in warm diseases. But since the knowledge of warm diseases is developed on the basis of cold-induced diseases, many terms are used for both, and so the terms of the two categories are put together in one section.

Proposed Standard Nomenclature

cold-induced disease 傷寒 [shāng hán][1]

sequential meridian transmission 循經傳 [xún jīng chuán][2]

direct attack 直中 [zhí zhòng][3]

combination of disease 合病 [hé bìng][4]

warm disease 温病 [wēn bìng][5]

contagion 傳染 [chuán rǎn][6]

adverse transmission 逆傳 [nì chuán][8]

warm pathogen invading the lung 温邪犯肺 [wēn xiè fàn fèi][9]

disharmony between nutrient and defense 營衛不和 [yíng wèi bù hé][10]

strong defense with weak nutrient 衛強營弱 [wèi qiáng yíng ruò][10]

heat transformation 熱化 [rè huà][12]

heat binding (in the interior) 熱結

meridian transmission 傳經 [chuán jīng][2]

skip-over meridian transmission 越經傳 [yuè jīng chuán][2]

double contraction 兩感 [liǎng gǎn][4]

overlapping of disease 並病 [bìng bìng][4]

sequential transmission 順傳 [shùn chuán][7]

adverse transmission to the pericardium 逆傳心包 [nì chuán xīn bāo][8]

weak defense with strong nutrient 衛弱營強 [wèi ruò yíng qiáng][10]

transmission of heat into the interior 熱邪傳裏 [rè xié chuán lǐ][11]

cold transformation 寒化 [hán huà][12]

heat binding in the bladder 熱結

[rè jié]; 熱邪內結 [rè xiè nèi jié][13]
fecal impaction with watery discharge 熱結旁流 [rè jié páng liú][13]
heat blockage 熱閉 [rè bì][14]
heat entering the pericardium 熱入心包 [rè rù xīn bāo][15]
heat entering blood 熱入血分 [rè rù xuè fèn][16]
stagnant heat in blood 血分瘀熱 [xuè fèn yū rè][16]
dual disease of defense and nutrient 衛營同病 [wèi yíng tóng bìng][17]
blaze in both *qi* and blood 氣血兩燔 [qì xuè liǎng fán][18]
heat scorching kidney yin 熱灼腎陰 [rè zhuó shèn yīn][20]
extreme heat producing wind 熱極生風 [rè jí shēng fēng][22]
mutual stirring-up of wnd and fire 風火相煽 [fēng huǒ xiāng shān][24]

膀胱 [rè jié páng guāng][13]
heat binding in the lower energizer 熱結下焦 [rè jié xià jiāo][13]
heat binding in the large intestine 熱結大腸 [rè jié dà cháng][13]
heat entering the blood chamber 熱入血室 [rè rù xuè shì][15]
heat entering nutrient-blood 熱入營血 [rè rù yíng xuè][15]
heat-toxin in blood 血分熱毒 [xuè fèn rè dú][16]
dual disease of defense and *qi* 衛氣同病 [wèi qì tóng bìng][17]
blaze in both *qi* and nutrient 氣營兩燔 [qì yíng liǎng fán][18]
heat damaging the mind 熱傷神明 [rè shāng shén míng][19]
exuberant heat consuming fluid 熱盛傷津 [rè shèng shāng jīn][21]
conjoint invasion of wind and damp 風濕相搏 [fēng shī xiāng bó][23]

Discussion

1. Externally contracted febrile diseases are generally called 傷寒 [shāng hán]. Literally, it means "cold damage", so some authors render it as "diseases caused by cold", but many authors would rather render it as "febrile diseases" or "exogenous febrile diseases". Since this term is closely related with the book 傷寒論 [shāng hán lùn] (*Treatise on Cold-induced Diseases*), translation of the title of the book should be seriously considered.

2. In the course of cold-induced diseases, the disease process is usually transmitted from one meridian to another with respective change of the clinical manifestation. This is called 傳經 [chuán jīng]. Regarding the English equivalent, different opinions exist in the rendering of the character 傳 [chuán]. "Transmission", "passage" and "transformation" have been used by different authors. "Transformation" seems inappropriate, for it refers to a complete change of the character of the disease. Most authors use the word "transmission".

Ordinarily the disease is transmitted from one meridian to another in the order of greater yang, bright yang, lesser yang, greater yin, lesser yin and reverting yin. Such a course of development is called 循經傳 [xún jīng chuán]. If the transmission is from one meridian to another with skipping of one or more meridians, it is called 越經傳 [yuè jīng chuán]. For the former, the words "orderly" and "sequential" have been suggested by different authors, and for the latter, "skipping" and "skip-over".

3. Attack of exogenous pathogens directly to the yin meridians instead of transmission from yang meridians is called 直中 [zhí zhòng]. Its English equivalent is generally recognized as "direct attack".

4. Besides sequential meridian transmission, there are several conditions in which two or more meridians are involved at the same time in a cold-induced disease. One is 合病 [hé bìng], in which two or more meridians (usually yang meridians) are attacked by a pathogen simultaneously. If both yin and yang meridians are attacked by a pathogen, this is called 兩感 [liǎng gǎn]. In meridian transmission, the involvement of two meridians, though occurring in succession, may co-exist. This is 並病 [bìng bìng]. As the equivalent of 兩感 [liǎng gǎn], "double contraction" seems to be better than "double infection" (which is too modernized) and "double-meridian febrile disease". For 合病 [hé bìng], most authors use the word "combination". For 並病 [bìng bìng], many authors use the word "complication", but it is not the proper word to reflect the original Chinese concept.

5. Acute febrile diseases, mostly infectious and epidemic, are called 溫病 [wēn bìng] in Chinese medicine. Many authors render it as "acute febrile diseases", "epidemic febrile disease" or "seasonal febrile diseases". These renderings are somewhat too Westernized, and they cause difficulty for the related terms. The literal translation "warm disease" seems appropriate, especially when the related terms are concerned, such as "warm pathogen" (溫邪 [wēn xié]), "warm-heat" (溫熱 [wēn rè]) and "warm-dryness" (溫燥 [wēn zào]).

6. 傳染 [chuán rǎn] refers to spreading of epidemic disease by contact, and so is equivalent to "contagion".

7. Ordinary proceeding of a febrile disease from the exterior to the interior, e.g., from defense system to *qi* system, is called 順傳 [shùn chuán]. Most authors render it as "sequential transmission", but some use "due transmission", "normal transmission", "normal passage", or "sequential transformation".

8. Extraordinary proceeding of a febrile disease, e.g., directly from

the defense system to the pericardium, is called 逆傳 [nì chuán]. This term has several different renderings, such as "reverse transmission", "abnormal transmission", "transmitting out of order", "disorderly transformation", and "abnormal passage". Although most authors prefer the first one, it may not precisely reflect the original concept. For example, it is not appropriate to say that transmission of an epidemic febrile disease from the exterior to the pericardium is "reverse transmission", for the ordinary transmission is not from the pericardium to the exterior. Therefore, the word "abnormal" or "adverse" seems better.

9. 溫邪犯肺 [wēn xiè fàn fèi] refers to the mechanism of the initial stage of an acute febrile disease that the warm pathogen invades the lung and the superficial defensive system. The term 溫邪 [wēn xiè] is discussed above in Note 5.

10. The defense system regulates the excretion of sweat while the nutrient system provides fluid for the formation of sweat. Disharmony between the two systems results in abnormal sweating, particularly spontaneous sweating in an exterior syndrome. This is called 營衛不和 [yíng wèi bù hé]. Most authors prefer the word "disharmony" for 不和 [bù hé]. Only a few authors use "disorder" or "dysfunction", which seem to be too general.

There are two common conditions of nutrient-defense disharmony. One is "weak defense with strong nutrient" (衛弱營強 [wèi ruò yíng qiáng]), the pathogenesis of spontaneous sweating without fever, and the other "strong defense with weak nutrient" (衛強營弱 [wèi qiáng yíng ruò]), the pathogenesis of sweating that occurs only during fever. Regarding these two English terminologies, there is practically no dispute, though they are often changed into sentences in writing.

11. It is proper to omit the character 邪 [xié] when the term 熱邪傳裏 [rè xié chuán lǐ] is rendered into English.

12. According to most authors, 熱化 [rè huà] and 寒化 [hán huà] are expressed as "transformation into heat" and "transformation into cold" or "heat transformation" and "cold transformation". Some authors prefer the word "conversion".

13. It is difficult to find an appropriate word to express the concept of 熱結 [rè jié]. The character 結 [jié] is rendered as "retention", "accumulation", and "stasis", but Nigel Wiseman proposes "binding". The verb "bind", when used as an intransitive verb, means "stick together". In addition, "binding" also has the meaning of "causing constipation". So it

is more appropriate than the other renderings. But for 熱結旁流 [rè jié páng liú], "fecal impaction with watery discharge" is succinct and easy to understand.

14. Most authors use "block" or "blockage" to express the concept of 熱閉 [rè bì], the mechanism of inadequate eruption in measles, severe cough and dyspnea in lung heat, and dysuria and suppression of urine in bladder heat.

15. The term 熱入血室 [rè rù xuè shì] is rendered into English in various ways, such as "invasion of the blood chamber by heat", "invasion of heat into the blood cavity", "attack of heat on the blood chamber", "heat attacking the blood chamber [uterus]", "pyretic invasion of the uterus", "heat invasion of the blood chamber", "attack of heat on the blood chamber", and "heat entering the blood chamber". The last one is selected for its direct and precise reflection of the Chinese orginal concept. For a similar reason, "heat entering the pericardium", "heat entering nutrient-blood" and "heat entering blood" are selected.

16. Regarding the term 血分 [xuè fèn], many authors render the character 分 [fèn] as "phase", "stage" or "level". This may be useful so far as the course of an acute epidemic disease is concerned. But the original meaning of 分 [fèn] is "division", so some authors use "sector", "aspect" or "portion". Other authors even use the word "system". In fact, when the term is not directly related to the division of a disease course, the character 分 [fèn] can be neglected. There is practically no difference between 熱入血 [rè rù xuè] and 熱入血分 [rè rù xuè fèn]. The only difference is that with the addition of 分 [fèn] the term will meet the required four-charactered structure. Whenever necessary, this character is deleted, as shown in 熱入營血 [rè rù yíng xuè].

17. As discussed elsewhere, the English equivalents of 衛 [wèi], 氣 [qì], 營 [yíng] and 血 [xuè] are "defense", "qi", "nutrient" and "blood", respectively. The translation of 同病 [tóng bìng] has several different patterns: "disease involving both…", "syndrome of both…", "affection of both…", "disorder involving simultaneously…", "coincidence of both…syndrome" and "dual disease of…". It is hard to say which one is the best. The last one is selected simply because of its literal coincidence with the Chinese original.

18. The English translation of 兩燔 [liǎng fán] has several patterns: "intense heat in both…", "dual blaze of…", "… both ablaze", "overabundant heat at both…", "flaming of heat at…", "vigorous heat of…". The

word "blaze" seems the proper one.

19. The character 傷 [shāng] in the term 熱傷神明 [rè shāng shén míng] is expressed commonly by the word "impair" or "damage". Comparatively speaking, "damage" corresponds more to the original concept. Some authors prefer "mental damage by heat". As a pathogenetic term the gerund form is selected.

20. Consumption of kidney yin by heat in febrile diseases is known as 熱灼腎陰 [rè zhuó shèn yīn]. Most authors use the word "consume" or "consumption", but Nigel Wiseman suggests using the word "scorch". The latter word better fits the Chinese original and has the meaning of "dry up", vividly describing the pathogenesis.

21. 熱盛傷津 [rè shèng shāng jīn] refers to the pathogenesis of fluid consumption in febrile diseases. It is not necessary to render 傷津 [shāng jīn] as "damage to fluid", for the full wording is 耗傷津液 [háo shāng jīn yè], equivalent to "consumption of fluid".

22. 熱極生風 [rè jí shēng fēng] is the mechanism referring to the occurrence of convulsions and opisthotonus in high fever. In this term, the key point is the selection of an appropriate expression for 生風 [shēng fēng]. The following renderings are frequently encountered: "produce wind", "generate wind", "engender wind", and "bring about wind", and each has its advocates. Among the verbs used in these terms, "produce" is the most popular one, "engender" is the most formal one, and both mean "cause to occur". Another way of expression is to put the resultant wind before the cause, e.g., "wind due to extreme heat". The latter is suitable for naming the syndrome.

23. 風濕相搏 [fēng shī xiāng bó] is a common pathological change that results in muscle ache and joint pain in wind-damp affliction. Different explanations of the phrase 相搏 [xiāng bó] lead to various English expressions of this term, e.g., "conjoint invasion of wind and dampness", "conjoint invasion of pathogenic wind-dampness", "wind-damp complication", "wind-damp combination", "wind and dampness contending with each other", "mutual contention of wind and dampness", and so on. The most authoritative dictionary of traditional Chinese medicine explains this term as follows: "Pathogenic wind and damp, invading the human body, cause disease in combination."* According to this explanation, the most

---

*"風邪與濕邪侵犯人體後，互相結合爲患。" （中醫大辭典）— cited form Zhong Yi Da Ci Dian (*Grand Dictionary of Traditional Chinese Medicine*) People's Health Publishing House, 1998, p.312.

appropriate English expression is "conjoint invasion of wind and damp".

24. 風火相煽 [fēng huǒ xiāng shān] is a pathological process that causes high fever and convulsions in the most advanced stage of an acute febrile disease. In the present publications there are two expressions for 相煽 [xiāng shān]: "fanning each other" and "stirring up each other".

DISORDERS OF *QI* AND BLOOD

Disorders of *qi* mainly include (1) insufficient generation of *qi* or excessive consumption of *qi*, resulting in *qi* defeciency, and (2) insufficient function or disordered movement of *qi*, leading to stangation, counterflow, sinking, blockage or collapse of *qi*. Disorders of the blood include (1) insufficient generation of blood or excessive consumption of blood, resulting in blood deficiency, and (2) disordered blood circulation, such as retarded flow, accelerated flow, adverse flow and frenetic flow.

Proposed Standard Nomenclature

qi deficiency 氣虛 [qì xū][1]

disorder of *qi* movement 氣機失調 [qì jī shī tiáo][3]

disturbance of *qi* movement 氣機不利 [qì jī bù lì][3]

qi depression 氣鬱 [qì yù][4]

qi stagnation 氣滯 [qì zhì][4]

qi sinking 氣陷 [qì xiàn][6]

qi collapse 氣脫 [qì tuō][8]

blood stasis 血瘀 [xuè yū][10]

bleeding due to blood heat 血熱妄行 [xuè rè wàng xíng][12]

(*qi*) collapse following hemorrhage 氣隨血脫 [qì suí xuè tuō][14]

blood stasis due to *qi* stagnation 氣滯血瘀 [qì zhì xuè yū][15]

insecurity of thoroughfare and conception [controller] vessels 衝任不固 [chōng rèn bù gù][16]

insecurity of superficial [defensive] *qi* 表[衛]氣不固 [biǎo [wèi] qì bù gù][2]

depression-stagnation of *qi* (movement) 氣機鬱滯 [qì jī yù zhì][4]

qi counterflow 氣逆 [qì nì][5]

qi block 氣閉 [qì bì][7]

blood deficiency 血虛 [xuè xū][9]

blood heat 血熱 [xuè rè][11]

disharmony of *qi* and blood 氣血失調 [qì xuè shī tiáo][13]

hemorrhage following *qi* sinking 血隨氣陷 [xuè suí qì xiàn][14]

blood stasis due to *qi* deficiency 氣虛血瘀 [qì xū xuè yū][15]

damage to thoroughfare and conception [controller] vessels 衝任損傷 [chōng rèn sǔn shāng][16]

Discussion

1. As discussed elsewhere, the most acceptable way of expressing 虛 [xū] in pathogenesis is "deficiency", hence "*qi* deficiency" for 氣虛 [qì xū].

2. 不固 [bù gù] is expressed as "dissipation", "weakness", "unconsolidation" and "insecurity" by different authors. The first two expressions are tortuous. "Consolidate" means "become more secure", and so "insecure" seems more appropriate than "unconsolidated".

3. The movement of *qi* plays an extremely important role in facilitating various physiological functions and maintaining life activity. Pathogenesis of disease is closely related to disorders of *qi* movement. There are various disorders of *qi* movement, including depression, stagnation, counterflow, sinking and penetration. They are generally called 氣機失調 [qì jī shī tiáo] or 氣機不利 [qì jī bù lì]. The term has been rendered in various ways such as "disorder of *qi*", "disorder of *qi* mechanism", "disorder of *qi* movement", "disturbance of *qi* function", "inhibited *qi* dynamic" and "visceral dysfunction". Since the proposed equivalent of 氣機 [qì jī] is "*qi* movement", it is better to render the whole term as "disorder (or disturbance) of *qi* movement".

4. Impeded *qi* movement is expressed as 氣機鬱滯 [qì jī yù zhì] in Chinese, and the term can be abbreviated as 氣鬱 [qì yù] or 氣滯 [qì zhì]. It should be noted that 鬱 [yù] and 滯 [zhì] are not exactly the same. Historically, 鬱 was used at first, and 氣鬱 [qì yù] was one of the six *yu* syndromes[*]. In the later times, 鬱 [yù] only refers to emotional depression. Contemporary Chinese medicine has made a distinct differentiation between 氣滯 [qì zhì] and 氣鬱 [qì yù]. The former refers to the stagnation of *qi* movement, and should be treated by freeing the *qi* flow; the latter refers to depression of *qi*, and should be relieved by dispersion. In fact, most authors render 滯 [zhì] as stagnation, and 鬱 [yù] as depression.

5. Another category of disordered *qi* movement is the disturbed direction of *qi* flow. Normally, lung *qi* and stomach *qi* move downwards, and liver *qi* spreads freely. If any pathogenic factor causes the *qi* of these organs to go adversely upward, there will be cough and asthma (when lung

---

[*]氣血衝和，百病不生，一有怫鬱，諸病生焉。其證有六：曰氣鬱、曰濕鬱、曰熱鬱、曰痰鬱、曰血鬱、曰食鬱。"（《醫學正傳》）

qi is involved), hiccups, belching, nausea, vomiting and regurgitation (when stomach *qi* is involved), headache and irascitablity (when liver *qi* is involved), and the pathological condition is called 氣逆 [qì nì]. How to properly render this term into English is a puzzling problem. The original sense of the term is easy to understand, but some of the translations have made the issue complex. The character 逆 [nì] is polysemous, but its primary meaning is demonstrated by the structure of the character. Its left and lower part means "go", and the whole character means "go against", referring to the direction of movement, particularly upward from below. The compound word 逆叛 [pàn nì] means "rebel against". However, many Western authors prefer "rebellious *qi*" or "rebellion of *qi*". In fact, "rebellious" or "rebellion" is the meaning of the character 叛 [pàn] but not 逆 [nì]. So this wording, though advocated by many Western authors, does not exactly reflect the original implication, nor does it conform with the Chinese language. Most Chinese authors render the term as "reversed flow of *qi*" or "adverse flow of *qi*". Nathan Sivin suggests "ch'i (*qi*) backflow", while Nigel Wiseman prefers "*qi* counterflow". Comparatively speaking, "*qi* counterflow" is probably the appropriate choice of words.

6. Another abnormal direction of *qi* flow is the failure of *qi* to ascend. This pathological change usually develops on the basis of *qi* deficiency, and is called 氣陷 [qì xiàn] in Chinese. Most authors render it in English as "*qi* sinking" or "sinking of *qi*", but some authors render it as "*qi* collapse", "collapsed *qi*", or "*qi* fall". "*Qi* collapse" or "collapsed *qi*" is more approriate for 氣脫 [qì tuō], a pathological condition characterized by massive escape of *qi*, often seen in a critical case manifested by sudden functional failure. "*Qi* sinking" is seen in chronic cases, without acute functional failure.

7. Blockage of *qi* movement leading to sudden loss of consciousness with trismus and clenched fists or abdominal colic with urinary and fecal stoppage is called 氣閉 [qì bì]. Among the various renderings "*qi* block" is the most succinct one.

8. The Chinese term 氣脫 [qì tuō] is an abbreviation of 元氣虛脫 [yuán qì xū tuō] (collapse of the original *qi*), and so the appropriate equivalent is "*qi* collapse".

9. For the term 血虛 [xuè xū] most authors use "deficiency" to express 虛 [xū]. There are three common forms: "deficiency of blood", "blood deficiency" and "deficient blood". All of them are appropriate, and

"blood deficiency" is selected as the proposed standard.

10. For expressing the concept 血瘀 [xuè yū] two English terms are commonly used: "congealed blood" and "blood stasis". Most authors use the latter, while the former is more appropriate for 瘀血 [yū xuè].

11. Heat in the blood causes increased blood flow, vascular dilation, or frenetic movement of the blood as the mechanism of hemorrhage. In Chinese it is called 血熱 [xuè rè], and the English equivalent is "blood heat".

13. Literally, 血熱妄行 [xuè rè wàng xíng] is translated as "frenetic movement of the blood due to heat in the blood". "Frenetic movement of the blood" is a metaphorical way of saying "bleeding" or "hemorrhage". So the term can be simplified as "bleeding due to blood heat".

13. Regarding the term 失調 [shī tiáo], "derangement", "disorder", "incoordination" and "disharmony" are used by different authors. For the selection, cf. "yin-yang disharmony".

14. 氣隨血脫 [qì suí xuè tu] is rendered in different ways: "hemorrhagic shock", which is too Westernized, and "qi deserting with the blood". In this term and also in 血隨氣陷 [xuè suí qì xiàn], 血 [xuè] refers to hemorrhage.

15. In the terms 氣滯血瘀 [qì zhì xuè yū] and 氣虛血瘀 [qì xū xuè yū] the functional character is omitted. When rendering it into English, the necessary joining word must be added.

16. Regarding 不固 [bù gù], cf. Note 2 of this section. For 任 [rèn], it is suggested to replace "conception" with "controller" (cf. page 262).

DISORDERS OF THE *ZANG-FU* ORGANS

The pathogenetic terms related to organ disorders can be classified into three overall categories: terms of deficiency conditions, terms of excess conditions, and terms of organ disharmonies. Deficiency conditions of the *zang-fu* organs chiefly involve insufficiency of *qi*, blood, essence, fluid, yin, and/or yang of the given organ(s). Terms relating to excess conditions of the *zang-fu* organs usually include the pathogen(s) and the organ(s) affected by the pathogen(s). Organ disharmonies are multifarious, usually manifested by functional disorders, occurring within an organ or between two or more organs.

Disorders of the Liver and Gallbladder

The liver in Chinese medicine is the *zang* organ that smoothes the flow of *qi*, particularly liver *qi*. So, besides various insufficiencies of the liver, disorders of the liver are mostly manifested as abnormal *qi* flow with the resultant changes, and hence the terminologies.

Proposed Standard Nomenclature

liver insufficiency 肝虛 [gān xū][1]

deficiency [insufficiency] of liver blood 肝血虛 [gān xuè xū]; 肝血不足 [gān xuè bù zú][1]

deficiency of liver and kidney yin 肝腎陰虛 [gān shèn yīn xū][1]

disharmony of liver *qi* 肝氣不和 [gān qì bù hé][2]

stagnation of liver *qi* 肝氣鬱結 [gān qì yù jié][3]

liver *qi* invading the stomach 肝氣犯胃 [gān qì fàn wèi][4]

upward counterflow of liver *qi* 肝氣上逆 [gān qì shàng nì][4]

transformation of liver yang into fire 肝陽化火 [gān yáng huà huǒ][6]

damp-heat in the liver and gallbladder 肝膽濕熱 [gān dǎn shī rè][10]

deficiency [insufficiency] of liver *qi* 肝氣虛 [gān qì xū]; 肝氣不足 [gān qì bù zú][1]

deficiency [insufficiency] of liver yin 肝陰虛 [gān yīn xū]; 肝陰不足 [gān yīn bù zú][1]

deficiency [insufficiency] of liver yang 肝陽虛[gān yáng xū]; 肝陽不足 [gān yīn bù zú][1]

transverse counterflow of liver *qi* 肝氣橫逆 [gān qì héng nì][4]

liver *qi* invading the spleen 肝氣犯脾 [gān qì fàn pí][4]

hyperactivity of liver yang 肝陽上亢 [gān yáng shàng kàng][5]

liver fire flaring up 肝火上炎 [gān huǒ shàng yán][7]

liver fire invading the lung 肝火犯肺 [gān huǒ fàn fèi][8]

liver stirring internally 肝風內動 [gān fēng nèi dòng][9]

Discussion

1. 虛 [xū] (deficiency) and 不足 [bù zú] (insufficiency) are interchangeable. It is suggested to take "deficiency [insufficiency] of liver *qi*, blood, yin or yang" as a pathogenetic term, and "liver *qi* [blood, yin or yang] deficiency" as a syndrome name.

"Deficiency of liver and kidney yin" is selected as a pathogenetic term for 肝腎陰虛 [gān shèn yīn xū], and "liver-kidney yin deficiency" as a syndrome name.

2. One of the basic mechanisms of liver diseases is the pathological change of the liver in its smoothing and discharging function, either insufficient or excessive. It is called 肝氣不和 [gān qì bù hé], which is rendered in English as "disorder of liver *qi*", "dysfunction of liver *qi*", and "disharmony of liver *qi*". Most authors prefer the last expression.

3. Emotional depression or upset often leads to stagnation of liver *qi* flow, known as 肝氣鬱結 [gān qì yù jié]. Most authors express the word 鬱結 [yù jié] as "stagnation", but a few individual authors prefer "depression", "stasis", "constraint" or "binding". A brief analysis of the Chinese term may be necessary. 肝氣鬱結 [gān qì yù jié] is often abbreviated as 肝鬱 [gān yù], but is not abbreviated as 肝結 [gān jié]; in addition, it can be renamed as 肝氣鬱滯 [gān qì yù zhì], in which the character 結 [jié] is no more used. So, 結 [jié] in this term is not the crucial character, and is added chiefly for rhetoric purpose.

4. There are two basic directions of 氣逆 [qì nì] (adverse flow or counterflow of *qi*) of the liver: transverse and upward. The pathological change in which hyperactive liver *qi*, running transversely, impairs the stomach or spleen function is known as 肝氣犯胃 [gān qì fàn wèi] or 肝氣犯脾 [gān qì fàn pí]. To express the concept of 犯 [fàn], the following words are frequently used: "invade", "attack", "affect", and "disrupt". Most authors prefer the first two words. Literal consideration is partial to the word "invade", for "attack" conforms to the character 襲 [xí]

5. The pathological change that explains symptoms such as dizziness, headache, tinnitus and blurred vision occurring in liver yin deficiency is known as 肝陽上亢 [gān yáng shàng kàng]. This term is rendered in various ways: "hyperactivity of liver-yang", "hyperactive liver yang", "liver-yang hyperactivity", "exuberance of liver yang", "ascendant liver yang", "sthenia of liver-yang", "excessive rise of liver-yang", "ascendant hyperactivity of liver yang", "hepatic system yang rising in excess", "liver yang rising", "hyper liver yang ascending", and "arrogant liver yang ascending". Based on the above renderings, "ascendant liver yang" and "liver yang ascending" are selected, the former serving as a syndrome name, and the latter as a pathogenetic term.

6. Further development of liver yang is its transformation into fire, called 肝陽化火 [gān yáng huà huǒ]. The main trend for rendering this into English is either "transformation of liver yang into fire" or "liver yang transforming into fire". The former is suitable for a syndrome name,

and the latter for a pathogenetic term.

7. "Up-flaming [up-flaring] liver fire", "flaming-up [flaring-up] of liver fire", and "liver fire flaming [flaring] up" can be selected as the equivalents of 肝火上炎 [gān huǒ shàng yán]. The first two are suitable for naming the syndrome, and the last one for describing the pathogenesis. The word "flare" is probably more suitable than "flame", as the former figuratively means "burst into sudden activity or anger".

8. 肝火犯肺 [gān huǒ fàn fèi] is both a syndrome name and a pathogenetic term. "Invasion of the lung by liver fire" and "liver fire invading the lung" are selected accordingly.

9. The term 肝風內動 [gān fēng nèi dòng] is often abbreviated to 肝風 [gān fēng]. The latter is rendered as "liver wind" without dispute. For expressing the concept of 動 [dòng], different words are used, but "stir" is the most common. Therefore, as a syndrome name "liver wind" is suggested, and as a term of pathogenesis "liver wind stirring internally is selected.

10. 肝膽濕熱 [gān dǎn shī rè] is a pathogenetic term and also a syndrome name. Since there is no verb in this term, it is difficult to make the distinction by using different grammatical patterns in its English equivalents. "Damp-heat in the liver and gallbladder" is selected for describing pathogenesis, and "liver-gallbladder damp-heat" as a syndrome name.

Disorders of the Heart

In Chinese medicine the heart is an organ that governs both blood circulation and mental activities. Disorders of the heart usaully involve both functional aspects. If the mental activity is mainly affected, the word "heart" is often replaced by "heart-mind" (心神 [xīn shén]) or simply "mind" (神 [shén]).

Proposed Standard Nomenclature

deficiency [insufficiency] of heart *qi* 心氣虛 [xīn qì xū]; 心氣不足 [xīn qì bù zú][1]

deficiency [insufficiency] of heart blood 心血虛 [xīn xuè xū]; 心血不足 [xīn xuè bù zú][1]

deficiency [insufficiency] of heart yin 心陰虛 [xīn yīn xū]; 心陰不足 [xīn yīn bù zú][1]

deficiency [insufficiency] of heart yang 心陽虛[xīn yáng xū]; 心陽不足 [xīn yáng bù zú][1] restlessness of heart-*qi* 心氣不寧 [xīn qì bù níng][2]

insecurity of heart *qi* 心氣不固 [xīn qì bù gù][3]

stasis of heart blood 心血瘀阻 [xīn xuè yū zhǔ][4]

over-consumption of heart nutrient 心營過耗 [xīn yíng guò hào][5]

heat damaging the mind 熱傷神明 [rè shāng shén míng][6]

phlegm misting the heart 痰迷心竅 [tán mí xīn qiào][7]

impaired nourishment of the heart 心神失養 [xīn shén shī yǎng][8]

mind failing to keep to its abode 神不守舍 [shén bù shǒu shè][9]

heart fire blazing 心火熾[亢]盛 [xīn huǒ chì [kàng] shèng][10]

heart fire flaring up 心火上炎 [xīn huǒ shàng yán][11]

heart fire deflagrating internally 心火內焚 [xīn huǒ nèi fén][12]

phlegm-fire agitating the mind [heart] 痰火擾神[心] [tán huǒ rǎo shén [xīn]][13]

heart transmitting heat to the small intestine 心移熱於小腸 [xīn yí rè yú xiǎo cháng][14]

Discussion

1. The Chinese word 不足 [bù zú] means "not sufficient". It is synonymous with 虛 [xū] when used in connection with any of the normal elements — *qi*, blood, yin or yang. In the past, particularly when rhythmical prose style was prevalent, the pathogenetic terms were usually formed with four characters, for example, either 心陰不足 [xīn yīn bù zú] or 心陰虧虛 [xīn yīn kuī xū] for expressing insufficiency or deficiency of heart yin. Only in recent decades has a small number of three-character pathogenetic terms such as 心陰虛 [xīn yīn xū] become popular in the Chinese medical literature.

The English expression certainly need not consider the literary impact on the wording. 心氣不足 [xīn qì bù zú] and 心氣虛 [xīn qì xū] are synonyms, and both can be rendered either as "insufficiency of heart *qi*" or as "heart *qi* deficiency". Most authors use the former as a pathogenetic term and the latter as a syndrome name. Similarly, "insufficiency of heart blood", "insufficiency of heart yin", and "insufficiency of heart yang" are used as pathogenetic terms, and "heart blood deficiency", "heart yin deficiency", and "heart yang deficiency" as syndrome names.

2. Impairment of heart *qi* may result in uneasiness, palpitations, susceptibility to fright, vexation, and insomnia. This pathological change is called 心氣不寧 [xīn qì bù níng]. It is actually the pathogenesis of the related symptoms. The corresponding English expressions include "un-

steadiness of heart-*qi*", "disquieting of heart *qi*", "restlessness of heart *qi*" and "disorder of heart *qi*". The word "disorder" is too general, and "unsteadiness" is appropriate for 不固 [bù gù] rather than 不寧 [bù níng]. The word "disquiet" is a transitive verb, signifying "to make somebody anxious". In the present case, one would ask whether the heart *qi* is disquieting or disquieted.

3. Symptoms such as floating astray of the mind, susceptibility to fright, forgetfulness, and spontaneous sweating are believed to result from a pathological change called 心氣不固[xīn qì bù gù]. This concept has been rendered into English in several ways: "unconsolidation of heart *qi*", "dissipation of heart *qi*", "weakness of heart *qi*", and "insecurity of heart *qi*". In all but the last one, the concept is expressed in a roundabout way. Therefore, the word "security" is selected.

4. The major disorder of heart blood flow is its impedement that causes precordial pain and a feeling suffocation. The pathological change is called 心血瘀阻 [xīn xuè yū zhǔ]. For this term, the rhetorical rules of the Chinese language should be seriously considered. Actually, 心血瘀 [xīn xuè yū] is sufficient for the expression, but it cannot be generally accepted because of the single-character ending. In order to make the phrase easy to read, one more character with a similar meaning should be added. When we render the Chinese term into English, there is no need to treat the two characters separately. So, the expressions available in recent publications — "stagnation of the heart blood", "heart blood stasis", "heart-blood stasis", "cardiac system blood coagulation", "heart blood stasis obstruction", "stagnant and obstructed heart blood", "heart static blood obstruction", etc. — can be classified into two categories. One is to take 瘀阻 [yū zhǔ] as one word with emphasis on 瘀 [yū] in meaning, and the other is to take the two characters as two separate words of equal importance. For translation, the second way might be necessary, but for the proposed standard nomenclature accurate reflection of the original concept is more important than the detailed reflection of each character. Therefore, "stasis of heart blood" is selected as the proposed standard pathogenetic term, and "heart blood stasis" as the syndrome name.

5. Excessive consumption of heart nutrient by heat causes emaciation, night fever and vexation. This pathological process is called 心營過耗 [xīn yíng guò hào] in Chinese. The disparity of English expression chiefly lies at the translation of the character 營 [yíng]. As discussed previously, some authors render 營 [yíng] as "construction", and hence

the term "excessive wearing of heart construction". According to the most recent edition of the national Chinese TCM textbook, it is clearly explained as "nutrition" or "nutrient". Therefore, "over-consumption of heart nutrient" is selected as the standard term.

6. The pathological process by which mental activity is impaired by heat is called 熱傷神明 [rè shāng shén míng]. Disparity in the English equivalent lies chiefly in the phrase pattern. The orginal Chinese is actually a complete sentence. There are mainly two ways to render it into English: "heat damaging the mind", and "mental disorder (caused) by heat". For indicating a process, use of the present participle is more popular.

7. Mental derangement, impaired consciousness or coma is often accompanied by phlegmatic sounds in the throat. In such cases it is believed that the morbid condition is caused by phlegm, and the pathological process is called 痰迷心竅 [tán mí xīn qiào] in Chinese. The statement is actually a complete sentence with the subject 痰 [tán], the predicate 迷 [mí], and the object 心竅 [xīn qiào]. 痰迷心竅 [tán mí xīn qiào] is also called 痰蒙心包 [tán méng xīn bāo]. So it is of no great significance whether the heart orifice or the pericardium is invaded by phlegm. The availabe choices in recent publications include "phlegm misting the heart", "phlegm clogging the orifices of the heart", "phlegm confusing the mind", "mucus confusing the heart openings", "heart confused by phlegm", "mental confusion due to phlegm", and "phlegm confounding the orifices of the heart". The most succinct one, "phlegm misting the heart", is selected as the standard term.

8. Patients with heart blood deficiency or heart yin deficiency usually suffer from palpitations, dysphoria, insomnia and amnesia. The symptoms are attributed to 心神失養 [xīn shén shī yǎng], which may be rendered as "impaired nourishment of heart-mind".

9. The basic mechanism of mental aberration or trance is called 神不守舍 [shén bù shǒu shè] in Chinese. It is a complete sentence with subject (神 [shén]), predicate (不守 [bù shǒu]) and object (舍 [shè]), but it is often used as a medical term. As a sentence, it can be rendered as "the mind fails to keep to its abode." As a medical term, many authors simply render it as "mental derangement", which is apart from the original wording and does not sound like a pathogenetic term. Nigel Wiseman suggests "spirit failing to keep to its abode". Since the character 神 [shén] in this term refers to the mind, so the word "spirit" is replaced by "mind", and

the whole term becomes "mind failing to keep to its abode" or "failure of the mind to keep to its abode".

10. Flaming of the heart fire may cause an excessive heat syndrome manifested by insomnia, dysphoria, or even impairment of consciousness and delirium. This pathological process is called 心火亢盛 [xīn huǒ kàng shèng]. The available expressions for selection are 'heart fire blazing", "flaring heart-fire", "exuberant fire due to hyperactivity of the heart", "exuberance of heart fire", "exuberant heart fire", "excessive heart fire", "excess heart fire", "hyperactivity of heart fire", "heart-fire hyperactivity" and "hyperactive and exuberant heart fire".

11. If the heart fire flares upward along the heart meridian, causing oral or lingual erosion, the pathological process is called 心火上炎 [xīn huǒ shàng yán]. Most authors use "flaring-up of heart fire" to express this process, but some render it as "heart fire flaming upward", "up-flaming heart fire", "uprising of heart fire", "upward flaming of heart fire", "heart fire blazing", or "heart fire rising".

12. 心火内焚 [xīn huǒ nèi fén] a pathological change in which intense heat disturbs the mental activity, causing vexation, insomnia, throbbing palpitations, restlessness, or even mania. Regarding the English equivalent, divergence exists in rendering the Han character 内 [nèi]. Some authors express it as "internal(ly)", while others omit it. It is better to keep this word because in this case there is no outer manifestation such as lingual erosion.

13. Agitation of the heart by phlegm-fire that causes mental derangement or mania is called 痰火擾心 [tán huǒ rǎo xīn]. It has several different renderings, and the disparity lies in the translation of 擾 [rǎo]. Most authors use the word "disturb", while some use "agitate", "stimulate" or "harass". Among these words, "agitate" may be the most appropriate so far as the mind is concerned.

14. In various renderings of 心移熱於小腸 [xīn yí rè yú xiǎo cháng], "transmit", "spread", "move", "transfer" and "pass" are used to express 移 [yí]. Since this pathological change is a type of meridian transmission, unification of the wording is preferable.

Disorders of the Spleen and Stomach

Proposed Standard Nomenclature

spleen insufficiency 脾虚 [pí xū][1]   deficiency [insufficiency] of spleen

deficiency [insufficiency] of spleen yin 脾陰虛 [pí yīn xū][1]

deficiency [insufficiency] of spleen yang 脾陽虛 [pí yáng xū][1]

spleen failing to transport 脾不[失]健運 [pí bù [shī] jiàn yùn][2]

spleen (qi) failing in up-sending 脾氣不升 [pí qì bù shēng][4]

middle qi sinking 中氣下陷 [zhōng qì xià xiàn][5]

upward counter-flow of stomach qi 胃氣上逆 [wèi qì shàng nì][7]

deficiency-cold of the spleen and stomach 脾胃虛寒 [pí wèi xū hán]

qi 脾氣虛 [pí qì xū]; 脾氣不足 [pí qì bù zú][1]

spleen failing to transport and transform 脾不運化 [pí bù yùn huà][2]

spleen failing to control the blood 脾不統血 [pí bù tǒng xuè][3]

spleen qi sinking 脾氣下陷 [pí qì xià xiàn][5]

stomach (qi) failing in down-sending 胃氣不降 [wèi qì bù jiàng][6]

deficiency of spleen and stomach yin 脾胃陰虛 [pí wèi yīn xū]

deficiency of spleen and kidney yang 脾腎陽虛 [pí shèn yáng xū]

Discussion

1. "Deficiency [insufficiency] of spleen qi [yin or yang]" are suggested to indicate pathogenesis, and "spleen qi [yin or yang] deficiency" as a syndrome name.

2. Dysfunction of the spleen in transporting and transforming nutrients and water is the main pathogenetic factor of spleen disorders. When both transportation and transformation are involved, the Chinese term is 脾不運化 [pí bù yùn huà]; when only transportation is involved, the Chinese term is 脾不健運 [pí bù jiàn yùn]. In the latter case, the attributive 健 is added to make the term into four characters, and nobody will say 脾不運 [pí bù yùn], but in the former case, 脾不健運化 [pí bù jiàn yùn huà] is never seen, simply for linguistic reasons. Therefore, the character 健 [jiàn] may be omitted when the term is rendered into English.

3. For the term 統血 [tǒng xuè], various expressions exist. It is commonly expressed in an explanatory way such as "keep the blood flowing within the vessels" and "keep the blood circulating within the vessels". As technical terms, both are too lengthy. Other expressions include "regulate the blood", "govern the blood", "manage the blood" and "control the blood". Among these terms most authors prefer the last one. Thus, the whole phrase 脾不統血 [pí bù tǒng xuè] can be rendered as "the spleen failing to control the blood" as a pathogenetic term, and "fail-

ure of the spleen to control the blood" as a syndrome name.

4. Dysfunction of the spleen in sending up nutrients is called 脾氣不升 [pí qì bù shēng]. The key question to be answered is whether the verb 升 [shēng] in this term is intransitive or transitive. According to the *Grand Dictionary of Traditional Chinese Medicine* it is transitive.[*] Therefore, the following expressions are to be considered: "spleen-*qi* failing to send up nutrients", "failure of spleen *qi* to send up nutrients" and "spleen *qi* failing to bear upward". Based on these expressions, "spleen *qi* failing in up-sending" is suggested. In fact, this term is also called 脾不升清 [pí bù shēng qīng]. So the character 氣 [qì] can be omitted when rendering the term into English.

5. 脾氣下陷 [pí qì xià xiàn] refers to weakness of the spleen with sinking of the middle *qi*, also called 中氣下陷 [zhōng qì xià xiàn]. Among various expressions, "spleen sinking", "sinking of spleen *qi*", "spleen *qi* fall", "spleen-*qi* collapse" and "collapse of spleen-*qi*", the word "sinking" is used by most of the authors.

6. 胃氣不降 [wèi qì bù jiàng] presents a similar problem to that of 脾氣不升 [pí qì bù shēng]. 降 [jiàng] is an abbreviation of 降濁 [jiàng zhuó], i.e. "to send the stomach contents downward". Therefore, the proper translation of this term is "stomach *qi* failing in down-sending". Furthermore, this term actually comes from the stomach function 胃主降濁 [wèi zhǔ jiàng zhuó], so the character 氣 [qì] can be omitted in the English rendering.

7. 胃氣上逆 [wèi qì shàng nì] is the pathogenesis of such stomach disorders as belching, hiccuping, regurgitation, and vomiting. There are various expressions: "adverse rising of stomach *qi*", "adverse rising of gastric *qi*", "stomach *qi* ascending counterflow", "stomach *qi* rebelling upward", "upward perversion of stomach *qi*", etc. As discussed in "*qi* counterflow", the word "rebelling" is not appropriate for medical use. The other expressions are practically the same as far as the term 上逆 [shàng nì] is concerned. "Upward counter-flow of stomach *qi*" is probably the most explicit.

---

[*]The definition of this term in Chinese is "脾氣衰弱不能升清的病機" (《中醫大辭典》) (a mechanism of disease in which the declined spleen *qi* is unable to send the clear upward — cited from the *Grand Dictionary of Traditional Chinese Medicine*. People's Health Publishing House, 1998, p.1535)

Disorders of the Lung

Proposed Standard Nomenclature

lung insufficiency 肺虚 [fèi xū][1]

deficiency [insufficiency] of lung yin 肺陰虛 [fèi yīn xū][1]

dysfunction of lung *qi* 肺氣不利 [fèi qì bù lì][2]

lung failing in purification 肺失清肅 [fèi shī qīng sù][4]

lung failing to distribute fluid 肺津不布 [fèi jīn bù bù][6]

wind-cold restraining the lung 風寒束肺 [fēng hán shù fèi][8]

deficiency [insufficiency] of lung *qi* 肺氣虛 [fèi qì xū]; 肺氣不足 [fèi qì bù zú][1]

obstruction of lung *qi* 肺氣不宣 [fèi qì bù xuān][3]

upward counter-flow of lung *qi* 肺氣上逆 [fèi qì shàng nì][5]

damage to lung vessels 肺絡損傷 [fèi luò sǔn shāng][7]

phlegm obstructing the lung 痰濁阻肺 [tán zhuó zǔ fèi][9]

Discussion

1. It is suggested to use "deficiency [insufficiency] of lung *qi* [yin or yang] as pathogenetic terms, and "lung *qi* [yin or yang] deficiency" as syndrome names.

2. It is extremely difficult to reflect all the implications of the term 肺氣不利 [fèi qì bù lì]. The character 利 [lì], when it is used singly in medicine, is often related to the promotion of urine secretion. Since the lung is believed to have such an important function as regulating the water passage, 肺氣不利 [fèi qì bù lì] refers particularly to the impairment of water metabolism, and is manifested by oliguria and edema. There are quite a few English expressions, such as "disturbance of lung *qi*", "dysfunction of lung *qi*", "inhibition of lung *qi*", "unsmoothness of lung *qi*", and "inaction of lung *qi*", but none of them can reflect this point. For the time being, "dysfunction of lung *qi*" is selected, and further discussion and revision is necessary.

3. Impediment of lung function resulting in nasal obstruction, sneezing and coughing is known as 肺氣不宣 [fèi qì bù xuān]. The difficulty in formulating the English expression lies in the understanding of the character 宣 [xuān]. When it is used in medicine, this character has two meanings: One is to scatter (宣散 [xuān sàn]), and the other, to keep unobstructed (宣通 [xuān tōng]). The given term refers to the latter one. That is why most authors use "obstruction of lung *qi*", "impediment of lung *qi*", "sluggishness of lung *qi*", "lung *qi* obstruction", "impaired cir-

culation of lung *qi*" or "impaired lung *qi*". Only a few authors prefer "non-diffusion of lung *qi*", "non-spreading of lung *qi*" or "non-diffusion of lung *qi*". As the proposed standard, "obstruction of lung *qi*" is selected.

4. 清肅 [qīng sù] and 肅降 [sù jiàng] are different in implication. The former refers to one function only, while the latter refers to two functions, i.e., 肅 [sù] (purify) and 降 [jiàng] (send downward). In the recent English-language publications, confusion is frequently encountered, for example, 肺失清肅 [fèi shī qīng sù] is rendered as "impairment of purifying and descending function of the lung". In fact, it only means "impaired purification of the lung".

5. 肺氣上逆 [fèi qì shàng nì] is one of the common mechanisms of lung disorders that cause coughing, dyspnea and asthma. Similar to "upward counter-flow of stomach *qi*" a series of different expressions exist for this term, such as "abnormal rising of lung *qi*", "upward perversion in the functioning of the lung", "adverse rising of lung *qi*", "lung *qi* ascending counterflow", "counter ascent of lung *qi*", "up-rising of lung *qi*", etc. For the selection of the appropriate expression, cf. the note on "upward counter-flow of stomach *qi*".

6. Failure of the lung to distribute fluid is known as 肺津不布 [fèi jīn bù bù]. Most authors express it as "failure of the lung to distribute fluid" or "lung failing to distribute fluid". The latter is selected in this scheme.

7. 肺絡損傷 [fèi luò sǔn shāng] is one of the pathogeneses that lead to hemoptysis. In this term, 絡 [luò] refers to blood vessels, and so "damage to lung vessels" is better than "damage to lung collaterals".

8. 風寒束肺 [fēng hán shù fèi] refers to the pathogenesis of colds and acute febrile diseases at the initial stage, with such symptoms as congested nose, sneezing, coughing, chills, and tense floating pulse. If only the superficies of the body is attacked by wind-cold, the designation is 風寒束表 [fēng hán shù biǎo]. In the Chinese terms it is appropriate to use the character 束 [shù], which, used in this term, means "bind up" or "restrain", so that the normal lung function is restricted or hampered. There are various expressions for the whole term, such as "wind-cold tightening the lung", "attack of wind-cold on the lung", "wind-cold attack of the lung", "wind-cold invasion of the lung", "wind-cold restricting the lung", wind-cold restraining the lung" and "wind-cold fettering the lung". Comparison of the expressions shows that "attack" is suitable for 襲 [xí], "invade" is suitable for 犯 [fàn], and "tighten" does not necessarily have

a pathogenetic sense (on the contrary, it may be corrective if something is loose). The proper words are "restrict" and "restrain".

9. Many authors render 痰濁阻肺 [tán zhuó zǔ fèi] as "phlegm turbidity obstructing the lung" or "obstruction of the lung due to phlegm turbid", but some authors neglect the character 濁 [zhuó] and prefer "phlegm obstructing the lung". The latter is more acceptable, as 濁 [zhuó] is inserted in the Chinese term chiefly for rhetorical purposes. The omission makes the English term more succinct.

Disorders of the Kidney and Bladder

Proposed Standard Nomenclature

kidney insufficiency 腎虛 [shèn xū][1]

deficiency [insufficiency] of kidney yin 腎陰虛 [shèn yīn xū][1]

insufficiency of kidney essence 腎精不足 [shèn jīng bù zú][1]

insecurity of kidney *qi* 腎氣不固 [shèn qì bù gù][2]

frenetic stirring of ministerial fire 相火妄動 [xiāng huǒ wàng dòng][4]

damp-heat in the bladder 膀胱湿热 [páng guāng shī rè]

deficiency [insufficiency] of kidney *qi* 腎氣虛 [shèn qì xū]; 腎氣不足 [shèn qì bù zú][1]

deficiency [insufficiency] of kidney yang 腎陽虛 [shèn yáng xū][1]

kidney failing to receive *qi* 腎不納氣 [shèn bù nà qì][2]

kidney insufficiency with flooding 腎虛水泛 [shèn xū shuǐ fàn][3]

decline of life gate fire 命門火衰 [mìng mēn huǒ shuāi][5]

deficiency-cold of the bladder 膀胱虛寒 [páng guāng xū hán]

Discussion

1. The dispute over the English equivalent of the term 腎精不足 [shèn jīng bù zú] lies in the translation of 不足 [bù zú]. Compared with "deficiency" and "vacuity", "insufficiency" seems most acceptable.

For other terms with 虛 [xū] or 不足 [bù zú], either "deficiency" or "insufficiency" is appropriate.

2. Regarding the translation of 納氣 [nà qì] and 不固 [bù gù], see page 54 and page 81 respectively.

3. Many authors use "edema" to express 水泛 [shuǐ fàn], but some authors prefer "flood". The latter fits the original concept better.

4. Most authors use "hyperactivity of ministerial fire" to express the concept of 相火妄動 [xiāng huǒ wàng dòng], but some suggest "fre-

netic stirring of ministerial fire". The latter is more accurate.

5. Most authors use "decline" or "declination" to express 衰 [shuāi] in 命門火衰 [mìng mén huǒ shuāi], while others use "debilitation". "Decline" better fits the orginal concept.

DIAGNOSTICS

The terms used in the diagnostics of traditional Chinese medicine can be generally classified into three groups: (1) terms related to diagnostic examinations, (2) terms related to syndrome differentiation or pattern identification, and (3) disease names. Before going into the standard nomenclature of the terms belonging to each group, some general terms used in diagnostics are discussed.

GENERAL DIAGNOSTIC TERMS

Proposed Standard Nomenclature

diagnostics 診斷學 [zhěn duàn xué][1]

diagnosis 診斷 [zhěn duàn][1]

syndrome 證 [zhèng][3]

diagnostic method 診法 [zhěn fǎ][2]

syndrome name 證名 [zhèng míng][3]

pattern 證 [zhèng][3]

syndrome manifestation 證候 [zhèng hòu][3]

pattern name 證名 [zhèng míng][3]

syndrome differentiation 辨證 [biàn zhèng][5]

syndrome pattern 證型 [zhèng xíng][4]

disease differentiation 辨病 [biàn bìng][6]

pattern identification 辨證 [biàn zhèng][5]

Discussion

1. In Chinese medicine both 診斷學 [zhěn duàn xué] (diagnostics) and 診斷 [zhěn duàn] (diagnosis) are newly developed terms, although recording of the related contents can be dated back to the *Canon of Medicine*.

2. The Chinese term 診法 [zhěn fǎ] or 四診 [sì zhěn] is not equivalent to "diagnosis". In both terms the major character 診 [zhěn] may be taken as an abbreviation of 診斷 [zhěn duàn] (diagnosis) or 診察 [zhěn chá] (examination). Most authors render 診法 [zhěn fǎ] as "diagnostic

method(s)", while others use "diagnostics", "examination(s)", "physical examination(s)", "method(s) of examination", and "technique(s) of diagnosis". "Diagnostics" is the science and practice of diagnosis of disease, and so it is too broad in sense. The word "technique" often refers to the skill in the diagnostic methods, and so it is somewhat too narrow in sense. The word "examination" is suitable, particularly when 診 [zhěn] is explained as 診察 [zhěn chá]. The only disadvantage is that it is a word with multiple senses, and is used in many fields other than diagnosis. But the meaning can certainly be deduced from the context. "Physical examination" seems too Westernized, and the examination in Chinese medicine is not limited to the patient's body. For example, the physician should also pay attention to the patient's environment. Therefore, either "diagnostic methods" or "examinations" can be selected as the standard term.

3. One of formidable obstacles in standardization of traditional Chinese medical terms is the determination of the equivalent of 證 [zhèng]. The Chinese term 證 [zhèng] itself is ambiguous, often causing controversial explanation and usage. In clinical medicine, 證 [zhèng] is an extremely important concept, by which most of the unique features of Chinese medical theory can be reflected. It should be noted that the Chinese term 證 [zhèng] has undergone a lot of changes. This medical term is a loan from ordinary language, and the primary meaning is "evidence". At first, it was widely used by Zhang Zhong-jing in his famous book *"Treatise On Cold-Induced and Miscellaneous Diseases"*. In this book, 證 [zhèng] was used in different senses even in the same sentence. For example, "柴胡證，但見一證便是 (For determining the indication of bupleurum, only one symptom is enough.)" In this sentence, the second 證 [zhèng] refers to symptoms of diagnostic significance. In the succeeding sentence, the author further equates 柴胡證 with 柴胡湯病證 (diseased conditions indicating bupleurum decoction). In other words, 證 [zhèng] can be replaced by 病證 [bìng zhèng].

Zhang Zhong-jing made a definite distinction between 病 [bìng] and 證 [zhèng]. In his *Synopsis of Prescriptions of the Golden Chamber*, he uses the three characters 病 [bìng], 脈 [mài] and 證 [zhèng] in the topic of each chapter, e.g., 黃疸病脈證並治 (The Pulse, Symptoms and Treatment of Icteric Diseases). In the text of each chapter, pulse conditions (脈 [mài]) and symptoms (證 [zhèng]) are considered separately. That the character 證 [zhèng] refers to "symptom" can be further demonstrated in the sayings of later generations: 舍脈從證 [shě mài cóng zhèng] and 舍

證從脈 [shě zhèng cóng mài] ("precedence of pulse over symptoms" and "precedence of symptoms over pulse").

The modern Chinese textbook of diagnostics clarifies this issue, and defines the related terms as follows: 證 [zhèng] is a unique concept, including 證名 [zhèng míng] and 證候 [zhèng hòu]. The former refers to the generalization of the cause, nature and location of the disease at a certain stage, and the latter refers to its specific clinical manifestations[*].

As for the equivalent of the term 證 [zhèng], no English word is exactly appropriate, and *pinyin* is not acceptable because: (1) the character 證 [zhèng] is widely used as a traditional medical term in Japan and Korea where the pronunciation is different from *zheng*, and (2) quite a few Chinese characters used in medicine have exactly the same sound and tone, for example, 正 [zhèng] and 症 [zhèng].

At first, 證 [zhèng] was translated as "symptom-complex" and then "syndrome", and even now many authors still prefer the translation "syndrome". Opposition chiefly lies in the fact that the word "syndrome" cannot fully reflect the characteristic features of the concept of 證 [zhèng] as it is used in Chinese medicine. In recent years, the word "pattern" has been held in high esteem by some authors. This word might have some advantage over the word "syndrome" if the disease diagnosis has already been made. However, "pattern" also has its disadvantages.

證 [zhèng] as a diagnostic entity, denotes a certain morbid or abnormal condition, but "pattern" simply means model or type, with no implication of a diseased condition. So, it is difficult to understand this word when it is used independently with no association with disease. As we know, Chinese medical treatment may be effectively applied simply under the syndrome differentiation. In many cases, disease diagnosis in Chinese medicine is based merely on the patient's chief complaint or the main symptom. In order to avoid dilemma, some authors assert that the word "pattern" is actually an abbreviation of "disease pattern" or "disharmony pattern". Anyway, neither "syndrome" nor "pattern" can fully reflect the whole picture of 證 [zhèng]. When we use the word "pattern", we have to think of the word in the light of Chinese medicine. If so, there is no reason to deny that the word "syndrome" can also be con-

---

[*]Zhu WF (editor-in-chief). Zhong Yi Zhen Duan Xue (*Diagnostics of Traditional Chinese Medicine*) (in Chinese), the Textbook Series for Programmed Courses of the TCM Univeristies and Colleges, Shanghai Science and Technology Press, 1998, p.186

sidered in a similar way.

According to *Webster's Comprehensive Dictionary of the English Language* (1996), syndrome is "an aggregate or set of concurrent symptoms together indicating the presence or nature of a disease." This definition is not at all contradictory to the concept of 證 [zhèng] in Chinese medicine. The number of syndromes of Western medicine listed in ICD-10 (WHO) (1994) is 475, and the number of 證 [zhèng] of Chinese medicine listed in the State Standard of the People's Republic of China (1997) is 800. So in both systems of medicine the word "syndrome" by no means refers to random combinations of symptoms.

In conclusion, the reason for avoiding the use of the word syndrome in Chinese medicine and replacing it with the word pattern is not adequate. Since the word syndrome has already been used by many authors for many years, particularly because in the official documents published in China "syndrome" is always used as the equivalent of 證 [zhèng] in the English translation or annotations, it is better not to make any change, so as to prevent new terminological confusion. Any reader who has a rudimentary knowledge of Chinese medicine will feel no difficulty in identifying the Western origin of "nephrotic syndrome" and the Chinese origin of "kidney yang deficiency syndrome". In reality, every English word used in the description of Chinese medicine should be comprehended in the light of Chinese medicine.

As for the word "pattern", since it has already been accepted by quite a few translators and writers it is also selected as another standard term, but it can only be used under the heading of a disease name.

4. 證型 [zhèng xíng] is a newly developed term, particularly useful when diagnosis is made in terms of both disease and syndrome. In this case, "syndrome pattern" is an appropriate term under the heading of disease diagnosis. The term "syndrome pattern" can be further abbreviated as "pattern". The authors who prefer "pattern" as the equivalent of 證 [zhèng] suggest "pattern type" for the present term. This wording may be far-fetched, showing the disadvantage of rendering 證 [zhèng] as "pattern" from another aspect.

5. To determine the syndrome or pattern is called 辨證 [biàn zhèng] in Chinese. Since the character 辨 [biàn] means "differentiate", many authors render the term as "syndrome differentiation", "syndrome discrimination" or even as "differential diagnosis". Those who prefer the word "pattern" mostly use "pattern identification", but others use "pattern

discrimination" or "pattern differentiation'. The words selected here are in accordance with most of the authors.

6. It is natural to render 辨病 [biàn bìng] as "disease differentiation" or "differential diagnosis of disease", because most authors take it for granted that "disease" and 病 [bìng] are equivalents. In reality, the Chinese concept of 病 [bìng] is quite different from that of disease from the Western point of view. A number of disease names in Chinese medicine are based on symptoms, for example, coughing, headache, vomiting, insomnia and edema.

TERMS OF DIAGNOSTIC METHODS

Many terms used in the diagnostic methods of traditional Chinese medicine are common to modern Western medicine, particularly the terms about symptoms such as pain, dizziness, headache, nausea, vomiting, diarrhea, coughing, palpitations, and so forth. In this scheme there is no need to collect all these terms, but on the basis of common symptoms some terms may be further developed with specific significance in traditional Chinese diagnosis. For example, "thirst" is a common term, but "thirst with preference for cold drinks" and "dryness in the mouth with no desire for drink" are special terms with diagnostic significance in Chinese medicine.

INSPECTION

Inspection is examination by using the eyes, including inspection of vitality, complexion, expression, posture, behavior, body surface, tongue, excreta, secretions, etc.

Inspection of the Patient's General Condition

Proposed Standard Nomenclature

inspection 望診 [wàng zhěn][1]   inspection of vitality 望神 [wàng
presence of vitality 得神 [dé shén][2]   shén][2]

false vitality 假神 [jiǎ shén][2, 4]

loss of vitality 失神 [shī shén][2, 3]

normal color 常色 [cháng sè][5]

inspection of color 望色 [wàng sè][5]

morbid color 病色 [bìng sè][5]

favorable color 善色 [shàn sè][5]

unfavorable color 惡色 [è sè][5]

complexion 面色 [miàn sè][6]

pale complexion 面色蒼白 [miàn sè cāng bái][7]

bright pale complexion 面色晄白 [miàn sè huǎng bái][7]

darkish complexion 面色黎黑 [miàn sè lí hēi][8]

flushed face 面紅 [miàn hóng][9]

bluish complexion 面青 [miàn qīng][11]

dusty complexion 面塵 [miàn chén][10]

sallow complexion 面色萎黃 [miàn sè wěi huáng][13]

yellow complexion 面黃 [miàn huáng][12]

squamous skin 肌膚甲錯 [jī fū jiǎ cuò][15]

puffy complexion 面浮 [miàn fú][14]

yellow puffiness 黃胖 [huáng pàng][16]

lying supine with the legs stretched 仰臥伸足 [yǎng wò shēn zú][17]

lying on the side with the knees drawn up 蹻臥縮足 [quán wò suō zú][17]

wriggling of extremities 手足蠕動 [shǒu zú rú dòng][18]

trembling of extremities 手足顫動 [shǒu zú chàn dòng][18]

twitching of muscles 筋惕肉瞤 [jīn tì ròu shùn][19]

deviated mouth 口喎 [kǒu wāi][20]

twitching of body 身瞤動 [shēn shùn dòng][19]

deviated eye and mouth 口眼喎斜 [kǒu yǎn wāi xiè][20]

lusterless eyes 兩眼無光 [liǎng yǎn wú guāng][21]

Spiritless eyes 神光耗散 [shén guāng hào sàn][21]

forward-staring eyes 瞪目直視 [dèng mù zhí shì][22]

sideways-staring eyes 橫目斜視 [hèng mù xié shì][22]

Discussion

1. For the term 望診 [wàng zhěn], various ways of expression have appeared in recent publications, such as "looking", "diagnosis by looking", "observation", "inspection", and "visual inspection". The word "inspection" is most appropriate and used by most authors, because "inspect" means to look at and examine carefully.

2. From these terms, it is apparent that the Chinese concept of 神 [shén] is better expressed by "vitality" than "spirit" (cf. the discussion on "vitality"). One's spirit includes feelings and thought that can hardly be examined merely by looking.

3. For 失神 [shī shén], there are various expressions in recent pub-

lications, such as "loss of spirit", "spiritlessness", "depletion of spirit", "out of sorts", "lack of vitality" and "loss of vitality". Some of these expressions are too general or vague. The word "vitality" is selected as discussed above.

4. For 假神 [jiǎ shén], the expressions include "false vitality", "false manifestation of vitality", and "false spiritedness". The word "vitality" is selected, as discussed above.

5. For 望色 [wàng sè], some authors prefer the term "inspection of complexion". Although complexion means the color of the skin, especially of the face, it may also imply the appearance of the face. For this term, the word "color" seems to be more appropriate than "complexion". Regarding the expression of 善 [shàn] versus 惡 [è], the following words are used by different authors: "favorable" versus "unfavorable", "benign" versus "malign", "kind" versus "unkind", "well-meaning" versus "ill-natured", etc. Since the attributives indicate the prognosis of the disease, the first two pairs are appropriate, and "favorable versus unfavorable" is more frequently used than "benign versus malign".

6. 面色 [miàn sè] refers not only to the color but also to the appearance of the skin of the face, so "complexion" is more appropriate than "color of the face".

7. Generally, a white complexion can be classified into three categories: 淡白 [dàn bái], 蒼白 [cāng bái] and 晄白 [huǎng bái], indicating blood deficiency, yang collapse with preponderant cold, and yang deficiency with water accumulation, respectively. 蒼白 [cāng bái] is more whitened than 淡白 [dàn bái]. Strictly speaking, 蒼 [cāng] has the meaning of bluish or grayish, and so 蒼白 [cāng bái] is the color of the face caused by cold with constricted blood vessels and sluggish blood flow. 晄白 [huǎng bái] differs from 淡白 [dàn bái] and 蒼白 [cāng bái] in luster. 晄白 [huǎng bái] is bright white, while 淡白 [dàn bái] is often described as pale and lusterless (淡白無華 [dàn bái wú huá]). Some authors suggest the following three phrases "pale white", "somber white" and "bright white" as the equivalents of 淡白 [dàn bái], 蒼白 [cāng bái] and 晄白 [huǎng bái], respectively. Except for bright white, the other two have not been widely accepted, and more authors simply use "pallid" for 淡白 [dàn bái] and "pale" for 蒼白 [cāng bái].

8. In Chinese medicine 面色黎黑 [miàn sè lí hēi] is a complexion with specific clinical significance indicating kidney insufficiency, cold syndromes, or blood stasis. For this term there are different expressions,

such as "dimmish black complexion", "dimmish and blackish complexion" and "soot-black facial complexion", but most authors simply use "darkish complexion". There is no such a word as dimmish in English. In the strict sense, 黧黑 [lí hēi] does not mean soot-black. ("Soot-black" is an appropriate equivalent for 黑如炱 [hēi rú tái].) The original meaning of the character 黧 [lí] is black mixed with a brownish color. In Chinese, 黧牛 [lí niú] is an ox with black hair mixed with some brownish hair.

9. If the entire face is red, it is called 面紅 [miàn hóng] in Chinese. There are different English expressions, such as "red facial complexion", "red complexion" and "flushed face". "Red complexion" is selected in order to keep consistency with other expressions concerning the color of the skin of the face.

10. A dark-gray complexion as if covered with dust is called 面塵 [miàn chén] in Chinese. It indicates latent pathogens in excess syndromes, and consumption of liver and kidney yin in deficiency syndromes. Most authors render it as "dusty complexion".

11. Bluish discoloration of the skin of the face resulting from stagnant blood circulation is seen in cold syndrome, severe pain, *qi* stagnation, blood stasis and convulsions. In Chinese it is called 面青 [miàn qīng]. As discussed elsewhere, the character 青 [qīng] may cause difficulty in translation as it denotes both green and blue. But when we deal with the issue in the reverse way, i.e., try to find an appropriate Chinese equivalent of the word bluish, there will not be any problem. To match the related terms, the proposed standard term is "bluish complexion".

12. Yellow discoloration of the skin of the face is called 面黃 [miàn huáng]. Some authors use the word "yellowish" to express this discoloration, but most authors prefer the word "yellow" because the latter includes various shades of yellow.

13. Sallow color of the skin of the face, usually occurring in spleen *qi* deficiency, is called 面色萎黃 [miàn sè wěi huáng]. Some authors render it as "sallow complexion", "withered-yellow facial complexion", or "sallow yellow facial complexion". "Sallow" is "of an unhealthy yellowish color", therefore "sallow complexion" with no addition of "withered" or "yellowish" is adequate.

14. A soft swollen face indicating retention of water-damp is called 面浮 [miàn fú]. Of its English equivalents, including "edema of the face", "facial edema" and "puffy face", the last one is the most appropriate choice, for puffiness is a sign that can be found upon inspection while

edema is a conclusion of examinations, indicating a pathological condition.

15. 肌膚甲錯 [jī fū jiǎ cuò] is a common sign indicating blood stasis. Various English equivalents have been suggested, such as "scaly skin", "scaly dry skin", "squamous skin", "squamous and dry skin" and "incrusted skin". The word "incrusted" or "encrusted" comes from "crust", which is defined as an outer layer of solid matter formed by the drying of a bodily exudate or secretion. In the case of blood stasis, the change of the skin is not related to exudation or secretion. The word "squamous" is derived from "squama", which is a general term in anatomical nomenclature for a scale or platelike structure. So, "squamous skin" is selected.

16. Yellow tinge of the skin with puffy face is called 黃胖 [huáng pàng], a term used in Chinese medicine to describe the general appearance of a patient with anylostomiasis. Direct literal translation of the Chinese term as "yellow obesity" is not recommendable because the character 胖 [pàng] does not always mean obesity. An appropriate equivalent of 胖 [pàng] is plumpness, which is not necessarily due to accumulation of fat. Some authors translate 黃胖 [huáng pàng] as "general edema with yellowish tinge of skin" or "general edema with sallow skin", which are actually explanations than translations. Other translations are "yellowish swelling" and "yellowish puffiness", the latter of which seems more appropriate. The word "yellowish" can be replaced by "yellow" for the latter includes all shades of yellow.

17. "Lying supine with the legs stretched" 仰臥伸足 [yǎng wò shēn zú] is a posture often taken by patients with excessive heat, and "lying on the side with the knees drawn up" 踡臥縮足 [quán wò suō zú], a posture often taken by patients with deficiency-cold.

18. Trembling (顫動 [chàn dòng]) and wriggling (蠕動 [rú dòng]) of the extremities are two types of involuntary movement, indicating stirring of internal wind. Some authors prefer "quivering" for 顫動 [chàn dòng].

19. 惕 [tì] and 瞤 [shùn] are synonymous, both signifying "tic" or "twitchings". Different characters are used in the term chiefly for rhetoric purposes.

20. For 喎 [wāi] and 喎斜 [wāi xié] there are several expressions, such as "oblique", "wry" and "deviated". Most authors prefer "deviated". Some authors turn it into "facial paralysis", which is too Westernized.

21. "Lusterless eyes" (兩眼無光 [liǎng yǎn wú guāng]) and "spiritless eyes" (神光耗散 [shén guāng hào sàn]) usually indicate that the patient is seriously ill.

22. A patient with loss of consciousness and eyes staring straight ahead (瞪目直視 [dèng mù zhí shì]) or staring sideways 橫目斜視 [hèng mù xié shì] is usually suffering from up-stirring of liver wind.

Inspection of Excreta

Proposed Standard Nomenclature

inspection of the sputum 望痰 [wàng tán][1]

scanty sticky sputum 痰少而粘 [tán shǎo ér nián][1]

white slippery sputum 痰白滑 [tán bái huá][1]

inspection of vomitus 望嘔吐物 [wàng ǒu tù wù][2]

watery stool 大便清稀 [dà biàn qīng xī][3]

loose stool 便溏 [biàn táng][3]

distant bleeding 遠血 [yuǎn xuè][3]

inspection of urine 望小便 [wàng xiǎo biàn][4]

long voiding of clear urine 小便清長 [xiǎo biàn qīng cháng][4]

turbid urine 小便渾濁 [xiǎo biàn hún zhuó][4]

white watery sputum 痰白清稀 [tán bái qīng xī][1]

yellow thick sputum 痰黃稠 [tán huáng chóu][1]

blood-stained sputum 痰中帶血 [tán zhōng dài xuè][1]

inspection of stool 望大便 [wàng dà biàn][3]

dry and hard stool 大便燥結 [dà biàn zào jié][3]

nearby bleeding 近血 [jìn xuè][3]

bloody stool 大便帶血 [dà biàn dài xuè][3]

short voiding of yellow urine 小便短黃 [xiǎo biàn duǎn huáng][4]

blood-stained urine 尿中帶血 [niào zhōng dài xuè][4]

Discussion

1. Two words are commonly used to express 望 [wàng] or 望診 [wàng zhěn]: "inspection" and "observation". For examining the excreta, "inspection" seems better.

For the character 痰 [tán] in the term 望痰 [wàng tán], it is better to use the word "sputum" instead of "phlegm", because what one can examine by the eyes is the visible phlegm, i.e., the sputum.

The attributives commonly used to describe the quality and quantity of sputum are as follows:

Chinese	Renderings by different authors	Word selected
白 [bái]	white, whitish, pale	white

黄 [huáng]	yellow, yellowish, purulent	yellow
稀 [xī]	thin	thin
清稀 [qīng xī]	watery, clear and thin,	watery
粘 [nián]	sticky, mucoid	sticky
粘稠 [nián chóu]	thick	thick
多 [duō]	abundant, copious, profuse, excessive	abundant
少 [shǎo]	scanty, little, a small amount of	scanty
带血 [dài xuè]	blood-stained, blood-tinged, bloody, containing blood, mixed with blood	blood-stained

2. Inspection of vomitus 望嘔吐物 [wàng ǒu tù wù] includes determination of its quality (watery, turbid, mucoid, containing undigested food), color (bile-stained, blood-stained), and smell (odorless, sour, fetid, or putrid).

3. In inspection of stools (望大便 [wàng dà biàn]), the attributives commonly used to describe the quality and quantity of stools are as follows:

Chinese	Renderings by different authors	Word selected
乾 [gān]	dry	dry
燥結 [zǎo jié]	dry bound, dry and hard	dry and hard
稀 [xī]	thin	thin
清稀 [qīng xī]	watery, clear and thin	watery
溏 [táng]	loose, sloppy	loose
带血 [dài xuè]	bloody, containing blood, blood-stained	bloody

近血 [jìn xuè], bleeding near the anus, is rendered as "proximal bleeding", "fresh blood in the stool", "nearby bleeding", and "near blood"; 遠血 [yuǎn xuè], bleeding far from the anus. is rendered as "distal bleeding", "distant bleeding", and "distant blood". The words "proximal" and "distal" are not appropriate, for customarily "proximal" means "near the center of the body" and "distal" means "away from the center of the body"

4. In inspection of urine (望小便 [wàng xiǎo biàn]), the following attributives are commonly used.

Chinese	Renderings by different authors	Word selected
清 [qīng]	clear, light-colored	clear

黃 [huáng]	yellow, dark-colored	yellow
渾濁 [hún zhuó]	turbid, cloudy, nebulous	turbid
長 [cháng]	long voiding of, profuse	long voiding of
短 [duǎn]	short voiding of, scanty	short voiding of
帶血 [dài xuè]	blood-stained, blood-tinged, bloody, mixed with blood, containing blood	blood-stained

Inspection of Finger Venules

Inspection of finger venules is a diagnostic method for children under 3, in which the extension and color of the superficial venules on the palmar side of the index finger are examined for determining the location, nature and severity of the disease as well as the prognosis. Some of the terms used in this examination have their own particularity.

Proposed Standard Nomenclature

inspection of finger venules 望指紋 [wàng zhǐ wén][1]

qi pass 氣關 [qì guān][3]

life pass 命關 [mìng guān][3]

three passes 三關 [sān guān][2]

wind pass 風關 [fēng guān][3]

extension to the nail 透關射甲 [tòu guān shè jiǎ][4]

Discussion

1. In the inspection of finger venules, the superficial venules on the palmar side of the index finger are examined. In traditional Chinese pediatrics these venules are called 指紋 [zhǐ wén]. There is no disagreement on this expression, but some authors prefer a detailed description such as "superficial venules of the index finger".

2. The three passes is a collective term for the three segments of the index finger for measuring the extension of the visible venules. The Chinese original is 三關 [sān guān]. As for the English equivalent of the character 關 [guān], words that have been used include "pass", "bar", "gate", "strategic pass", etc. Most authors prefer the word "pass".

3. The three passes are 風關 [fēng guān], 氣關 [qì guān], and 命關 [mìng guān] corresponding to the proximal segment, middle segment and distal segment of the index finger respectively. Most of the authors render them as "wind pass", "qi pass" and "life pass". Some authors insist on

using *pinyin*, i.e., "*fengguan*", "*qiguan*" and "*mingguan*". This is not generally accepted, for *pinyin* gives no information, only meaningless sounds. Rendering 風 [fēng] as "wind" and 命 [mìng] as "life" is rational, because in the course of an externally contracted disease, "wind" usually refers to the initial stage when only the exterior portion of the body is involved, and "life" indicates the seriousness of the disease with the life endangered.

4. Extension of visible venules through all the passes to the nails is called 透關射甲 [tòu guān shè jiǎ]. Various renderings appear in the publications: "appearance of the superficial veins extending through the three passes toward the finger nail", "extending of the superficial venules through the three passes toward the tip of the index finger", "extension of visible veins through all the bars to the nail", "shooting through strategic passes to the nail", "extending of the superficial veins through the three passes toward the tip of index finger", etc. All of them are explanatory. For the standard nomenclature a shortened phrase is required, and thus "extension (through passes) to the nail".

TONGUE DIAGNOSIS

Examination of the tongue, chiefly by inspection, is crucial to diagnosis. It gives information about the condition of both health *qi* and pathogenic *qi*. Many terms used in this field have their own characteristic features

Proposed Standard Nomenclature

tongue diagnosis 舌診 [shé zhěn][1]

presentation of the tongue 舌象 [shé xiàng][2]

sides of the tongue 舌邊 [shé biān][3]

central part of the tongue 舌心 [shé xīn][3]

tongue body 舌體 [shé tǐ][4]

tongue color 舌色 [shé sè][5]

pale tongue 淡白舌 [dàn bái shé][7]

paleness of the tongue 舌淡 [shé dàn][7]

inspection of the tongue 望舌 [wàng shé][1]

tip of the tongue 舌尖 [shé jiān][3]

middle part of the tongue 舌中 [shé zhōng][3]

root of the tongue 舌根 [shé gēn][3]

base of the tongue 舌本 [shé běn][3]

tongue proper 舌質 [shé zhì][4]

pale-red tongue 淡紅舌 [dàn hóng shé][6]

redness of the tongue 舌紅 [shé

red tongue 紅舌 [hóng shé][8]

purple tongue 紫舌 [zǐ shé][10]

cyanotic tongue 青紫舌 [qīng zǐ shé][10]

enlarged tongue 胖大舌 [pàng dà shé][12]

indented tongue 齒痕舌 [chǐ hén shé][14]

cracked tongue 裂紋舌 [liè wén shé][16]

trembling tongue 顫動舌 [chàn dòng shé][18]

deviated tongue 歪斜舌 [wāi xié shé][20]

protruding and moving tongue 吐弄舌 [tǔ nòng shé][22]

tongue coating color 苔色 [tāi sè][24]

black coating 黑苔 [hēi tāi][24]

curdy coating 腐苔 [fǔ tāi][26]

slippery coating 滑苔 [huá tāi][28]

dry coating 燥苔 [zào tāi][30]

rough coating 糙苔 [cāo tāi][30]

peeled tongue 光剝舌 [guāng bō shé][32]

rooted coating 有根苔 [yǒu gēn tāi][34]

hóng][8]

crimson tongue 絳舌 [jiàng shé][9]

blue tongue 青舌 [qīng shé][10]

thin tongue 瘦薄舌 [shòu báo shé][11]

swollen tongue 腫脹舌 [zhǒng zhàng shé][13]

prickled tongue 芒刺舌 [máng cì shé][15]

stiff tongue 強硬舌 [jiàng yìng shé][17]

flaccid tongue 痿軟舌 [wěi ruǎn shé][19]

shortened tongue 短縮舌 [duǎn suō shé][21]

tongue coating 舌苔 [shé tāi][23]

white coating 白苔 [bái tāi][24]

yellow coating 黃苔 [huáng tāi][24]

gray coating 灰苔 [huī tāi][24]

stained coating 染苔 [rǎn tāi][25]

greasy coating 膩苔 [nì tāi][27]

moist coating 潤苔 [rùn tāi][29]

peeling of tongue coating 舌苔脫落 [shé tāi tuó luò][31]

mirror tongue 鏡面舌 [jìng miàn shé][33]

rootless coating 無根苔 [wú gēn tāi][35]

Discussion

1. The two Chinese terms 舌診 [shé zhěn] and 望舌 [wàng shé] are closely related but have different meanings. The former is rendered into English in various ways, such as "tongue diagnosis", "lingual diagnosis", "tongue inspection", "inspection of the tongue", "observation of the tongue", and "tongue examination". Strictly speaking, the term "tongue examination" or "tongue inspection" is more appropriate, but many authors render it as "tongue diagnosis" to stress its special role in Chinese diagnostics. To date, the term "tongue diagnosis" is widely accepted. It is selected as the standard term for its frequency in usage.

望舌 [wàng shé] is different. It refers to the procedure of inspecting the tongue for diagnostic purposes, but does not include diagnosis-making. The procedure of diagnosis-making based on inspecting the tongue is "tongue diagnosis" 舌診 [shé zhěn]. The distinction might be arbitrary, but it tallies with the practical use.

2. "Tongue presentation" is a newly developed Chinese medical term. It has been rendered into English in various ways, such as "picture of the tongue", "tongue picture", "tongue demonstration", "tongue image", and "tongue presentation". The last one seems the best choice for it hardly causes misunderstanding.

3. The partition of the tongue is one of the characteristic features of tongue diagnosis in Chinese medicine. Generally, a tongue can be divided into the following areas: tip, borders, root and middle part. Each area reflects the pathological change of one or two *zang-fu* organs. Therefore, it is important to standardize the name of the parts.

The distal end of the tongue is called 舌尖 [shé jiān], which reflects the condition of the heart and lung. Most authors use the word "tip" to nominate this part. Some use the word "apex", which is not widely accepted because "apex" usually refers to the top or highest point.

The lateral side of the tongue is called 舌邊 [shé biān], which reflects the condition of the liver and gallbladder. Several expressions have been used for nominating this part of the tongue: "sides of the tongue", "edges of the tongue", "margins of the tongue", and "borders of the tongue". They are similar but not exactly the same in meaning. "Edge" refers to the narrowest part along the outside of something, especially of a cutting instrument or along the outside of a solid flat object. 'Border" is the edge or side(s) of anything but especially of the land belonging to two countries. "Margin" is the blank space round the written or printed matter on a page or anything like this. Therefore, "side" which refers to the area near the edge or boundary, is probably the most appropriate word.

The "central or middle part of the tongue" that often reflects the condition of the spleen and stomach corresponds to 舌中 [shé zhōng] or 舌心 [shé xīn]. There are some other expressions such as "center of the tongue", "tongue center" and "middle surface of the tongue", but with no significant difference.

舌根 [shé gēn] or 舌本 [shé běn] is the part of the tongue that often reflects the condition of the kidney. Two English equivalents, "root" and "base" of the tongue, are often used, and more authors prefer the first one.

4. The tongue itself, excluding its coating, is called 舌體 [shé tǐ] or 舌質 [shé zhì]. The former is ordinarily rendered as tongue body, but the latter has various expressions such as "tongue substance", "tongue material", "tongue tissue", and "tongue proper". Among these terms, "tongue proper" seems appropriate, suiting the original concept best, and is more frequently used than others.

5. Color of the tongue proper reflects the condition of *qi* and blood as well as the functional state of *zang-fu* organs. It is called 舌色 [shé sè] in Chinese, and the English equivalent is "tongue color" or "color of the tongue". Some authors render it over-scrupulously as "tongue-body color". In fact, no misunderstanding will happen if the word "body" is omitted.

6. A normal tongue is pale red. In Chinese it is called 淡紅舌 [dàn hóng shé]. Most authors use "pale red tongue" as the equivalent, but some other authors prefer "pink tongue", "light-red tongue", or "slightly red tongue". The proposed standard term is selected according to the frequency of use. Some authors insert hyphen between "pale" and "red". This is not recommended.

7. A tongue paler than normal is called 淡白舌 [dàn bái shé]. It is usually seen in *qi* and blood deficiency or yang deficiency. Most of the authors render it as "pale tongue". For emphasizing the pale color of the tongue, 舌淡 [shé dàn] in Chinese and paleness of the tongue in English are ordinarily used.

8. A tongue redder than normal, indicating the presence of heat, is called 紅舌 [hóng shé]. The corresponding English expressions include "red tongue", "reddened tongue" and "reddish tongue". Among these terms "red tongue" is most point-blank, and is used by most authors.

If the expression is emphasized on the color that the tongue possesses, "redness of the tongue" (舌紅 [shé hóng]) is used

9. If the tongue is deep red, indicating the presence of intense heat, it is called 絳舌 [jiàng shé] in Chinese. As the equivalent, "crimson tongue", "scarlet tongue", "dark red tongue" and "deep red tongue" are used.

10. A tongue purple in color indicates stagnation of circulating *qi* and blood, and a tongue blue in color indicates the presence of congealing cold with blood stasis. They are designated 紫舌 [zǐ shé] and blue tongue

青舌 [qīng shé], respectively. The corresponding English equivalents are "purple tongue" and "blue tongue". Some authors prefer "purplish" and "bluish", and some even use both "purple" and "purplish" or "blue" and "bluish" in the same writing. In daily English, such statements as "go purple with rage" and "hands blue with cold" are quite similar with the Chinese concepts. So it is unnecessary to use the words "purplish" and "bluish".

A tongue bluish purple in color is called 青紫舌 [qīng zǐ shé]. Since the word "cyanosis" used in Western medicine is translated into Chinese as 青紫 [qīng zǐ], it is generally acceptable to use cyanosis as the equivalent of 青紫 [qīng zǐ], and hence the term "cyanotic tongue".

11. A tongue thinner than normal is called 瘦薄舌 [shòu báo shé]. It indicates deficiency of *qi* and blood if it is pale, and indicates deficiency of yin if it is red. The English equivalent is "thin tongue" with no controversy.

12. A tongue larger than normal due to accumulation of fluid is called 胖大舌 [pàng dà shé]. There are several different expressions in English: "enlarged tongue", "bulgy tongue", "plump tongue", "flabby tongue", and "corpulent tongue". The most popular one is "enlarged tongue". The word "bulge" is a rounded swelling with an outward curve. So "bulgy" is not an exact description. The rest ones may be more lively descriptions, but most of them are related to accumulated fat or fatty flesh. This is probably why most authors would rather use the commonest word "enlarged".

13. 腫脹舌 [zhǒng zhàng shé] is also an abnormally enlarged tongue, but it is usually reddened, often caused by exuberant fire of the heart and spleen or externally contracted damp-heat. Most authors use "swollen tongue" as the equivalent, but some others suggest glossocele and glossoncus. Glossocele means swelling and protrusion of the tongue, and glossoncus refers to a swelling or mass of the tongue. Both of them are rarely used words, and not exactly in conformity with the original sense of the Chinese term.

14. A tongue with dental indentations on its margins is called 齒痕舌 [chǐ hén shé] in Chinese. It is seen in retention of water-damp when the tongue is enlarged as well. In the recent publications in English there are various expressions such as "indented tongue", "tooth-marked tongue", "teeth-printed tongue", "dental indentations on tongue edges", "tongue bearing dental impressions", "tongue with teeth marks on its margins", etc. Some of them are explanations rather than technical terms.

The term "indented tongue" is selected for its succinctness.

15. A tongue with thorn-like protrusions on its surface, indicating the presence of exuberant heat, is called 芒刺舌 [máng cì shé]. For this term there are two common expressions: "prickled or prickly tongue", and "thorny tongue". More authors prefer "prickled tongue".

16. A tongue with cracks on its surface often indicates consumption of fluids or yin. It is called 裂紋舌 [liè wén shé] in Chinese. Two terms are commonly used as its English equivalents: "cracked tongue" and "fissured tongue". Terms such as "split tongue" and "cleft tongue" are used only occasionally. Fissure is a long deep crack. Since the crack on the tongue is not necessarily long and deep, "cracked tongue" is hence selected.

17. In patients suffering from high fever with impairment of consciousness and also in cases of apoplexy, the tongue may be difficult to move freely. In Chinese, the tongue is called 強硬舌 [jiàng yìng shé]. As the English equivalent, most authors prefer "stiff tongue", while a few authors use "rigid tongue".

18. An involuntarily quivering tongue is a sign of endogenous wind. The English equivalents for the Chinese term 顫動舌 [chàn dòng shé] are "trembling tongue", "tremulous tongue", and "quivering tongue". For the selection of the term as the standard, consideration of its synonym 舌顫 [shé chàn] is helpful. The latter is most frequently rendered as "trembling tongue" or "tremor of the tongue".

19. A flabby tongue unable to move easily is seen in impairment of yin or deficiency of *qi* and blood. It is called 痿軟舌 [wěi ruǎn shé] and rendered into English as "flaccid tongue" by most of the authors. Some other terms such as "atrophy of tongue", "atrophic and soft tongue", and "limpness of the tongue" have been suggested, but none is widely accepted.

20. A tongue that deviates to one side when extended is known as 歪斜舌 [wāi xié shé]. The English equivalents include "deviated tongue", "wry tongue" and "crooked tongue". "Deviated tongue" is most frequently used.

21. A tongue that cannot be fully extended from the mouth and appears to be contracted is known as 短縮舌 [duǎn suō shé]. Most authors render it as "shortened tongue", and some others as "short tongue", "contracted tongue", "retracted tongue" and "curving tongue".

22. A tongue that extends out of the mouth with repeated licking of the lips or incessant moving is called 吐弄舌 [tǔ nòng shé] in Chinese.

It is a combined expression of protruding tongue (吐舌 [tǔ shé]) and moving tongue (弄舌 [nòng shé]). Various expressions have appeared in recent publications, such as "protrusion of tongue", "frequent protrusion of tongue" and "wagging tongue" for 吐舌 [tǔ shé], "wagging tongue", "moving tongue", "worrying tongue", "playing with tongue" and "sticking out the tongue" for 弄舌 [nòng shé], and "wagging tongue", "wagging of the tongue", "playing with the tongue", "protrusion of tongue" and "protrusion and worrying of the tongue" for 吐弄舌 [tǔ nòng shé]. In short, the following verbs or their present participles are used to express 吐弄 [tǔ nòng]: "protrude", "move", "wag", "play with", "worry" and "stick out". The word "wag" may cause misunderstanding because "tongues wag" refers to gossip or rumor. "To play with the tongue" may be just a childish behavior, not indicating disease. "To stick out the tongue" is not a sign of disease, either. "To worry" means to seize something with the teeth and shake or pull it about, not exactly equivalent to the Chinese concept. Therefore, the only choice is "protruding and moving".

23. The layer of moss-like material covering the tongue is called 舌苔 [shé tāi], inspection of which can provide information about the nature, depth and location of the pathogenic factor, the strength and integrity of the normal *qi*, and the degree of fluid consumption. The character 苔 (pronounced tái) means "moss". When it is used in the term 舌苔 [shé tāi] it refers to something like moss, and is pronounced [tāi]. The English equivalents are: tongue coating, fur, and moss. "Tongue coating" is the most popular one.

24. The color of the tongue coating reflects the heat or cold nature of the syndrome. Generally, the tongue coating can be classified into "white coating" 白苔 [bái tāi], "yellow coating" 黄苔 [huáng tāi], "black coating" 黑苔 [hēi tāi] and "gray coating" 灰苔 [huī tāi]. Some authors prefer the words "whitish", "yellowish", "blackish" and "grayish", but these words are not widely accepted as the equivalents of the above-mentioned Chinese terms, for they do not exactly reflect the original meaning. For example, "yellowish" is equivalent to 微黄 [wēi huáng] or 淡黄 [dàn huáng], which is also commonly used to describe the color of the tongue coating.

25. A tongue coating stained by food, medicine, etc. is known as 染苔 [rǎn tāi]. It is often rendered as "stained coating" or "colored coating". The former is more exact, and is used by more authors.

26. 腐苔 [fǔ tāi] is a form of tongue coating consisting of coarse

granules, looking like curds, capable of being wiped off and reflecting retention of food in the stomach. For this term there are various English expressions: "curdy coating", "curdy fur", "bean curd tongue fur", "spongy curdy tongue coat", "crusty tongue coating", "moldy coating", "decant fur", "residue-like fur", etc. The most commonly used one is "curdy coating".

27. 膩苔 [nì tāi] is a dense, sticky, slimy tongue coating, thick in the center, thin on the sides, and hard to wipe off. It indicates the presence of phlegm-damp or retained food. Three adjectives are often used to describe this form of tongue coating: "greasy", "slimy", and "sticky". Most authors prefer the word "greasy", as this form of tongue coating looks more like grease (thick semi-solid oily substance) than slime (thick liquid substance), and the word "sticky" is equivalent to 粘 [nián] rather than 膩 [nì].

28. A moist tongue coating with excessive fluid and an oily appearance is known as 滑苔 [huá tāi]. It indicates the presence of dampness. For expressing this form of tongue coating in English, the following adjectives are used: "slippery", "smooth", and "glossy". The word "slippery" is the most appropriate one because it means "smooth, wet and polished", fully describing the features of this form of tongue coating. In reality, most authors use this word.

29. 潤苔 [rùn tāi] is moderately moistened tongue coating, seen either in normal persons or in patients with no damage to the body fluids. Most authors prefer the word "moist". A few authors use the word "wet", which, referring to containing too much water, differs from the Chinese original.

30. Dry coating 燥苔 [zào tāi] is a sign generally indicative of damage to the body fluids, and rough coating 糙苔 [cāo tāi] is so dry a tongue coating that looks rough, indicating severe damage to the body fluids. There is no disagreement on the wording of the two terms.

31. Complete or partial peeling of the tongue coating is known as 舌苔脫落 [shé tāi tuó luò]. Many authors use the word "exfoliation", such as "exfoliated tongue coating" or "exfoliative fur". This word is used in Western medicine, specifically defined as falling off in scales. But in the peeling process of tongue coating, no scales can be found. So it is better to express this term in a more general way, and "peeling of tongue coating" is thus selected.

32. A completely peeled tongue resembling a mirror is called 鏡面舌

[jìng miàn shé]. Its English equivalents include "mirror-like tongue", "mirror tongue", and "glossy tongue". The term "mirror tongue" is selected for its direct conformity with the Chinese original.

33. A tongue coating that is firmly attached to the tongue surface is known as 有根苔 [yǒu gēn tāi], and that can be easily wiped or scraped off is known as 無根苔 [wú gēn tāi]. Most authors render 有根 [yǒu gēn] and 無根 [wú gēn] as "rooted" or "with root" and "rootless" or "without root", respectively. Terminologically, a single-worded attribute is better than a phrase, and so "rooted coating" and "rootless coating" are selected.

AUSCULTATION

In Chinese medicine, auscultation refers to listening to the patient's voice, sounds of breath, coughing, etc., with the ear without using a stethoscope.

Proposed Standard Nomenclature

auscultation 聞聲音 [wén shēng yīn][1]

deep harsh voice 語聲重濁 [yǔ shēng zhòng zhuó][2]

faint low voice 語聲低微 [yǔ shēng dī wēi][3]

hoarseness 嘶嗄 [sī shà][4]

loss of voice 失音 [shī yīn][5]

dyspnea 喘 [chuǎn][6]

panting 喘促 [急] [chuǎn cù [jí]][6]

asthma 哮喘 [xiào chuǎn][6]

shortage of *qi* 少氣 [shǎo qì][7]

shortness of breath 短氣 [duǎn qì][7]

wheezing dyspnea 喘鳴 [chuǎn míng][8]

wheezing 哮 [xiào][8]

phlegm rattle 痰鳴 [tán míng][9]

coughing 咳嗽 [ké sòu][10]

vomiting 嘔吐 [ǒu tù][10]

retching 乾嘔 [gān ǒu][10]

hiccoughing 呃逆 [è nì][10]

belching 噯氣 [ài qì][10]

sighing 太息 [tài xī][10]

sneezing 噴嚏 [pēn tì][10]

yawning 呵欠 [hē qiàn][10]

borborygmi 腸鳴 [cháng míng][10]

Discussion

1. Many authors use the word "listening" to express the Chinese concept of 聞聲音 [wén shēng yīn]. In order to collocate with other diagnostic methods such as inspection and palpation, the word "auscultation" is thus selected. In addition, "listening" may be misunderstood as

"paying attention to what the patient complains of".

2. 語聲重濁 [yǔ shēng zhòng zhuó] is a change of voice due to nasal congestion, usually occurring in colds. There are different expressions for this symptom: "low voice speaking", "low raucous voice", "deep and harsh voice", "harsh voice", "deep and stuffy sound" and "heavy voice". More authors prefer "deep and harsh voice".

3. 語聲低微 [yǔ shēng dī wēi] is a change of voice in deficiency conditions, particular *qi* deficiency. It is rendered as "weak voice", "low and weak voice", "faint low voice", etc., with not much discrepancy.

4. Rough and harsh voice is known as 嘶嗄 [sī shà]. Its English equivalent is "hoarseness of voice", "hoarseness", "huskiness", etc. Most authors use "hoarseness", and so it is selected as the proposed standard.

5. Failure to utter with the voice and only whispered speech is known as 失音 [shī yīn]. It is rendered either as "loss of voice" or as "aphonia". The former is more popular.

6. In Chinese medicine, the common patterns of disordered respiration are dyspnea 喘 [chuǎn], wheezing 哮 [xiào], shortage of *qi* 少氣 [shǎo qì], and shortness of breath 短氣 [duǎn qì]. 喘 [chuǎn] is difficult or labored breathing, and so it is usually rendered as dyspnea. But there are other expressions, such as "panting", "asthma", "breathlessness", and "rapid respiration". "Panting" means labored breathing with rapid short breaths, corresponding to 喘促 [chuǎn cù] or 喘急 [chuǎn jí]. "Asthma" is dyspnea accompanied by wheezing, and so it corresponds to 哮喘 [xiào chuǎn], a symptom and also a disease name in Chinese medicine. "Breathlessness" is a common word synonymous with dyspnea or panting. Rapid respiration has not much significance in Chinese medicine, unless it is accompanied by other manifestations such as coarse breathing.

7. 少氣 [shǎo qì] refers to feeble breathing with a lack of *qi*. It is rendered as "lack of *qi*", "asthenic breathing", "shortage of *qi*", "deficiency of *qi*", etc. Most authors prefer "shortage of *qi*". It simulates "shortness of breath" (短氣 [duǎn qì]) but differs in that "shortage of *qi*" only occurs in deficiency conditions while "shortness of breath" may be seen either in deficiency conditions or in excess conditions.

As for 短氣 [duǎn qì], most authors render it as "shortness of breath", a few prefer "short breath" or "short breathing"

8. "Wheezing" is a continuous sound consisting of a whistling noise generated from the airway. It corresponds to 哮 [xiào] in Chinese. This is

generally accepted by most authors, but a few prefer "bronchial wheezing". The latter expression is too Westernized, and in reality, addition of the word "bronchial" is not necessary. From the perspective of Chinese medicine, wheezing comes from the airway, but not necessarily from the bronchus.

Closely related to 哮 [xiào] is the term 哮喘 [xiào chuǎn], also called 喘鳴 [chuǎn míng], referring to difficult and labored breathing with a continuous sound in the airway. 哮喘 [xiào chuǎn] as a disease name refers to "asthma", but it is also a symptom, synonymous with 喘鳴 [chuǎn míng], which means dyspnea with wheezing, and is rendered as "wheezing dyspnea".

9. Rattling sound caused by phlegm in the airway is called 痰鳴 [tán míng]. For this term there are various expressions: "rale", "phlegm rale", "wheezy phlegm", "phlegm wheezing", "rattling in the throat", and "phlegm rattle". In Western medicine, "rale" and "rattle" are different. Rale is an abnormal sound heard accompanying the normal respiratory sounds on auscultation of the chest, usually with the help of a stethoscope, while rattle is a throat noise caused by air passing through mucus, audible at a certain distance. So the latter is more suitable for the Chinese medical concept.

10. Other sounds from the patient that may be helpful for the diagnosis are coughing 咳嗽 [ké sòu], vomiting 嘔吐 [ǒu tù], retching 乾嘔 [gān ǒu], hiccoughing 呃逆 [è nì], belching 噯氣 [ài qì], sighing 太息 [tài xī], sneezing 噴嚏 [pēn tì], yawning 呵欠 [hē qian], and borborygmi 腸鳴 [cháng míng]. All these terms, both English and Chinese, are generally recognized, and no discussion is needed.

INTERROGATION

Inquiring of the patient the complaints and the history of the illness is an important way of gaining information for diagnosis. It is called 問診 [wèn zhěn] in Chinese medicine. Among its renderings "interrogation", "inquiry or inquiring", "asking" or "diagnosis by asking", the first one is selected as the proposed standard due to its common use by many authors, and also due to its collocation with inspection, auscultation, and palpation.

Inquiry about Chills and Fever

Proposed Standard Nomenclature

intolerance of cold 畏寒 [wèi hán][1]

shivering chill 寒戰 [hán zhàn][2]

aversion to heat 惡熱 [wù rè][4]

fever without chills 但熱不寒 [dàn rè bù hán][5]

alternating chills and fever 寒熱往來 [hán rè wǎng lái][6]

slight fever 微熱 [wēi rè][8]

Late afternoon fever 日晡潮熱 [rì bū cháo rè][10]

feverish sensation in the palms and soles 手足心熱 [shǒu zú xīn rè][11]

aversion to cold 惡寒 [wù hán][1]

chill 惡寒 [wù hán][1]

aversion to wind 惡風 [wù fēng][3]

fever 發熱 [fā rè][4]

chills without fever 但寒不熱 [dàn hán bù rè][5]

high fever without chills 壯熱 [zhuàng rè][7]

tidal fever 潮熱 [cháo rè][9]

vexing heat in the chest, palms and soles 五心煩熱 [wǔ xīn fán rè][11]

unsurfaced fever 身熱不揚 [shēn rè bù yáng][12]

Discussion

1. 畏寒 [wèi hán] refers to a sensation of cold which can be relieved by wearing more clothes or warming near a source of heat, and 惡寒 [wù hán] is a disagreeable sensation of cold which cannot be relieved by warmth. The former is usually rendered as "intolerance of cold", and the latter as "aversion to cold". Differentiation between them is of great significance in Chinese diagnosis. The former usually indicates insufficiency of yang-*qi* in the body, while the latter, often accompanied or followed by fever, is a symptom caused by exogenous pathogens that invade the exterior portion of the body. For the former, some alternatives are used, such as "fear of cold", "chilly sensation", but "intolerance of cold" seems most popular. "Chill" is synonymous with "aversion to cold", both being equally commonly used.

2. "Shivering chill" is a chill accompanied by involuntary muscular twitching. It corresponds to 寒戰 [hán zhàn] in Chinese medicine. There are other renderings of 寒戰 [hán zhàn]: "chill", "rigor", "shivering", "shivering with cold", etc. "Shivering chill" seems to be most explicit, and is hence selected as the proposed standard.

3. Strong dislike of wind is known as 惡風 [wù fēng]. Most of the authors render it as "aversion to wind".

4. In Chinese medicine, 發熱 [fā rè] is not confined to a rise of body temperature. General and localized feverish sensation is also included in

this symptom. This causes difficulty for the translation of Chinese into English. But to find a corresponding term from Chinese medicine for the term "fever", there is no problem at all. The word "fever" is a commonly used term in Chinese medicine, and its Chinese equivalent is naturally 發熱 [fā rè].

5. Fever without chills (但熱不寒 [dàn rè bù hán]) and chills without fever (但寒不熱 [dàn hán bù rè]) are two symptoms indicating interior heat and interior cold, respectively. Some authors prefer the literal translation "heat without cold" and "cold without heat". But the latter expressions are somewhat vague and ambiguous, because the words cold and heat are not customarily used to describe the patient's complaint.

6. 寒熱往來 [hán rè wǎng lái] is not a term difficult to express in English, but the expressions are multifarious, such as "alternate chills and fever", "alternating chills and fever", "alternate attacks of chills and fever", "alternate spells of fever and chills", "alternate episodes of chills and fever", "alternating episodes of chills and fever", "alternating cold and heat", "alternation of fever and chills", "hot-cold alternation", and "chill-heat alternating". Since this term refers to a symptom, and 寒 [hán] and 熱 [rè] are abbreviations of 惡寒 [wù hán] and 發熱 [fā rè], rendering them as "chills and fever" is better than "cold and heat". In addition, the words "attacks", "episodes" and "spells" are not absolutely necessary, nor are they included in the original term, and so can be deleted. Therefore, either "alternate chills and fever" or "alternating chills and fever" is selected as the proposed standard.

7. In Chinese medicine, 壯熱 [zhuàng rè] is defined as persistent high fever without chills. It is well defined and easy to understand, but it is difficult to find an appropriate English equivalent. In recent publications the available translations include "vigorous fever", "ardent fever", "sthenic fever", and "strong heat", none of them being really satisfactory. Therefore, most authors just use the simplest term "high fever". A better translation needs to be found, but as a standard English term "high fever" is applicable. If the fever is accompanied by chills or is persistent, the writer may add attributives whenever necessary.

8. Most authors render 微熱 [wēi rè] as "slight fever". "Low-grade fever" suggested by some authors seems to be too modernized.

9. 潮熱 [cháo rè] is a fever with periodic rise and fall of body temperature at fixed hours of a day like a tide. The common English expressions for this symptom are "tidal fever", "hectic fever", "recurring

fever", and "afternoon fever". "Tidal fever" is the most appropriate one, and is used by most authors. "Hectic fever" is a fever that occurs each day with profound sweating and chills. "Recurring fever" does not necessarily refer to a fever that recurs daily, and "afternoon fever" gives the limitation that the fever only occurs in the afternoon.

10. Many authors translate 日晡潮熱 [rì bū cháo rè] as "afternoon fever", but Nigel Wiseman proposes "late afternoon fever". The latter is selected as the standard term because it precisely reflects the original concept. In ancient China, the day and night were divided into twelve watches, and the period from noon to evening was divided into the following sections: 日中 [rì zhōng], i.e., midday watch, 11 a.m. – 1 p.m., 日昃 [rì zè], i.e., early afternoon watch, 1 p.m. – 3 p.m., 日晡 [rì bū], i.e., late afternoon watch, 3 p.m.– 5 p.m., and 日入 [rì rù], i.e., sunset watch, 5 p.m.– 7 p.m.

11. 五心煩熱 [wǔ xīn fán rè] is a very common symptom. Its significance is stressed by Chinese medicine, but is often neglected by Western medicine, and so no corresponding English term is available. There are various expressions, all of which are translated from the Chinese. Disparities exist in the translation of 五心 [wǔ xīn], which literally means "five centers". Such a literal translation will inevitably cause misunderstanding because the inner side of the hand and the underside of the foot are not called "centers" in English. Therefore, from the expressions suggested by different authors "dysphoria with feverish sensation in the chest, palms and soles" "five feverish centers", "feverish sensation of five centers", "burning sensation in the five centers", "feverish sensation in the chest, palms and soles", and "vexing heat in the five centers", the term "vexing heat in the chest, palms and soles" is selected as the proposed standard. Another wording of this term is 手足心熱 [shǒu zú xīn rè], equivalent to "feverish sensation in the palms and soles".

12. 身熱不揚 [shēn rè bù yáng] is a pattern of fever in which the physician feels the patient's skin hot only on extended palpation. For this term available expressions include "recessive fever", "obscured fever", "unsurfaced fever" and "dull fever". Among these terms, "unsurfaced fever" is the nearest to the original sense.

Inquiry about Sweating

Abnormal sweating gives information about the property of pathogens and the condition of the yin-yang balance.

Proposed Standard Nomenclature

spontaneous sweating 自汗 [zì hàn][1]

night sweats 盜汗 [dào hàn][2]

hot sweats 熱汗 [rè hàn][3]

cold sweats 冷汗 [lěng hàn][4]

profuse sweating 大汗 [dà hàn][5]

shiver sweating 戰汗 [zhàn hàn][6]

exhaustion sweating 絕汗 [jué hàn][7]

sweating head 頭汗 [tóu hàn][8]

sweating palms and soles 手足心汗 [shǒu zú xīn hàn][8]

sweating forehead 額汗 [é hàn][8]

genital sweating 陰汗 [yīn hàn][8]

half-body sweating 半身汗出 [bàn shēn hàn chū][9]

Discussion

1. 自汗 [zì hàn] is excessive sweating during the daytime with no apparent cause (such as hot weather, thick clothing) or at the slightest physical exertion. Almost all authors render it as "spontaneous perspiration" or "spontaneous sweating".

2. 盜汗 [dào hàn] refers to sweating during sleep, a symptom frequently occurring in yin deficiency with endogenous heat. Many authors render it as "night sweating", but the term used in Western medicine with the same sense is "night sweats".

3. Sweating accompanied by fever, occurring in a yang syndrome such as exterior wind-heat or internal heat is called 熱汗 [rè hàn]. Most authors use "hot sweat" as its equivalent, while some use "hot sweating", and "febrile perspiration".

4. Profuse sweating accompanied by cold body and limbs is known as 冷汗 [lěng hàn]. As the equivalent, most authors prefer "cold sweat", while some use "cold sweating" and "clammy perspiration". As the terms used in history taking (interrogation), the common expression is the best choice.

5. Most authors prefer the popular wording "profuse sweating" to show the Chinese concept of 大汗 [dà hàn], while some express it as "excessive perspiration", "hyperhidrosis" or "polyhidrosis".

6. Sweating following shivering in the course of a febrile disease is called 戰汗 [zhàn hàn]. From the available expressions "perspiration after shivering", "sweating with rigor", "perspiration following chills", "chilly sweating" and "shiver sweating", the last one is the most common.

7. According to the national textbook of Chinese medicine in Chinese, 絕汗 [jué hàn] is described as "incessant profuse sweating of a critically

ill patient, often leading to exhaustion"[*] The expressions used by different authors include "sweating of the dying", "depleting sweat", "sweating from exhaustion", "expiry sweating", "sweating at critical stage", "dying sweating", etc. The conditions described in some of these terms seem too serious.

8. Sweating occurring in localized areas is often nominated according to the area of the body. For example, sweating chiefly or only on the head is called 頭汗 [tóu hàn], sweat on forehead, 額汗 [é hàn], on palms and soles, 手足心汗 [shǒu zú xīn hàn], in the genital region, particularly the scrotum, 陰汗 [yīn hàn]. Most authors render these as "sweating head", "sweating forehead", "sweating palms and soles", and "genital sweating", respectively.

9. There are several different ways to express the concept of 半身汗出 [bàn shēn hàn chū]: "hemihidrosis", "hemilateral sweating", "half-body sweating", "sweating on half of the body", "sweating on either side of the body". Most authors use the term "hemihidrosis", but this is too Westernized and professional. As a patient's complaint, "half-body sweating" seems more appropriate.

Inquiry about Pain

The terms used for inquiring about pain include those indicating the property or severity and those indicating the location of pain.

Proposed Standard Nomenclature

distending pain 脹痛 [zhàng tòng][1]

stabbing pain 刺痛 [cì tòng][2]

wandering pain 遊走痛 [yóu zǒu tòng][3]

scurrying pain 竄痛 [cuàn tòng][3]

fixed pain 固定痛 [gù dìng tòng][4]

burning pain 灼痛 [zhuó tòng][6]

cold pain 冷痛 [lěng tòng][5]

dull pain 隱痛 [yǐn tòng][8]

colicky pain 絞痛 [jiǎo tòng][7]

pulling pain 掣痛 [chè tòng][10]

pain with heaviness sensation 重痛 [zhòng tòng][9]

pain with emptiness sensation 空痛 [kōng tòng][11]

oppressive pain 悶痛 [mèn tòng][12]

soreness 痠[酸]痛 [suān tòng][13]

aching pain 痠[酸] [suān][13]

chest pain 胸痛 [xiōng tòng][14]

headache 頭痛 [tóu tòng][14]

[*]Zhu WF (editor-in-chief). Zhong Yi Zhen Duan Xue (*Diagnostics of Traditional Chinese Medicine*) (in Chinese), the Textbook Series for Programmed Courses of the TCM Univeristies and Colleges, Shanghai Science and Technology Press, 1998, p.64.

epigastric pain 脘痛 [wǎn tòng][14]   hypochondriac pain 脅痛 [xié tòng][14]
abdominal pain 腹痛 [fù tòng][14]   back pain 背痛 [bèi tòng][14]
lumbar pain 腰痛 [yāo tòng][14]   body pains [周]身[疼]痛 [(zhōu) shēn (téng) tòng][15]

Discussion

1. Pain associated with feeling of distension is a common type of pain, called 脹痛 [zhàng tòng] in Chinese, and is rendered as distending pain by most authors.

2. A sharp pain as if caused by a stab is called 刺痛 [cì tòng] in Chinese, and "stabbing pain" in English. Some authors call it "prickle pain", which is not so widely used as "stabbing pain".

3. A pain that repeatedly changes its location is called 竄痛 [cuàn tòng] if it occurs in the chest and abdomen, and called 遊走痛 [yóu zǒu tòng] if it occurs in the joints of the extremities. The two terms are often expressed in English as "scurrying pain" and "wandering pain", respectively. For the former one, some authors suggest "moving pain". This is not recommended in this scheme for it might be misunderstood as pain occurring during motion.

4. A pain fixed in location is called 固定痛 [gù dìng tòng]. It is a modernized Chinese medical term. Traditionally this type of pain is described as 痛有定處 [tòng yǒu dìng chù]. No matter what the Chinese term is, the English equivalent "fixed pain" is acceptable.

5. Pain accompanied by a cold sensation is called 冷痛 [lěng tòng]. It is rendered as "cold-pain" "cold pain", "cold-type pain", and even "crymodynia". Among these, "cold pain" is widely accepted.

6. Pain accompanied by a burning sensation is described as 灼痛 [zhuó tòng]. Some authors render it as "scorching pain", but more authors prefer "burning pain".

7. The description of 絞痛 [jiǎo tòng] in Chinese medicine and colic in Western medicine are the same, and the word is translated into Chinese as 絞痛 [jiǎo tòng], and so it is reasonable to render 絞痛 [jiǎo tòng] in Chinese medicine as "colicky pain". Some authors suggest "gripping pain", but more authors prefer "colicky pain".

8. 隱痛 [yǐn tòng] is a pain often continuous but not felt sharply. It is rendered as "dull pain", "faint pain" and "vague pain", of which the first one is widely accepted.

9. As Chinese medicine describes, when the *qi* movement is obstruc-

tion by damp a pain occurs that is often accompanied by a sensation of heaviness. Such a pain is called 重痛 [zhòng tòng]. This term is rendered as "heavy pain" or "pain with heaviness sensation" in English. Since the former might be mistaken as a serious pain or intense pain, the latter is selected as the proposed standard.

10. Pain in one part involving another part as if pulled or drawn along a meridian is known as 掣痛 [chè tòng]. It is rendered as "pulling pain" or "contracting pain". The former is more widely accepted.

11. Pain accompanied by a sensation of emptiness is known as 空痛 [kōng tòng]. The renderings include "empty pain" and "hollow pain". Since neither can give a clear-cut concept without causing misunderstanding, it is suggested that a term like the English equivalent of 重痛 [zhòng tòng], namely "pain with emptiness sensation" be used.

12. Pain accompanied by an oppressive sensation is known as 悶痛 [mèn tòng]. It is rendered as "oppressive pain", "obtuse pain" or "suffocating pain". Comparatively speaking, "oppressive pain" seems the most appropriate, for "obtuse" is ambiguous, and "suffocating" is too serious.

13. 痠 [suān] is a continuous dull pain, often related to overstrain, and occurring in the locomotive parts of the body such as the back, limbs, knees and other joints. According to most authors, 痠[酸]痛 [suān tòng] is rendered as "aching pain" and "soreness". Because of their frequent use, both are selected as the proposed standard.

14. Terms of various pains nominated according to location are usually common to both Chinese and Western medicine, e.g., headache 頭痛 [tóu tòng], chest pain 胸痛 [xiōng tòng], hypochondriac pain 脅痛 [xié tòng], epigastric pain 脘痛 [wǎn tòng], abdominal pain 腹痛 [fù tòng], back pain 背痛 [bèi tòng], and lumbar pain 腰痛 [yāo tòng]. Some of them may have more special terms in English such as gastralgia and lumbago. These terms are recommended as disease names rather than symptoms.

15. The term 身痛 [shēn tòng] is an abbreviation of 周身疼痛 [zhōu shēn téng tòng], referring to pain or ache over the whole body. It may be rendered as "body pain", "generalized pain", "general aching" or "body aches".

Inquiry about Discomfort in the Head, Chest and Abdomen

Besides pain, various discomforts occurring in the head, chest and abdomen are often important symptoms with diagnostic significance.

Proposed Standard Nomenclature

heavy-headedness 頭重 [tóu zhòng][1]

palpitations 心悸 [xīn jì][3]

fearful throbbing 怔忡 [zhēng chōng][3]

epigastric stuffiness 脘痞 [wǎn pǐ][4]

abdominal distention 腹脹 [fù zhàng][4]

generalized heaviness 身重 [shēn zhòng][5]

dizziness 頭暈 [tóu yūn][2]

vertigo 眩暈 [xuán yūn][2]

fright palpitations 驚悸 [jīng jì][3]

vexation 心煩 [xīn fán][3]

thoracic oppression 胸悶 [xiōng mèn][4]

abdominal fullness 腹滿 [fù mǎn][4]

numbness 麻木 [má mù][6]

insensitivity 不仁 [bù rén][6]

Discussion

1. 頭重 [tóu zhòng] refers to a subjective feeling of heaviness in the head. Many authors express it as "heaviness in the head" or "heaviness of the head", but "heavy-headedness" is the most succinct.

2. 頭暈 [tóu yūn] is a sensation of unsteadiness with a feeling of movement within the head, and vertigo 眩暈 [xuán yūn] is an illusory sense that either the environment or one's own body is revolving. They are rendered as "dizziness" and "vertigo", respectively, by most authors.

3. 心悸 [xīn jì] is a subjective feeling of the heart beat, equivalent to "palpitations". Palpitations caused by fright are called 驚悸 [jīng jì], and continuous severe palpitations are called 怔忡 [zhēng chōng]. 心煩 [xīn fán] is different from palpitations; it is a feeling of unrest or irritability focused on the heart area, and most authors render it as "vexation".

4. 痞 [pǐ], 脹 [zhàng], 滿 [mǎn], 悶 [mèn] are synonyms, but have some difference in meaning. 痞 [pǐ] is a polysemant. It means "mass" when it is used as an abbreviation for 痞積 [pǐ jī] or 痞塊 [pǐ kuài], but as a subjective feeling it refers to a sensation of stuffiness. In the latter case, 痞 [pǐ] is very close to 脹 [zhàng] in meaning, and is often used in combination with 滿 [mǎn] or 悶 [mèn] as 痞滿 [pǐ mǎn] or 痞悶 [pǐ mèn]. Some authors propose "glomus" as the equivalent of 痞 [pǐ], and "glomus and fullness" as the equivalent of 痞滿 [pǐ mǎn]. This is apparently not acceptable, because the Latin word "glomus" has already been defined in Western medicine as "a small, histologically recognizable body, composed of fine arterioles connecting directly with veins, and possessing a rich nerve supply".*

*Cited from *Dorland's Illustrated Medical Dictionary*, 29th ed., 2000, p.753.

According to most authors, as a subjective feeling, "stuffiness" is equivalent to 痞 [pǐ], "distension" equivalent to 脹 [zhàng], "fullness" equivalent to 滿 [mǎn], and "oppression" equivalent to 悶 [mèn].

5. 身重 [shēn zhòng] is often rendered as "heavy sensation of the body". This is apparently explanatory. As a medical term, "generalized heaviness" or "heavy body" is more appropriate.

6. 麻木 [má mù] refers to reduced sensitivity or loss of sensitivity to touch, and is rendered as "numbness" by most authors. Loss of sensitivity to touch is also called 不仁 [bù rén]. The two terms are often used together as 麻木不仁 [má mù bù rén] and simply rendered as "numbness".

Inquiry about the Ears and Eyes

Inquiry about the ears and eyes is not only significant for getting information about local conditions, but also helpful for determining the pathological changes of the related internal organs.

Proposed Standard Nomenclature

tinnitus 耳鳴 [ěr míng][1]

deafness 耳聾 [ěr lóng][2]

impaired hearing 重聽 [chóng tíng][3]

eye pain 目痛 [mù tòng][3]

blurred vision 目昏 [mù hūn][5]

dizzy vision 目眩 [mù xuàn][4]

night blindness 雀盲 [què máng][6]

Discussion

1. Most authors believe that tinnitus and 耳鳴 [ěr míng] are equivalents. Others prefer "ringing in the ear".

2. According to most authors, "deafness" and 耳聾 [ěr lóng] are natural equivalents.

3. Some authors suggest "hypoacusia" for 重聽 [chóng tíng], and "ophthalmalgia" for 目痛 [mù tòng]. These terms are too professional. As patients' complaints, it is better to select popular terms such as "impaired hearing" or "hearing impairment" and "eye pain".

4. Some authors render 目眩 [mù xuàn] simply as "dizziness" or "giddiness", but the original Chinese term is closely related to the eyes or vision. "Dizzy vision" or "visual dizziness" is more appropriate.

5. "Dysopia" and "asthenopia" are too professional for a patient's complaint. "Blurred vision" or "blurring of vision" may be better than "clouded vision".

6. "Nyctalopia" is too professional. "Night blindness" is more acceptable than "sparrow blindness".

Inquiry about Thirst and Fluid Intake

Information about the condition of body fluid can be obtained by inquiry about thirst and fluid intake.

Proposed Standard Nomenclature

thirst 口渴 [kǒu kě][1]

thirst with preference for cold drinks 口渴喜冷（飲）[kǒu kě xǐ lěng (yǐn)][2]

vexing thirst 煩渴 [fán kě][4]

thirst with desire to drink 口渴欲飲 [kǒu kě yù yǐn][1]

dryness in the mouth with no desire to drink 口乾不欲飲 [kǒu gān bù yù yǐn][3]

Discussion

1. Most authors translate 口渴 [kǒu kě] and 口渴欲飲 [kǒu kě yù yǐn] as "thirst" and "thirst with desire to drink".

2. 口渴喜冷(飲) [kǒu kě xǐ lěng (yǐn)] indicates consumption of body fluids by excessive heat. It is rendered as "thirst with preference for cold drinks", "thirst with liking for cold drinks" and "thirst and fondness for cold drink". They are practically alike.

3. "Dryness in the mouth with no desire to drink" 口乾不欲飲 [kǒu gān bù yù yǐn] is a unique description in Chinese medicine. It is also called 渴不欲飲 [kě bù yù yǐn], which is usually translated as "thirst with no desire to drink". Neither 渴不欲飲 [kě bù yù yǐn] nor its English equivalent are logical. In Chinese 渴 [kě] means 口乾 [kǒu gān] (dryness in the mouth) + 思飲 [sī yǐn] (desire to drink), and in English the word thirst also refers to the feeling caused by a desire to drink. The present selection has no such flaw.

4. 煩渴 [fán kě] is a symptom indicating consumption of body fluids. How to explain the Chinese term 煩渴 [fán kě] is an interesting question. From the renderings it can be seen that the term is explained in two different ways. One is that the two characters are placed side by side, each having independent meanings. Thus, the rendering is "vexation and thirst", "fidgeting and thirst" or "restlessness and thirst". The other way is that the two characters are considered as a single term with the first

character as an attributive; hence "polydipsia", "frequent thirst" and "excessive thirst".

Inquiry about Appetite and Food Intake

Inquiry about the appetite and food intake is particularly important for determining the condition of the spleen and stomach.

Proposed Standard Nomenclature

anorexia 納呆 [nà dāi]; 厭食 [yàn shí][1]

anorexia despite hunger 饑不欲食 [jī bù yù shí][1]

Polyphagia with frequent hunger 多食善饑 [duō shí shàn jī][2]

dietary partiality 飲食偏嗜 [yǐn shí piān shì][3]

vomiting of sour putrid matter 嘔吐酸腐 [ǒu tù suān fǔ][4]

vomiting of clear mucus 嘔吐清涎 [ǒu tù qīng xián][4]

belching 噯氣 [ài qì][5]

vomiting of retained food 嘔吐宿食 [ǒu tù sù shí][4]

putrid belching 噯腐 [ài fǔ][5]

acid regurgitation 吞酸 [tūn suān][6]

heartburn 燒心 [shāo xīn][6]

Discussion

1. Lack or loss of appetite for food is known as 納呆 [nà dāi] and 厭食 [yàn shí]. Both can be expressed by "anorexia".

"Anorexia despite hunger" (饑不欲食 [jī bù yù shí]) is a symptom that usually indicates deficiency of stomach yin with endogenous fire. There are various expressions: "anorexia with hunger", "hunger without appetite", "hunger with no desire to eat", "hunger with disinclination to eat", "no desire to eat despite hunger", etc. In this term, the point that needs stressing is not "hunger" but "no desire to eat", i.e., anorexia.

2. A patient with exuberant stomach fire may have increased digestion manifested by excessive eating with frequent hunger, known as 多食善饑 [duō shí shàn jī] or 消穀善饑 [xiāo gǔ shàn jī]. For this term, "polyphagia" is better than "hyperorexia", "polyrexia", "insatiable appetite" or "ravenous appetite", as suggested by some authors because "polyphagia" refers to both appetite and eating to excess.

3. Partiality for certain kinds of food is called 飲食偏嗜 [yǐn shí piān shì], which is often rendered as "dietary partiality".

4. According to the vomitus, vomiting can be classified into vomiting of clear mucus (嘔吐清涎 [ǒu tù qīng xián]), vomiting of sour putrid

matter (嘔吐酸腐 [ǒu tù suān fǔ]) and vomiting of retained food (嘔吐宿食 [ǒu tù sù shí]). Different expressions are used for 清涎 [qīng xián], 酸腐 [suān fǔ] and 宿食 [sù shí], but the disparity is chiefly based on the variation of the Chinese original, e.g., "vomiting of clear water" for 嘔吐清水 [ǒu tù qīng shuǐ].

5. 噯氣 [ài qì] is rendered as "belching" or "eructation". More authors prefer the popular word, though both are definitely correct. There are different opinions about rendering 腐 [fǔ] as "fetid" or "putrid". The latter may be more appropriate, for it refers to the foul smell coming from something that has become decomposed.

6. Heartburn and 燒心 [shāo xīn] are natural equivalents. Acid regurgitation is known as 吞酸 [tūn suān], which literally means acid swallowing. Since the acid contents swallowed are regurgitated from the stomach, it is reasonable to use the term "acid regurgitation".

Inquiry about Bowel Movements

The two main symptoms related to bowel movements are constipation and diarrhea.

Proposed Standard Nomenclature

constipation 便秘 [biàn bì][1]
loose bowels 便溏 [biàn táng][2]
watery diarrhea 水瀉 [shuǐ xiè][3]
early morning diarrhea 五更泄 [wǔ gēng xiè][5]
purulent and bloody stools 膿血便 [nóng xuè biàn][7]

diarrhea 泄瀉 [xiè xiè][1]
loose stools 溏便 [táng biàn][2]
diarrhea with fecal incontinence 滑瀉(失禁) [huá xiè (shī jìn)][4]
undigested food in stools 完穀不化 [wán gǔ bù huà][6]
tenesmus 下墜 [xià zhuì]; 裏急後重 [lǐ jí hòu zhòng][8]

Discussion

1. Diarrhea 泄瀉 [xiè xiè] and constipation 便秘 [biàn bì] are two common terms used both in Chinese and Western medicine. The English and Chinese terms are mutually translatable. In Chinese 泄 [xiè] and 瀉 [xiè] are synonymous, but have a minor difference in meaning. In modern Chinese medicine, however, 泄瀉 [xiè xiè] is taken as one single term, and so it is not necessary to render them as two words.

2. Soft or semiliquid unformed stool is known as 溏便 [táng biàn]

and discharge of soft, unformed stools is known as 便溏 [biàn táng]. The renderings include "loose stool(s)", "loose bowel(s)", "sloppy stool" and "sloppy diarrhea". The word "sloppy" means "too liquid" when it refers to a semi-liquid substance, more than the original term signifies.

3. "Watery diarrhea" 水瀉 [shuǐ xiè] is a term used at present. Some other terms such as 洞泄 [dòng xiè] and 注泄 [zhù xiè] also refer to "watery diarrhea", but since they use different characters, the literal translation should differ from "watery diarrhea". There are many renderings, e.g., "cold diarrhea", "thoroughflux diarrhea" and "damp diarrhea" for 洞泄 [dòng xiè], and "drenching diarrhea", "spouting diarrhea", "watery diarrhea" and "outpour diarrhea" for 注泄 [zhù xiè]. In reality, they are all alternative translations for 水瀉 [shuǐ xiè]*.

4. 滑瀉 [huá xiè] refers to diarrhea with inability to control the evacuation of stools. In modern texts, the term is revised as 滑瀉失禁 [huá xiè shī jìn]. There are many equivalents suggested by different authors for 滑瀉 [huá xiè], such as "efflux diarrhea", "lingering diarrhea", "frequent diarrhea", "incessant diarrhea" and "involuntary diarrhea", but none of them is satisfactory. The problem can be solved with reference to the revised term. "Diarrhea with fecal incontinence" is easy to understand, and concordant with the Chinese original.

5. 五更泄 [wǔ gēng xiè] is a special pattern of diarrhea characterized by its occurrence daily early in the morning. Several renderings have appeared in recent publications: "diarrhea before dawn", "morning diarrhea", "early morning diarrhea", "fifth-watch diarrhea", "fifth-hour diarrhea" and "cock-crow diarrhea". The character 更 [gēng] is an ancient unit for measuring time, referring to one of the five two-hour periods into which the night was divided, and is often translated as "watch". Rendering the term into English, "fifth-watch diarrhea" is a literal translation. As a proposed standard term, it might not be appropriate, because at present even the Chinese people can hardly define the time period of the fifth watch. Therefore, "early morning diarrhea" is selected.

6. 完穀不化 [wán gǔ bù huà] refers to the presence of undigested food in stools. Although it often occurs during diarrhea, the term itself does not necessarily mean that the stools must be loose. The correspond-

---

*"洞泄，一名濡瀉，瀉下多水也"。《醫宗必讀》("洞泄 [dòng xiè], also called 濡瀉 [rú xiè], is discharge of watery stools." cited from *Essential Readings in Medicine*, 1637)

"注泄，水瀉的古稱"《中醫大辭典》("注泄 [zhù xiè] is an ancient name for 水瀉 [shuǐ xiè]. cited from the *Grand Dictionary of Traditional Chinese Medicine* 1998, p.983.)

ing expressions include "non-transformation of food", "loose stool with undigested grains", and "loose stools with undigested food". A more succinct one, i.e., "undigested food in stools" is proposed as the standard term.

7. In dysentery, the stools usually contain mucus and blood. This is called 膿血便 [nóng xuè biàn] in Chinese medicine. The character 膿 [nóng] is pus. Although Chinese medicine gives names to various fluids in the body, there is no such concept as mucus. So, the renderings of 膿血便 [nóng xuè biàn] are "stool with blood and pus", "stool containing pus and blood", "purulent and bloody stool", "bloody purulent stool", etc. They are practically the same.

8. 下墜 [xià zhuì] refers to incessant but ineffectual desire to defecate. It is equivalent to "tenesmus", and also called 裏急後重 [lǐ jí hòu zhòng].

Inquiry about Urination

Inquiry about urination covers the amount of urine, frequency of urination, difficulty in urination, and discomfort during urination.

Proposed Standard Nomenclature

long voiding of clear urine 小便清長 [xiǎo biàn qīng cháng][1]

turbid urine 小便渾濁 [xiǎo biàn hún zhóu][2]

difficult and painful urination 小便澀痛 [xiǎo biàn sè tòng][4]

dribbling urination 小便淋漓 [xiǎo biàn lín lí][6]

short voiding of dark urine 小便短赤 [xiǎo biàn duǎn chì][1]

frequent urination 小便頻數 [xiǎo biàn pín shuò][3]

urinary incontinence 小便失禁 [xiǎo biàn shī jìn][5]

dribbling after voiding 餘瀝不盡 [yú lì bù jìn][7]

Discussion

1. 小便清長 [xiǎo biàn qīng cháng] and 小便短赤 [xiǎo biàn duǎn chì] are common symptoms indicating cold syndrome and heat syndrome, respectively. Many authors render them as "clear [light-colored] profuse [copious] urine" and "scanty reddish [dark-colored] urine". The expressions do not fully reflect the original Chinese concept. The characters used in the Chinese terms are 長 [cháng] (long) and 短 [duǎn] (short) but not 多 [duō] (profuse) and 少 [shǎo] (scanty). This indicates the urine vol-

ume of each voiding rather than the total urine volume. Therefore, "long voidings of clear urine" and "short voidings of reddish urine" are selected.

2. There are two common expressions for 小便渾濁 [xiǎo biàn hún zhóu]: "turbid urine" and "cloudy urine". The first is more commonly used.

3. For expressing 小便頻數 [xiǎo biàn pín shuò], either "frequent urination" or "frequent micturition" is commonly used.

4. 小便澀痛 [xiǎo biàn sè tòng] is the major symptom of stranguria. Most authors render it as "difficult and painful urination".

5. Failure of voluntary control of urination is called 小便失禁 [xiǎo biàn shī jìn]. Most authors use "urinary incontinence" or "incontinence of urine" as its equivalent, and some abbreviate it as "incontinence".

6. Dribbling discharge of urine with inability to achieve a full stream is known as 小便淋漓 [xiǎo biàn lín lí]. Most authors render it as "dribbling urination" or "dribbling of urine".

7. Continual dribbling discharge of urine after voiding is known as 餘瀝不盡 [yú lì bù jìn].

Abnormal Tastes in the Mouth

Chinese medicine puts special emphasis on inquiring the patients about abnormal tastes in the mouth, for they give important clues to the diagnosis of *zang-fu* organ disorders.

Proposed Standard Nomenclature

taste (in the mouth) 口味 [kǒu wèi][1]

sweet taste (in the mouth) 口甜 [kǒu tián][3]

sour taste (in the mouth) 口酸 [kǒu suān][3]

sticky slimy sensation in the mouth 口粘膩 [kǒu nián nì][4]

bland taste (in the mouth) 口淡 [kǒu dàn][2]

bitter taste (in the mouth) 口苦 [kǒu kǔ][3]

salty taste (in the mouth) 口鹹 [kǒu xián][3]

Discussion

1. In Chinese medicine, 口味 [kǒu wèi] refers to subjective abnormal tastes or flavors in the mouth. Most authors render it as "taste in the mouth", but in writing the single word "taste" is enough. Therefore, the proposed standard term is "taste (in the mouth)", indicating that the words

in parentheses can be omitted.

2. Diminished sensitivity of taste is called 口淡 [kǒu dàn] in Chinese medicine. It is rendered as "tastelessness", "tastelessness in the mouth", "a tasteless mouth", "absence of taste", "inability to taste", "flat taste in the mouth", "dysgeusia" and "bland taste in the mouth". The last one is selected so as to conform to other related terms.

3. Subjective sweet, bitter, sour, or salty tastes in the mouth are called 口甜 [kǒu tián], 口苦 [kǒu kǔ], 口酸 [kǒu suān] or 口鹹 [kǒu xián], respectively. The equivalents used by different authors are "sweet [bitter, sour, or salty] taste in the mouth", "sweetness [bitterness, sourness, or saltiness] in the mouth", "sweetness [bitterness, sourness, or saltiness] of mouth", and "a sweet [bitter, sour, or salty] mouth". The most unmistakable one is "sweet [bitter, sour, or salty] taste in the mouth", but in actual writing the phrase "in the mouth" may be omitted. So, the proposed standard term is "sweet [bitter, sour, or salty] taste (in the mouth)".

4. Sticky slimy sensation in the mouth (口粘膩 [kǒu nián nì]) is also a subjective sensation in the mouth. Some authors present it as "greasy taste in the mouth" or "stickiness in the mouth", partially reflecting the original concept of the term.

Menstrual Complaints

The common menstrual complaints include abnormal menstrual cycles, cessation of menstruation, and painful menstruation. In Western medicine, abnormal menstrual cycles are expressed by change of the menstrual cycle, but in Chinese medicine, abnormal menstrual cycles are expressed in terms of the date of menstruation.

Proposed Standard Nomenclature

shortened menstrual cycles 月經先期 [yuè jīng xiān qī][1]

early periods 月經提前 [yuè jīng tí qián][1]

lengthened menstrual cycles 月經後期 [yuè jīng hòu qī][2]

late periods 月經錯後 [yuè jīng cuò hòu][2]

irregular menstrual cycles 經行先後無定期 [jīng xíng xiān hòu wú dìng qī][3]

irregular periods 經行先後無定期 [jīng xíng xiān hòu wú dìng qī][3]

absence of menstruation 經閉 [jīng bì][4]

cessation of menstruation 經斷[絕] [jīng duàn [jué]][4]

painful periods 經行腹痛 [jīng

dysmenorrhea 痛經 [tòng jīng][5]   xíng fù tòng][5]

Discussion

1. A variety of expressions are used for 月經先期 [yuè jīng xiān qī] and 月經提前 [yuè jīng tí qián]. "Preceded menstrual cycle", "preceded menorrhea", "early menses", "advanced menstruation" and "menstruation ahead of the time" are apt to cause misunderstanding that the first appearance of menstruation is ahead of the due age. "Shortened menstrual cycles" as a professional term does not cause such a problem, and "early periods", as a popular term, fits the patient's complaint better.

2. A variety of expressions are used for 月經後期 [yuè jīng hòu qī] and 月經錯後 [yuè jīng cuò hòu]. "Delayed menses", "delayed menorrhea", "delayed menstruation", "retarded menstruation" and "late menstruation" cannot completely avoid misunderstanding that the first appearance of menstruation is delayed beyond the due age. "Lengthened menstrual cycle" as a professional term does not cause such a problem, and "late periods", as a popular term fits the patient's complaint better.

3. Most authors use "irregular periods" or "irregular menstrual cycles" to express the concept of 經行先後無定期 [jīng xíng xiān hòu wú dìng qī]. The former is popular, and the latter professional. Both are selected as standard terms.

4. 經閉 [jīng bì] and 經斷[絕] [jīng duàn [jué]] are two different terms, but have some common meaning. The former term means no experience of menstruation in a woman beyond the age of 18, and the latter, the natural cessation of menstruation occurring around the age of 50 in the female. However both refer to absence of menstruation for more than three months not related to pregnancy, lactation or menopause.

5. 經行腹痛 [jīng xíng fù tòng] means abdominal pain during menstruation, a popular translation of 痛經 [tòng jīng] (dysmenorrhea).

PALPATION

Palpation is examination of the surface of the body by feeling with the hand or fingers, including taking the pulse. Because of its special importance in Chinese medical diagnosis, pulse taking is often regarded as independent of body palpation

Proposed Standard Nomenclature

palpation 切診 [qiè zhěn]

palpation on the epigastrium and abdomen 按脘腹 [àn wǎn fù][1]

skin palpation 按肌膚 [àn jī fū][1]

palpation on the extremities 按手足 [àn shǒu zú][1]

cardiac apical examination 診虛裏 [zhěn xū lǐ][2]

palpation on the chest and hypochondria 按胸脅 [àn xiōng xié][1]

abdominal palpation diagnosis 腹診 [fù zhěn][1]

acupoint palpation 按腧穴 [àn shù xué][1]

Discussion

1. Most of these terms are newly developed in the modern textbooks of traditional Chinese medicine. The character 按 [àn] means both "palpate" and "press".

2. 虛裏 [xū lǐ] is the traditional Chinese name of the cardiac apex. 診虛裏 [zhěn xū lǐ] is rendered by different authors as "palpating the cardiac apex", "palpation on the apex of the heart", "feeling the apex", "apical pulse examination", etc.

PULSE DIAGNOSIS

The common terms related to pulse diagnosis include the descriptions of pulse positions, finger technique, and pulse conditions.

Proposed Standard Nomenclature

pulse diagnosis 脈診 [mài zhěn][1]

inch (cun), bar (guan), cubit (chi) 寸、關、尺 [cùn guān chǐ][2]

pushing 推循 [tuī xún][3]

individual palpation 單按 [dān àn][3]

radial pulse at the wrist 寸口脈 [cùn kǒu mài][4]

abnormal pulse 病脈 [bìng mài][6]

superficial pulse 浮脈 [fú mài][7]

deep pulse 沉脈 [chén mài][8]

rapid pulse 數脈 [shuò mài][10]

pulse taking 切脈 [qiè mài][1]

lifting, pressing, and searching 舉、按、尋 [jǔ、àn、xún][3]

total palpation 總按 [zǒng àn][3]

radial artery at the wrist 寸口 [cùn kǒu][4]

pulse (condition) 脈象 [mài xiàng][5]

floating pulse 浮脈 [fú mài][7]

sunken pulse 沉脈 [chén mài][8]

hidden pulse 伏脈 [fú mài][9]

slow pulse 遲脈 [chí mài][11]

moderate pulse 緩脈 [huǎn mài][12]

relaxed pulse 緩脈 [huǎn mài][12]

empty pulse 虛脈 [xū mài][13]

full pulse 實脈 [shí mài][14]

surging pulse 洪脈 [hóng mài][15]

thready pulse 細脈 [xì mài][16]

thin pulse 細脈 [xì mài][16]

faint pulse 微脈 [wēi mài][17]

weak pulse 弱脈 [ruò mài][18]

soggy pulse 濡脈 [rú mài][19]

soft pulse 軟脈 [ruǎn mài][20]

slippery pulse 滑脈 [huá mài][21]

choppy pulse 澀脈 [sè mài][22]

tympanic pulse 革脈 [gé mài][23]

firm pulse 牢脈 [láo mài][24]

long pulse 長脈 [cháng mài][25]

short pulse 短脈 [duǎn mài][25]

swift pulse 疾脈 [jí mài][26]

racing pulse 疾脈 [jí mài][26]

hurried pulse 促脈 [cù mài][27]

hasty pulse 促脈 [cù mài][27]

knotted pulse 結脈 [jié mài][28]

intermittent pulse 代脈 [dài mài][29]

tense pulse 緊脈 [jǐn mài][30]

tight pulse 緊脈 [jǐn mài][30]

scattered pulse 散脈 [sǎn mài][31]

wiry pulse 弦脈 [xiàn mài][32]

hollow pulse 芤脈 [kōu mài][33]

large pulse 大脈 [dà mài][34]

small pulse 小脈 [xiǎo mài][34]

throbbing pulse 動脈 [dòng mài][35]

dorsally located pulse 反關脈 [fǎn guān mài][36]

slantingly located pulse 斜飛脈 [xié fēi mài][37]

pulse bereft of stomach *qi* 脈無胃氣 [mài wú wèi qì][38]

calm pulse 脈靜 [mài jìng][39]

agitated pulse 脈躁 [mài zào][40]

Discussion

1. There are various translations of 脈診 [mài zhěn], such as "pulse diagnosis", "pulse taking", "pulse examination", "pulse feeling", "feeling of the pulse", and "diagnosis by feeling the pulse". All of them are acceptable. The most popular one is "pulse diagnosis", and the rest are equivalent to 切脈 [qiè mài].

As for 切脈 [qiè mài], most authors render it as "pulse taking".

2. The three sections over the radial artery for feeling the pulse are called 寸 [cùn], 關 [guān] and 尺 [chǐ]. The bar (*guan*) is just over the eminent head of the radius at the wrist, where the tip of the physician's middle finger is placed; the inch (*cun*) is next to it on the distal side, where the tip of the physician's index finger rests, and the cubit (*chi*) is on the proximal side where the tip of the physician's ring finger is placed. The difficulty in translating the names of the pulse position lies in the difference of the length unit between China and the Western world, as well as between the ancient past and the present. However, in body measurement the length unit is always proportional. Therefore, the use of inch and

cubit is still suitable for 寸 [cùn] and 尺 [chǐ]. Some authors use "foot" for 尺 [chǐ]. This might not be appropriate, for this position is on the wrist, not on the ankle. Most authors use both *pinyin* and English, i.e., inch (*cun*), bar (*guan*), and cubit (*chi*). Some other expressions include "front, middle and rear (pulse position)", "inch section, pass section and cubit section".

3. The basic manipulations in pulse taking are touching, pressing, and searching (舉、按、尋 [jǔ àn xún]). By touching is meant lightly resting the fingers on the patient's wrist; by pressing is meant, feeling the pulse with proper force; and by searching is meant varying the force or moving the fingers to get a more distinct pulse reading. There are different renderings of 舉 [jǔ], such as "lifting" or "releasing pressure". Considering that the finger technique of 舉 [jǔ] is also called 浮取 [fú qǔ] (feeling the superficial level), more authors prefer the word "touching".

Other terms related to manipulation in pulse taking are pushing the finger tip along the artery, called 推循 [tuī xún] (pushing), palpating the three sections of pulse with the three fingers simultaneously, called 總按 [zǒng àn] (total palpation), and taking the pulse at each of the three sections individually, called 單按 [dān àn] (individual palpation). There are different renderings such as "side-to-side sliding of the fingers during pulse feeling" for 推循 [tuī xún], "feeling the pulse with three fingers" for 總按 [zǒng àn], and "feeling the pulse with one finger" for 單按 [dān àn].

4. 寸口 [kǒu mài] is the portion of the radial artery whose pulsation can easily be felt at the wrist. To render it into English, many authors suggest *pinyin* and some authors use literal translation such as "inch-mouth" or "inch opening". Since the radial pulse at the wrist is also examined in Western medicine, there is no need to use *pinyin*, making pulse taking unnecessarily complicated and mysterious. The characteristic features of pulse taking in Chinese medicine chiefly lie in the differentiation of various pulse patterns and their diagnostic significance for disorders of the internal organs, and not in the nomenclature of the artery examined. For any anatomical structure, the corresponding English name, if there is one, should be used, no matter how big the difference in the recognition of functional activities or clinical significance between Chinese and Western systems of medicine. Creation of a new anatomical name for a known anatomical structure, even in *pinyin*, will mislead as to a new discovery. Therefore, "radial artery (at the wrist)" is used as the

proposed standard, with 寸口 [cùn kǒu] or 寸口脉 [cùn kǒu mài] as the reference.

5. The condition of the pulse felt on examination is called "pulse condition" 脉象 [mài xiàng]. It includes the following elements: depth, rate, length, force, breadth, smoothness, tension, and rhythm, on which the classification of pulses is based, and hence the nomenclature of pulses. Besides "pulse condition", many related words have been used to express this concept, such as "pulse image", "pulse phenomena", "pulse presentation", "type of pulse", "pulse manifestation" and "pulse picture". However, the most practical way is to render 脉象 [mài xiàng] simply as "pulse".

6. 病脉 [bìng mài] refers to a pulse indicating pathological change. It is rendered as "abnormal pulse" by most authors. Some other expressions are occasionally used, such as "pathological pulse", "morbid pulse" and "diseased pulse".

7. "Floating pulse" is a pulse that can be felt by a light touch, and grows faint on hard pressure, corresponding to 浮脉 [fú mài] in Chinese. It is also frequently rendered as "superficial pulse". Because of their common use, both "floating pulse" and "superficial pulse" are collected in the proposed standard nomenclature.

8. A pulse that can only be felt while pressing hard is 沉脉 [chén mài]. It has been rendered in English in several ways: "deep pulse", "sunken pulse", "sinking pulse" and "submerged pulse". Most authors prefer "deep pulse", but strictly speaking, the word "sunken" is more concordant with the original Chinese. So, both are recommended as the standard terms. The word "sinking" may lead to some misunderstanding of a progressive change, indicating that the pulse gradually becomes deeper and deeper.

9. A pulse which can only be felt on pressing to the bone, situated even deeper than deep pulse, is called 伏脉 [fú mài]. Most authors render it as "hidden pulse". A few authors use the words "deep-sited" or "stealthy" to describe this pulse

10. A pulse of more than 90 beats per minute is called a rapid pulse 數脉 [shuò mài]. Most authors prefer "rapid pulse", and only a few use the word "accelerated" or "fast" to describe the feature of this pulse. In ancient China, the pulse rate was measured with reference to the physician's respiration, but in modern textbooks, the rate is counted per minute.

11. 遲脈 [chí mài] is a pulse with less than 60 beats per minute. As its English equivalent, most authors prefer "slow pulse", but a few use the word "retarded".

12. The Chinese character 緩 [huǎn] is polysemous. It means "moderate", and a pulse with a moderate rate and moderate tension indicates a normal pulse. It also means "relaxed" and "retarded", in opposition to 緊 [jǐn] (tense) and 急 [jí] (hurried). As early as more than a thousand years ago, Wang Bin (c710–805), well-known for his rearrangement and revision of the *Su Wen* (*Plain Questions*), one of the two component parts of the *Canon of Medicine*, made a special note on this pulse as follows: "緩謂縱緩，非動之遲緩也". ("The word 緩 [huǎn] means relaxed, and does not refer to slowness of the pulsation.") This is also emphasized in modern Chinese textbooks. Therefore, other expressions such as "slow pulse" and "retarded pulse" are not recommendable.

13. The Chinese term 虛脈 [xū mài] may have two meanings. One is used as a collective term referring to all kinds of pulses that indicate deficiency conditions. The other is used in its narrow sense, referring to a pattern of abnormal pulse characterized by insufficient filling and diminished force. The present scheme of proposed standard nomenclature only includes the term in the latter sense. To render it into English, there are two ways: (1) empty or vacuous pulse, and (2) feeble pulse. Since this term is used in parallel with 實脈 [shí mài], most authors prefer the first wording. Between "empty" and "vacuous", the latter is too serious as it means "completely empty", and so the former is more frequently used. Some other renderings such as "discrete pulse", "empty and forceless pulse" and "asthenic pulse", are not widely accepted.

14. The Chinese term 實脈 [shí mài] also represents a dual concept. On the one hand, it is taken as a collective term for all kinds of pulses indicating the presence of excess conditions; and on the other hand, it is regarded as a discrete pulse pattern. In the present scheme only the term in the narrow sense is included. Various expressions have been suggested by different authors: "full pulse", "replete pulse", "forceful pulse", "substantial pulse", "substantive pulse", "sthenic pulse", "solid pulse", etc. Among them, "full pulse" and "replete pulse" are the ones used by the majority of authors. However, the use of the word "replete" is open to discussion. It means "full to the utmost", and so seems too serious. In addition, it is often used as a predicative adjective rather than an attribu-

tive adjective.

15. A pulse beating like dashing waves with forceful rising and gradual decline is known as 洪脈 [hóng mài]. The renderings include "surging pulse", "full pulse", "flooding pulse", "bounding pulse", "overflowing pulse", etc. Most authors prefer "surging pulse", which figuratively describes the feature of this pulse. "Full pulse" is not so suitable, because the character only describes the breadth or amplitude of the pulse, but not its fullness. A full pulse always indicates excessiveness, while a surging pulse may occur in either excess conditions or deficiency conditions. The opposite of 洪脈 [hóng mài] is 細脈 [xì mài] (thin pulse), but not 虛脈 [xū mài] (empty pulse).

16. 細脈 [xì mài] is a pulse as thin as a silk thread, straight and soft, feeble yet always perceptible on hard pressure. The renderings include "thready pulse", "thin pulse" and "fine pulse". Each term has its advocates, but only the former two are selected in this scheme. The meaning of the word "fine" is somewhat equivocal as the description of the pulse. Some authors render the term as "small pulse", but the latter is more appropriate for 小脈 [xiǎo mài].

17. 微脈 [wēi mài] is a pulse felt thready and soft, scarcely perceptible, showing exhaustion to the extreme. Several words are used to express the quality of this pulse: "faint", "indistinct", "minute" and "subtle". The selection of the most appropriate one depends upon the reference of the description: the size, force or tension of the pulse. According to the Chinese textbook, the description refers to the force or strength of the pulse.[*] "Indistinct" means vague, and "subtle" means "not easy to detect". Both describe this pulse in certain respects, but an indistinct or subtle pulse may occur in other cases such as abnormal location of the artery. "Minute" means very small in size, but not in strength. "Faint" is probably the best word, because it refers to something that cannot be clearly perceived, and at the same time it means lacking strength.

18. A pulse felt deep, soft and thin is 弱脈 [ruò mài]. Most authors render it as "weak pulse". There are other renderings, such as "frail pulse" and "feeble pulse". The word "frail" means physically weak and easily

---

[*]Zhu WF (chief editor). Zhong Yi Zhen Duan Xue, *Diagnostics of Traditional Chinese Medicine* (in Chinese), The Textbook Series for Programmed Courses of the TCM Universities and Colleges, Shanghai Science and Technology Press, 1995, p.96.

broken, and "feeble" is weak and faint. So they are not widely accepted.

19. In Chinese medicine, 濡脈 [rú mài] is described as a pulse which feels on light pressure like a thread floating on water, but grows faint on hard pressure. There are two expressions widely used: "soggy pulse" and "soft pulse". The latter is used by more authors, but it is not a direct translation of the original term. It comes from an annotation revealing that a soggy pulse is also called soft pulse (濡脈又稱軟脈). In this scheme they are collected as two entries. Other expressions such as "weak-floating pulse", "soft and floating pulse", "sluggish pulse", and "melting pulse" are not widely accepted.

20. Soft pulse 軟脈 [ruǎn mài] is synonymous with soggy pulse 濡脈 [rú mài]. Both terms are collected in this scheme, because of their frequent use.

21. In Chinese medicine, 滑脈 [huá mài] is described as a pulse coming and going smoothly like beads rolling on a plate. Most authors use the word "slippery" to describe this pulse. A small number of authors use the word "smooth", and even fewer authors use the word "rolling".

22. 澀脈 [sè mài] is described as a pulse coming and going unsmoothly with a small, fine, slow joggling tempo like scraping bamboo with a knife. Most authors prefer the word "choppy", which means slightly rough, moving in short broken waves. It figuratively describes the quality of this pulse. In addition, the word "choppy" comes from "chop" which means to cut something into pieces with a knife, very similar to the description in Chinese. Some authors use "rough pulse", "unsmooth pulse" and "uneven pulse", which are not as satisfactory as "choppy pulse". A few authors use the word "hesitant" or "irregular", which may lead to misunderstanding, as disordered rhythm.

23. 革脈 [gé mài] is a pulse felt hard and hollow as if touching the surface of a drum. In this term the character 革 [gé] does not simply mean leather or animal skin. It actually refers to a drum with skin stretched tightly across the open ends of a hollow, round frame. The renderings include "tympanic pulse", "leather pulse", "drumskin pulse", "drumhead pulse", "wiry and hollow pulse", etc. The word tympanic means "like or of the nature of a drum", figuratively describing the feature of the pulse and so more authors prefer this word,

24. According to the national TCM textbook, 牢脈 [láo mài] is defined as a pulse deeply seated, full, large, wiry and long, but cannot be detected by touch with light or moderate force. It can only be detected by

heavy pressing, and it is "firm and non-movable (堅著不移)"*. Therefore, most authors render it as "firm pulse". It is incorrect to take 牢 [láo] as an abbreviation for 牢獄 [láo yù] (prison), and so the renderings "prison pulse" and "confined pulse" are not acceptable.

25. A pulse with a large extent exceeding the inch (*cun*), bar (*guan*) or cubit (*chi*) sections is called "long pulse" 長脈 [cháng mài] and a pulse with a shorter extent, only felt at the inch (*cun*) or bar (*guan*) section, but not perceptible at the cubit (*chi*) section is called "short pulse" 短脈 [duǎn mài]. Almost all authors render the two terms in the same way.

26. A pulse felt hasty and swift, with 120-140 beats per minute is called 疾脈 [jí mài]. Renderings for this term are "swift pulse", "racing pulse", "rapid pulse", "fast pulse", "hurried pulse" and "short and quick pulse". "Rapid pulse" and "hurried pulse" are not recommended, because many authors use them to express 數脈 [shuò mài] or 促脈 [cù mài] respectively. "Swift pulse" and "racing pulse" are equally suitable, and hence both are selected.

27. A rapid pulse with irregular intermittence is called 促脈 [cù mài]. Various words have been used to describe this pattern of pulse: "hurried", "hasty", "skipping", "running", "abrupt", "irregularly abrupt", "rapid irregularly interrupted", etc. Some are explanatory. "Hurried" and "hasty" seem more concordant with the Chinese original.

28. A pulse of moderate rate, pausing at irregular intervals is called 結脈 [jié mài]. Different authors express the term in various ways: "knotted pulse", "irregular pulse", "slow and irregular pulse", "irregularly intermittent pulse", "bound pulse", "hesitant pulse", etc. The one that is accepted and used by most authors is "knotted pulse".

29. A pulse pausing at regular intervals is called 代脈 [dài mài]. "Intermittent pulse" is generally accepted as its equivalent. Some authors render it as "regularly intermittent pulse" or "regularly interrupted pulse". The modifications are explanatory, and are not adopted in the proposed standard.

30. 緊脈 [jǐn mài] is a pulse which feels like a tightly stretched cord. Both the words "tense" and "tight" well reflect the original meaning, and the authors using either one are approximately equal in number. So, both

---

*Zhu WF (chief editor). Zhong Yi Zhen Duan Xue, *Diagnostics of Traditional Chinese Medicine* (in Chinese). The Textbook Series for Programmed Courses of the TCM Universities and Colleges, Shanghai Science and Technology Press, 1995, p.93.

are selected as the proposed standard.

31. In Chinese medicine, 散脈 [sǎn mài] is defined as a pulse that feels diffuse and feeble upon a light touch and faint upon hard pressure, indicating exhaustion of *qi* in critical illnesses. Most authors agree with the word "scattered".

32. 弦脈 [xián mài] is a pulse which feels straight and long, like a musical string. As its equivalent, "wiry pulse" is used by most authors, and so is selected as the proposed standard. Other expressions include "taut", "stringy", "strung", "string-like", and "string-tight" to describe the pulse.

33. 芤脈 [kōu mài] is described as a pulse that feels as if it is floating, large, soft and hollow, like a scallion stalk, formed by sudden decrease of circulating blood volume Some authors prefer "scallion-stalk pulse" or "onion-stem pulse" to keep consistency with the Chinese term. It is an excellent word-to-word translation, but "scallion stalk" or "onion stem" may give different impressions to different persons. So, most authors prefer "hollow pulse" in order to avoid misunderstanding.

34. 大脈 [dà mài] is a pulse with a high wave which lifts the examiner's finger to a greater height than normal, either forceful or weak. Most authors prefer "large pulse" as its equivalent, and some others use "big pulse". A few authors suggest "gigantic pulse", but they also use "large pulse" at the same time.

As for 小脈 [xiǎo mài], most authors render it as "small pulse".

35. The classical description of 動脈 [dòng mài] is "a rapid pulse occurs at the bar (*guan*) section, imperceptible at the proximal and distal sections, and throbbing like a bean at the fixed position"* There are disparities in the English expression: "moving pulse", "stirred pulse", "stirring pulse", "tremulous pulse", "shaking pulse", "strong and rapid pulse", "throbbing pulse", etc. It is difficult to select the most appropriate one because the character 動 [dòng] used in this term does not simply mean "moving". The word "shaking" or "tremulous" may refer to too high a frequency. The characteristic features of this pulse are rapid, short (limited to the bar (*guan*) section) and slippery like a bouncing bean. The

---

*"若數脈見於關上，上下無頭尾，大如豆，厥厥動搖者，名曰動也。"（《傷寒論·辨脈法》 Method of Pulse Differentiation in *Treatise on Cold-Induced Diseases*）"動脈見於關上，無頭尾，大如豆，厥厥然動搖。"（《脈經》 *Pulse Classic*）In the above two citations, the same adverb 厥厥 or 厥厥然 is used. It means that the pulse is rooted with no change of position (Jian Ming Zhong Yi Zi Dian, *Concise Dictionary of Charaters in Chinese Medicine*, Guizhou People's Publishing House, 1985, p.349).

word "throbbing" probably describes all the features.

36. 反關脈 [fǎn guān mài] is due to anatomic anomaly of the radial artery that makes the pulse beat felt on the dorsal aspect of the wrist. Many authors render it as "ectopic radial pulse", but the wording is not precise because a slantingly located pulse is also ectopic. Some authors express it as "pulse on the back of the wrist". It is correct but explanatory, unlike a technical term. Between "dorsally located pulse" and "contralateral radial pulse", the first on is selected.

37. 斜飛脈 [xié fēi mài] is due to an anatomic anomaly of the radial artery that makes the pulse run from the cubit (*chi*) section outward and slantwise to the back of the hand. Some authors also use "ectopic radial pulse" for this pulse, obliterating its difference from dorsally located pulse. Other expressions include "slantingly-located pulse", "slantingly located radial artery", "oblique pulse", and "oblique-running pulse", among which the first one is selected.

38. A pulse that has lost its usual rhythm, frequency and evenness, usually indicates a critical lack of stomach *qi*, and so is called 脈無胃氣 [mài wú wèi qì]. Most authors express this concept as "pulse without stomach *qi*". However, Nigel Wiseman's suggestion—"pulse bereft of stomach *qi*"— can better reflect the real meaning of this term.

39. 脈靜 [mài jìng] refers to a pulse that becomes gentle and even in the course of illness, usually indicating incipient improvement. Most authors express this concept as "calm pulse" or "pulse calmed". Some others describe it as "tranquil pulse", "gentleness of pulse", or "mild and even pulse".

40. 脈躁 [mài zào] refers to a pulse that becomes rapid and rushing, usually indicating deterioration of the patient's condition. Compared with "rapid and rushing pulse" and "rash pulse", the term "agitated pulse" is more appropriate.

SYNDROME NAMES
(PATTERN NAMES)

Syndrome differentiation plays a major role in Chinese medical diagnosis. Since the syndrome usually involves the location, cause, pathogenesis and nature of the disease, the syndrome names may include related terms such as parts of the body or internal organs, the six excesses and other pathogens, and the pathogenetic terms. Terminologically, when the syndrome [pattern] name is short, deriving merely from the location, nature or pathogen individually, the suffix 證 [zhèng] is always added, for example, 表證 [biǎo zhèng], 寒證 [hán zhèng]. In these terms deletion of the suffix will cause confusion. So in both Chinese and English, 證 [zhèng] or "syndrome [pattern]" is an indispensable element of these short terms. In the cases of syndrome [pattern] names deriving from pathogenetic terms, no such a suffix was added in the Chinese nomenclature in the past, but recently *the State Standard of P.R. China: the Clinical Terminology of Traditional Chinese Medical Diagnosis and Treatment — Syndromes* promulgated in 1997 makes a regulation that all the syndrome names should have the character 證 [zhèng] at the end. For example, 肝火上炎 [gān huǒ shàng yán] was both a pathogenetic term and a syndrome name, but now it is only a pathogenetic term indicating a pathological change, and the corresponding syndrome name is 肝火上炎證 [gān huǒ shàng yán zhèng]. The addition of the character 證 [zhèng] in the syndrome name is necessary because the other characters are exactly the same as those in the pathogenetic terms. Without the suffix, one can not make the differentiation. The English terminology, however, is different. It is easy to differentiate a syndrome name from the relevant pathogenetic term by modifying the grammatical structure, and it is difficult to add "syndrome [pattern]" at the end of a long phrase indicating the pathogenesis.

Grammatically, all pathogenetic terms in Chinese are derived from complete sentences. There are three sentence patterns: I. subject + transitive verb + direct object, II. subject + intransitive verb + adjunct, and III. subject + linking verb + subject complement. In most terms the sentences are in the active voice, but occasionally they are in the passive voice.

Pattern I is quite common when the term includes the pathogenic factor, for example, 痰火擾心 [tán huǒ rǎo xīn] (Phlegm-fire agitates the heart). In Chinese, the four characters 痰火擾心 [tán huǒ rǎo xīn] as a phrase are good enough to form a pathogenetic term, but in English some modification is necessary. The sentence can be turned into: "phlegm-fire agitating the heart", "agitation of the heart by phlegm-fire", "phlegm-fire agitation of the heart", and "heart agitated by phlegm-fire".

There are adequate options for expressing the pathogenesis or pathological change and the syndrome in different ways. The phrase containing a gerund is suggested as the proposed standard of a pathogenetic term, and one of the others may be the syndrome [pattern] name. It would be verbose if the word "syndrome [pattern]" were added at the end of any of such phrase.

Pattern II can be exemplified by 心火上炎 [xīn huǒ shàng yán] (Heart fire flares up.), in which 心火 [xīn huǒ] (heart fire) is the subject, 炎 [yán] (flares) is an intransitive verb term, and 上 [shàng] (up) is an adjunct, an adverb of direction. The sentence can be turned into a phrase such as "heart fire flaring up", "flaring-up of heart fire", and "up-flaring heart fire", with the word "flaring" as a present participle, noun and adjective. The first one is suitable for designating the pathogenesis, and one of the others as a syndrome name. However, not all pathogenetic terms of this pattern can be treated as such, and the wording may be flexible to meet the majority opinion.

Pattern III is probably most commonly encountered but easy to be mistaken as a noun. For example, in 心火亢盛 [xīn huǒ kàng shèng] (Heart fire becomes exuberant.) there is actually a hidden linking verb. (In the classical Chinese language the linking verb is often omitted.) The sentence can be turned into a phrase such as "exuberance of heart fire", "heart fire exuberance" or "exuberant heart fire".

Since the differentiation between the pathogenetic terms and syndrome names can be made by grammatical modification, it is preferable to avoid the addition of the word "syndrome [pattern]" at the end of a long phrase. In the above examples, "phlegm-fire agitation of the heart", "up-flaring of heart fire" and "heart fire exuberance" are selected as the syndrome names.

EIGHT-PRINCIPLE SYNDROME DIFFERENTIATION (EIGHT-PRINCIPLE PATTERN IDENTIFICATION)

Proposed Standard Nomenclature

eight principles 八綱 [bā gāng][1]
eight-principle pattern identification 八綱辨證 [bā gāng biàn zhèng][1]

eight-principle syndrome differentiation 八綱辨證 [bā gāng biàn zhèng][1]

yin-yang pattern identification 陰

yin-yang syndrome differentiation 陰

陽辨證 [yīn yáng biàn zhèng][2]
yin syndrome 陰證 [yīn zhèng][3]
exterior and interior 表裏[biǎo lǐ][4]
exterior syndrome 表證 [biǎo zhèng][5]
cold and heat 寒熱 [hán rè][7]
cold syndrome 寒證 [hán zhèng][7]
heat syndrome 熱證 [rè zhèng][7]
deficiency syndrome 虛證 [xū zhèng][8]
excess syndrome 實證 [shí zhèng][8]
exterior heat syndrome 表熱證 [biǎo rè zhèng][9]
exterior excess syndrome 表實證 [biǎo shí zhèng][9]
interior heat syndrome 裏熱證 [lǐ rè zhèng][10]
interior excess syndrome 裏實證 [lǐ shí zhèng][10]
deficiency-heat syndrome 虛熱證 [xū rè zhèng][11]
excess-heat syndrome 實熱證 [shí rè zhèng][11]
interior deficiency-heat syndrome 裏虛熱證 [lǐ xū rè zhèng][12]
exterior-heat and interior-cold syndrome 表熱裏寒證 [biǎo rè lǐ hán zhèng][13]
exterior-excess and interior-deficiency syndrome 表實裏虛證 [biǎo shí lǐ xū zhèng][13]
upper-cold (and) lower-heat syndrome 上寒下熱證 [shàng hán xià rè zhèng][14]
upper-excess (and) lower-deficiency syndrome 上實下虛證 [shàng shí xià xū zhèng][14]
true heat with false cold 真熱假寒 [zhēn rè jiǎ hán][15]
true deficiency with false excess

陽辨證 [yīn yáng biàn zhèng][2]
yang syndrome 陽證 [yáng zhèng][3]
interior syndrome 裏證 [lǐ zhèng][5]
half-exterior (and) half-interior syndrome 半表半裏證 [bàn biǎo bàn lǐ zhèng][6]
deficiency [insufficiency] and excess [excessiveness] 虛實 [xū shí][8]
exterior cold syndrome 表寒證 [biǎo hán zhèng][9]
exterior deficiency syndrome 表虛證 [biǎo xū zhèng][9]
interior cold syndrome 裏寒證 [lǐ hán zhèng][10]
interior deficiency syndrome 裏虛證 [lǐ xū zhèng][10]
deficiency-cold syndrome 虛寒證 [xū hán zhèng][11]
excess-cold syndrome 實寒證 [shí hán zhèng][11]
interior deficiency-cold syndrome 裏虛寒證 [lǐ xū hán zhèng][12]
exterior-cold and interior-heat syndrome 表寒裏熱證 [biǎo hán lǐ rè zhèng][13]
exterior-deficiency and interior-excess syndrome 表虛裏實證 [biǎo xū lǐ shí zhèng][13]
upper-heat (and) lower-cold syndrome 上熱下寒證 [shàng rè xià hán zhèng][14]
upper-deficiency (and) lower-excess syndrome 上虛下實證 [shàng xū xià shí zhèng][14]
true cold with false heat 真寒假熱 [zhēn hán jiǎ rè][15]
true excess with false deficiency 真實假虛 [zhēn shí jiǎ xū][15]
yin deficiency syndrome 陰虛證

真虛假實 [zhēn xū jiǎ shí][15]

yang deficiency syndrome 陽虛證 [yáng xū zhèng][16]

yin exhaustion syndrome 亡陰證 [wáng yīn zhèng][17]

yang exhaustion syndrome 亡陽證 [wáng yáng zhèng][17]

[yīn xū zhèng][16]

yin collapse syndrome 陰脫證 [yīn tuō zhèng][17]

yang collapse syndrome 陽脫證 [yáng tuō zhèng][17]

Discussion

1. In Chinese medicine the guiding principles of syndrome differentiation are differentiating the location of disease between exterior and interior, distinguishing the nature of disease between cold and heat, identifying the patient's condition as deficiency or excess, and generalizing the syndrome or pattern as yin or yang. These principles are collectively called 八綱 [bā gāng]. In recent publications the following expressions are used as its equivalent: "eight principal syndromes", "eight principles", "eight guiding principles", "eight parameters", "eight guiding parameters", "eight rubrics", "eight indicators", etc. It is hard to say which one is definitely the best. Since the term "eight principles" is the most commonly used, it is selected as the proposed standard.

As for the term 八綱辨證 [bā gāng biàn zhèng], the English equivalent depends on the rendering of 辨證 [biàn zhèng]. In this scheme both "eight-principle syndrome differentiation" and "eight-principle pattern identification" are proposed as the standard terms.

2. In syndrome differentiation, yin and yang are two basic principles for categorizing all the syndromes (or patterns), including the other principles, namely, interior, cold, and deficiency pertaining to yin, and exterior, heat, and excess to yang. Since the terms yin and yang are generally accepted, the appropriate equivalent of 陰陽辨證 [yīn yáng biàn zhèng] is naturally "yin-yang syndrome differentiation" or "yin-yang pattern identification".

3. All syndromes, according to their yin-yang nature, can be grossly classified into two general categories: "yin syndrome" or "yin pattern" 陰證 [yīn zhèng] and "yang syndrome" or "yang pattern" 陽證 [yáng zhèng].

4. 表裏 [biǎo lǐ] is used to indicate the location of a disease, or, more precisely, the depth of the disease. 表 [biǎo] refers to the skin, subcutaneous tissues, muscles and superficial meridians, while 裏 [lǐ] refers to

the internal organs and bone marrow. For expressing 裏 [lǐ], most authors use "interior", and for expressing 表 [biǎo], some authors use "superficial", but more authors prefer "exterior". The word "exterior" has more advantages because it is both an adjective and a noun, and particularly because it is more concordant with the Chinese concept than "superficial". "Exterior" can be used to denote the outer portion of the body including the afore-mentioned tissues, while "superficial" or "superficies" refers only to the body surface.

5. 表證 [biǎo zhèng] is a general term for syndromes affecting the exterior part of the body, and 裏證 [lǐ zhèng], a general term for syndromes indicating that the interior part of the body is diseased. Their equivalents, therefore, are "exterior syndrome" or "exterior pattern" and "interior syndrome" or "interior pattern" respectively.

6. There are different ways to express 半表半裏 [bàn biǎo bàn lǐ], such as "meso-exterior-interior", "midstage", "half-superficies and half-interior", "half-exterior/half-interior", "half-interior half-exterior". Since this term is often discussed together with exterior and interior syndromes, it is better that it be concordant with the words exterior and interior.

7. 寒熱 [hán rè] is used to indicate the nature of a disease. There is no disagreement about the equivalent "cold" vs. "heat", and hence "cold syndrome" or "cold pattern" as the equivalent of 寒證 [hán zhèng], and "heat syndrome" or "heat pattern" as the equivalent of 熱證 [rè zhèng].

8. There has been much dispute over the equivalent of 虛 vs. 實. Even at present there is still considerable discrepancy. Tracing it to its source, the dispute comes from the effort to search for a word-to-word equivalent, or, more precisely, for a character-to-word equivalent.

There are four main pairs of translations of 虛 [xū] vs. 實 [shí] as the names of syndromes (or patterns): asthenia vs. sthenia, vacuity vs. repletion, emptiness vs. fullness, deficiency vs. excess. Before making the selection, the primary elements of these two terms should be considered. Firstly, they are technical terms indicating different morbid conditions. So they only indicate diseased states, excluding healthy conditions. Secondly, according to traditional Chinese medicine, the definition of 虛證 [xū zhèng] is "consumption of essential *qi*", and that of 實證 [shí zhèng] is "exuberance of pathogenic *qi*". It should be noted that essential *qi* includes yin, yang, *qi*, blood, etc., and exuberance of pathogenic *qi* is entirely different from exuberance of normal *qi*. Thirdly, "consumption of essential *qi*" does not necessarily mean total deprivation of essential *qi*. The latter only serves as an extreme example, but is by no means of universal significance. "Asthenia" means lack of strength. This word is only suitable for describing the condition of *qi*, and can not be assigned to yin, blood, essence or other substances. So is "sthenia", which means unusual energy or vigor. In addition, asthenia and sthenia are very unkind to the ears, particular when differentiating between "asthenia syndrome" and "sthenic syndrome". Vacuity means lack of purpose, meaning or intelligence. This has nothing to do with the original meaning of 虚 [xū]. Another meaning of vacuity is the state of being a vacuum or emptiness. Nobody can remain alive if any of the essential *qi* is completely lost. Repletion is also inappropriate, because it often denotes a normal state. In comparison with the above terms, deficiency and excess are the best, because deficiency means "state of lacking something essential", excess means "going beyond the normal limits". Both indicate abnormal conditions, but do not necessarily go to extremes. Most authors accept "deficiency" and "excess" as names of syndromes (or patterns), but some authors criticize these words for their invalidity in other terms. It is true that to render 虚脈 [xū mài] as deficiency pulse or deficient pulse is confusing. However, the key issue is that many Chinese characters are polysemous. Each Chinese character may have different meanings when it is used in different terms, and it is impractical, impossible and unnecessary to search for one and only one equivalent for each Chinese character. As for the above-mentioned translations, all of them have their use in Chinese medicine. Deficiency is good for naming the syndrome (deficiency syndrome 虚證 [xū zhèng]), empty for describing the pulse (empty pulse 虚脈 [xū mài]), vacuity for describing the state of mental quiescence in *qigong* (vacuity quiescence 虚靜 [xū jìng]), and in some (but not all) instances asthenic for the fire symptom in a deficiency state (asthenic fire 虚火 [xū huǒ]).

The above discussion deals with English translation of Chinese medical terms. As for the standardized nomenclature, the problem will be easier to solve because not every term has to strictly accord with the original term in the Chinese language word for word.

In conclusion, the most widely accepted equivalents of 虚證 [xū zhèng] and 實證 [shí zhèng] are "deficiency syndrome" and "excess syndrome", respectively.

9. Exterior syndromes are classified in terms of cold vs. heat and deficiency vs. excess, as 表寒證 [biǎo hán zhèng], 表熱證 [biǎo rè zhèng],

表虛證 [biǎo xū zhèng] and 表實證 [biǎo shí zhèng]. In accordance with the above discussions on 寒 [hán], 熱 [rè], 虛 [xū] and 實 [shí], the proposed standard nomenclature of these terms should respectively be "exterior cold syndrome" or "exterior cold pattern", "exterior heat syndrome" or "exterior heat pattern", "exterior deficiency syndrome" or "exterior deficiency pattern", and "exterior excess syndrome" or "exterior excess pattern".

10. Similar to exterior syndromes, interior syndromes can also be classified into 裏寒證 [lǐ hán zhèng] 裏熱證 [lǐ rè zhèng] 裏虛證 [lǐ xū zhèng] and 裏實證 [lǐ shí zhèng] with the corresponding English equivalents "interior cold syndrome", "interior heat syndrome", "interior deficiency syndrome" and "interior excess syndrome", respectively. Some authors use "internal" instead of "interior", but in this scheme "interior" is suggested as the only word used to express the concept of the Chinese medical term 裏 [lǐ].

11. Even when the word "deficiency" is used as the equivalent of 虛 [xū], there are still different expressions for 虛寒 [xū hán]: "deficiency cold", "deficiency-cold" and "deficient cold", and for 虛熱 [xū rè]: "deficiency heat", "deficiency-heat" and "deficient heat". It should be noted that "cold", "heat", "deficiency" and "excess" all indicate the nature of the syndrome, while "exterior" and "interior" signify the gross location of the illness. "Exterior cold syndrome" will not cause confusion, and it is easily understood as a cold syndrome occurring in the exterior part of the body. But "deficient cold syndrome" may be misleading; it may be understood as meaning that the cold is deficient. In Chinese medicine, "deficiency" refers to health *qi*, but not to pathogenic *qi*. In the syndrome name, "cold" means that the syndrome is caused by cold and manifested by cold symptoms. So the syndrome can be considered a combination of deficiency syndrome and cold syndrome. Therefore, "deficiency-cold syndrome" is probably the best expression. There is a similar problem with "excess". "Excessive cold syndrome" and "excessive heat syndrome" are misleading, as they indicate extremely serious conditions.

12. Syndromes of deficiency-cold and deficiency-heat usually occur in the interior, and are called "interior deficiency-cold syndrome" and "interior deficiency-heat syndrome", respectively. They further show that "deficiency-cold" and "deficiency-heat" are superior to "deficient cold" and "deficient heat" terminologically.

13. Clinically, complicated conditions of exterior, interior, cold and heat are not infrequently encountered, such as exterior-cold and interior-heat syndrome, exterior-heat and interior-cold syndrome, exterior-deficiency and interior-excess syndrome, and exterior-excess and interior-deficiency syndrome. Terminologically, they are simple additions of proposed standard terms, and so no further discussion is necessary.

14. For expressing 上 [shàng] and 下 [xià] most authors use "upper and lower", while some authors prefer "above and below". The real meanings of 上 [shàng] and 下 [xià] in these terms are in the upper portion of the body and in the lower portion of the body, respectively.

15. The presence of seeming and deceptive cold symptoms in diseases caused by heat is called 假寒 [jiǎ hán] (false cold), and presence of seeming and deceptive heat symptoms in diseases caused by cold is called 假熱 [jiǎ rè] (false heat). 真熱假寒 [zhēn rè jiǎ hán] (true heat with false cold) refers to a heat syndrome with seeming and deceptive cold symptoms, and 真寒假熱 [zhēn hán jiǎ rè] (true cold with false heat) refers to a cold syndrome with seeming and deceptive heat symptoms. In recent publications, two different ways are used to express 真 vs. 假: "real vs. pseudo-" and "true vs. false". "Pseudo-" is a Greek prefix. Generally, Greek prefixes are often combined with Greek or Latin elements, but "cold" and "heat" are not Greek- or Latin-origined words. Therefore, "true vs. false" is adopted in this scheme. This is also available for 真虛假實 [zhēn xū jiǎ shí] (true excess with false deficiency) and 真實假虛 [zhēn shí jiǎ xū] (true deficiency with false excess).

16. In the eight principles of syndrome differentiation, classification of yin and yang is the guiding program, on which exterior, heat and excess syndromes can classified as yang syndromes, and interior, cold and deficiency syndromes as yin syndromes. But generalized deficiency, exhaustion and collapse of yin or yang are also included in the eight-principle syndrome differentiation.

17. According to the State Standard Terminology of Traditional Chinese Medical Diagnosis and Treatment, P.R. China, 1997, 陰脫證 [yīn tuō zhèng] and 亡陰證 [wáng yīn zhèng] are synonyms with the same implication, and so are 陽脫證 [yáng tuō zhèng] and 亡陽證 [wáng yáng zhèng]. In recent publications on Chinese medicine in English, 亡陰 [wáng yīn] is rendered as "yin exhaustion (or exhaustion of yin)", "yin depletion (depletion of yin)" and "yin collapse (of collapse of yin)", and

陰脫 [yīn tuō] is also rendered as "yin exhaustion (or exhaustion of yin)", "yin depletion (depletion of yin)" and "yin collapse (of collapse of yin)", in addition, "yin desertion". The words used to express the yang cases are the same: "exhaustion", "depletion" and "collapse". The word "exhaustion" is most frequently used, and the next is the word "collapse". These two words have some difference in meaning. Generally speaking, collapse occurs suddenly, while exhaustion does not. The Chinese terminology refers to both. Therefore, it is better to give consideration to both renderings.

SIX-MERIDIAN SYNDROME DIFFERENTIATION (SIX-MERIDIAN PATTERN IDENTIFICATION)

Six-meridian syndrome differentiation is chiefly used for diagnosing different stages of febrile diseases.

Proposed Standard Nomenclature

six-meridian syndrome differentia-tion 六經辨證 [liù jīng biàn zhèng][1]

meridian syndrome 經證 [jīng zhèng][3]

greater yang syndrome 太陽病證 [tài yáng bìng zhèng][1, 2]

greater yang fu-organ syndrome 太陽腑證 [tài yáng fǔ zhèng][1, 3]

bright yang meridian syndrome 陽明經證 [yáng míng jīng zhèng][1, 3]

lesser yang syndrome 少陽病證 [shào yáng bìng zhèng][1, 2]

lesser yin syndrome 少陰病證 [shào yīn bìng zhèng][1, 2]

six-meridian pattern identification 六經辨證 [liù jīng biàn zhèng][1]

syndromes of the six meridians 六經病證 [liù jīng bìng zhèng][2]

fu-organ syndrome 腑證 [fǔ zhèng][3]

greater yang meridian syndrome 太陽經證 [tài yáng jīng zhèng][1, 3]

bright yang syndrome 陽明病證 [yáng míng bìng zhèng][1, 2]

bright yang fu-organ syndrome 陽明腑證 [yáng míng fǔ zhèng][1, 3]

greater yin syndrome 太陰病證 [tài yīn bìng zhèng][1, 2]

reverting yin syndrome 厥陰病證 [jué yīn bìng zhèng][1, 2]

Discussion

1. The traditional names of the meridians in the framework of yin and yang are not necessarily used in acupuncture, but they cannot be avoided

in six-meridian syndrome differentiation. Besides the use of Romanized Chinese, each term has several different expressions:

太陽— *taiyang*, greater yang, yang major

陽明— *yangming*, yang brightness, bright yang, splendid yang

少陽— *shaoyang*, lesser yang, yang minor

太陰— *taiyin*, greater yin, yang major

少陰— *shaoyin*, lesser yin, yin minor

厥陰— *jueyin*, terminal yin, reverting yin, shrinking yin

From the above terms, the following are selected "greater yang", "bright yang", "lesser yang", "greater yin", "lesser yin", and "reverting yin".

2. About 病 [bìng] and 病證 [bìng zhèng]: Syndrome differentiation in accordance with the theory of the six meridians was initiated in the book *Treatise on Cold-induced Diseases*, and the terms 六經病 [liù jīng bìng] appeared even earlier, in the *Canon of Medicine*. It should be noted that in ancient times the character 病 [bìng] meant serious illness, different from the modern concept of disease. To date, the Chinese terms 六經病 [liù jīng bìng] (including 太陽病 [tài yáng bìng], 陽明病 [yáng míng bìng], 少陽病 [shào yáng bìng], 太陰病 [tài yīn bìng], 少陰病 [shào yīn bìng] and 厥陰病 [jué yīn bìng]) seem to be ambiguous, because they are six stages of febrile diseases but not six febrile diseases. So, in modern Chinese textbooks, they are changed to 六經病證 [liù jīng bìng zhèng] (including 太陽病證 [tài yáng bìng zhèng], 陽明病證 [yáng míng bìng zhèng] etc.). There are probably two reasons to designate these terms as 病證 [bìng zhèng] instead of the single character 證 [zhèng] . One is that they have been called 病 [bìng] traditionally, and the other and predominant one is that a four-character term is better than a three-character term both in rhetoric and in pronunciation. So far as the English equivalents are concerned, there is no need to keep the translation of the character 病 [bìng].

3. About 經證 [jīng zhèng] and 腑證 [fǔ zhèng]: When an attack by a pathogen on any of the three yang meridians is confined to the meridian itself, the morbid condition is called 經證 [jīng zhèng]. When the related *fu*-organ is also affected, the condition is called 腑證 [fǔ zhèng]. As discussed previously, the standard nomenclature of 經 [jīng] is "meridian", and the recommended equivalent of 腑 [fǔ] is "*fu*-organ", therefore the proposed standard terms are "meridian syndrome" and "*fu*-organ syndrome".

DEFENSE-QI-NUTRIENT-BLOOD SYNDROME DIFFERENTIATION (PATTERN IDENTIFICATION)

The regime of defense, *qi*, nutrient and blood syndrome differentiation was developed for the diagnosis of different stages of the course of acute febrile diseases, usually epidemic. It is still used at present.

Proposed Standard Nomenclature

defense-*qi*-nutrient-blood syndrome differentiation 衛氣營血辨證 [wèi qì yíng xuè biàn zhèng]

four-aspect pattern identification 衛氣營血辨證 [wèi qì yíng xuè biàn zhèng]

syndrome of defense system 衛分證 [wèi fèn zhèng]

defense-aspect pattern 衛分證 [wèi fèn zhèng]

syndrome of *qi* system 氣分證 [qì fèn zhèng]

qi-aspect pattern 氣分證 [qì fèn zhèng]

syndrome of nutrient system 營分證 [yíng fèn zhèng]

construction-aspect pattern 營分證 [yíng fèn zhèng]

syndrome of blood system 血分證 [xuè fèn zhèng]

blood-aspect pattern 血分證 [xuè fèn zhèng]

Discussion

For the standard English nomenclature of 衛分 [wèi fèn], 氣分 [qì fèn], 營分 [yíng fèn] and 血分 [xuè fèn], the following issues are to be discussed: (1) How to express 分 [fèn] in these terms? It is rendered as "level", "aspect", "system", and "phase" by different authors. Each word has its own grounds. This regime of syndrome differentiation, as a rule, is for diagnosing warm diseases (epidemic febrile diseases), and indicating the development of the disease from the superficial portion to the deep portion of the body. The word level seems to be appropriate, if it is preceded by an adjective such as "defensive". But if the preceding word is a noun, confusion can result, e.g., blood level may be misunderstood as the level of something in the blood, and *qi* level as the level or content of *qi*. "Phase" is the most appropriate word if 分 [fèn] is regarded as a division of the disease process. However, the original meaning of 分 [fèn] is "component" or "portion", indicating the location of the disease, i.e., the portion of the body. In fact, 衛分 [wèi fèn] refers to the superficial portion of the body, and is also called 衛表 [wèi biǎo], namely the defensive superficies. At the initial stage of an epidemic disease, the superficial defensive portion of the body is affected, and the morbid condition is called 衛分證 [wèi fèn zhèng]. The term 氣分 [qì fèn] refers to the middle portion of the body including the lung, stomach, spleen, gallbladder and large intestine. When this portion of the body is invaded in an epidemic disease, there is high fever with other manifestations of exuberant heat. 營分 [yíng fèn] and 血分 [xuè fèn] refer to the nutrient and blood parts, invasion of which usually causes fever with rashes, bleeding and impairment of consciousness. Among the present renderings, "system" signifying a group of parts and "aspect" signifying a particular part are appropriate expressions.

TRIPLE-ENERGIZER SYNDROME DIFFERENTIATION (TRIPLE-ENERGIZER PATTERN IDENTIFICATION)

Triple-energizer syndrome differentiation was also developed for the diagnosis of different syndromes occurring in acute febrile diseases. It is less commonly used than defense-*qi*-nutrient-blood syndrome differentiation at present.

Proposed Standard Nomenclature

triple-energizer syndrome differentiation 三焦辨證 [sān jiāo biàn zhèng]

triple-energizer pattern identification 三焦辨證 [sān jiāo biàn zhèng]

upper-energizer syndrome 上焦病證 [shàng jiāo bìng zhèng]

upper-energizer pattern 上焦病證 [shàng jiāo bìng zhèng]

middle-energizer syndrome 中焦病證 [zhōng jiāo bìng zhèng]

middle-energizer pattern 中焦病證 [zhōng jiāo bìng zhèng]

lower-energizer syndrome 下焦病證 [xià jiāo bìng zhèng]

lower-energizer pattern 下焦病證 [xià jiāo bìng zhèng]

Discussion

For the proposed standard nomenclature of 三焦 [sān jiāo], please see Note 4 of *Zang-fu* Organs (p. 37)

QI-BLOOD SYNDROME DIFFERENTIATION
(QI-BLOOD PATTERN IDENTIFICATION)

Disorders of *qi* and blood include inadequacy and abnormal movement of *qi* and/or blood. Inadequacy of *qi*, blood, and both belong to deficiency conditions, and abnormal movements such as *qi* stagnation and blood stasis usually indicate excess conditions. The related terms have already been discussed in the chapter on pathogenetic terms. In the names of syndromes, the word "syndrome" or "pattern" is added at the end of each term. But practically, the abbreviated form with omission of such an ending is more commonly used.

Proposed Standard Nomenclature

qi-blood syndrome differentiation 氣血辨證 [qì xuè biàn zhèng]

qi deficiency (syndrome [pattern]) 氣虛證 [qì xū zhèng]

qi-blood (dual) deficiency (syndrome [pattern]) 氣血兩虛證 [qì xuè liǎng xū zhèng]

blood stasis (syndrome [pattern]) 血瘀證 [xuè yū zhèng]

qi deficiency and blood stasis (syndrome [pattern]) 氣虛血瘀證 [qì xū xuè yū zhèng]

blood cold (syndrome [pattern]) 血寒證 [xuè hán zhèng]

qi-blood pattern identification 氣血辨證 [qì xuè biàn zhèng]

blood deficiency (syndrome [pattern]) 血虛證 [xuè xū zhèng]

qi depression (syndrome [pat- tern]) 氣鬱證 [qì yù zhèng]

qi stagnation (syndrome [pattern]) 氣滯證 [qì zhì zhèng]

qi-stagnation and blood-stasis (syndrome [pattern]) 氣滯血瘀證 [qì zhì xuè yū zhèng]

blood heat (syndrome [pattern]) 血熱證 [xuè rè zhèng]

Discussion

For the proposed standard nomenclature of the above syndrome names, please see the corresponding pathogenetic terms in the section Disorders of Qi and Blood (p.80-83).

BODY-FLUID SYNDROME DIFFERENTIATION
(BODY-FLUID PATTERN IDENTIFICATION)

The condition of body fluids is another important aspect of Chinese diagnosis. The related syndromes include fluid insufficiency and fluid excess, and the terminologies are thus derived.

Proposed Standard Nomenclature

body-fluid syndrome differentiation 津液辨證 [jīn yè biàn zhèng][1]

lung fluid insufficiency (syndrome [pattern]) 肺燥津虧證 [fèi zào jīn kuī zhèng][3]

intestine fluid insufficiency (syndrome [pattern]) 腸燥津虧證 [cháng zào jīn kuī zhèng][3]

water retention syndrome [pattern] 水停證 [shuǐ tíng zhèng][5]

wind-phlegm syndrome 風痰證 [fēng tán zhèng][6]

heat-phlegm syndrome 熱痰證 [rè tán zhèng][6]

body-fluid pattern identification 津液辨證 [jīn yè biàn zhèng][1]

fluid insufficiency (syndrome [pattern]) 津液虧虛證 [jīn yè kuī xū zhèng][2]

stomach fluid insufficiency (syndrome [pattern]) 胃燥津虧證 [wèi zào jīn kuī zhèng][3]

fluid retention syndrome [pattern] 飲證 [yǐn zhèng][4]

phlegm syndrome [pattern] 痰證 [tán zhèng][6]

cold-phlegm syndrome 寒痰證 [hán tán zhèng][6]

dryness-phlegm syndrome 燥痰證 [zào tán zhèng][6]

Discussion

1. For the English equivalent of 津液 [jīn yè], please see Note 14 of Basic Physiological Substances (p. 48).

2. The characters 虧 [kuī], 虛 [xū], 耗 [hào], 傷 [shāng], 損 [sǔn], though they have some minor differences in meaning, are actually synonymous, and can replace each other. Their common meaning is "inadequacy" or "insufficiency". In addition, a series of double-character words can be formed if they are preferable to single-character words from the linguistic point of view. For example, 津液虧 [jīn yè kuī] is clear enough, but 津液虧虛 [jīn yè kuī xū] is more readable. 肺燥津虧 [fèi zào jīn kuī] is better than 肺燥津虧虛 [fèi zào jīn kuī xū], for the latter is long-winded and difficult to pronounce. All these points are issues of the Chinese language that need not be reflected in the proposed standard nomenclature.

Standardization of the Chinese terms is prerequisite for the proposed standard English nomenclature. The term 肺燥津虧證 [fèi zào jīn kuī zhèng] is also expressed as 肺燥津傷證 [fèi zào jīn shāng zhèng], but in the State Standard Terminology of Traditional Chinese Medical Diagnosis and Treatment, P.R. China, 1997, only the former is regarded as the standard term. 胃燥津虧證 [wèi zào jīn kuī zhèng] is also collected in the State Standard, and 腸燥津虧證 [cháng zào jīn kuī zhèng] is cited from the Chinese national textbook *Chinese Medical Diagnostics*.

4. Most authors render 飲證 [yǐn zhèng] as "fluid retention syndrome". Their disagreement is on the insertion of a hyphen between "fluid" and "retention". Some authors prefer the word "rheum" for 飲 [yǐn]. About the use of the word "rheum", please see the discussion on page 66.

5. 水停證 [shuǐ tíng zhèng] is a newly developed term in the Chinese national textbook Chinese Medical Diagnostics. In the past it was called 水氣 [shuǐ qì] (water *qi*) or simply 水 [shuǐ] (water). Since neither is bound to be considered as abnormal unless it is retained in the body, 水停 [shuǐ tíng] (water retention) is more reasonable to indicate the morbid condition.

6. "Phlegm syndrome [pattern]" (痰證 [tán zhèng]) is a general term including 痰飲 [tán yǐn] (phlegm-fluid), 痰濕 [tán shī] (phlegm-damp), 濕痰 [shī tán] (damp-phlegm), etc.

Regarding the English equivalent of 痰 [tán], please see the discussion on page 66. "Wind-phlegm" 風痰 [fēng tán], "cold-phlegm" 寒痰 [hán tán], "heat-phlegm" 熱痰 [rè tán], and "dryness-phlegm" 燥痰 [zào tán] are pathogens in combination with phlegm.

DISEASE-CAUSE SYNDROME DIFFERENTIATION (DISEASE-CAUSE PATTERN IDENTIFICATION)

In Chinese medicine the theoretical knowledge of the cause of disease is the basis of diagnosis, but disease cause determined in clinical diagnosis may or may not be identical with the theoretical cause. The disease causes thus determined are chiefly the six excesses as pathogens and certain pathological products that turn into pathogenic factors.

Terminologically, the composition of the syndrome names purely related to the cause of disease is usually as follows: a single or combined pathogenic factor + syndrome (e.g., "external wind syndrome", "wind-damp syndrome"). The pathogenic factors commonly include the six excesses, either external or endogenous, and other endogenous factors due to dysfunction of *zang-fu* organs such as phlegm, retained fluid, etc.

Emotional factors and various pathogenic factors originating from life style are usually not mentioned in syndrome names, though they may be discussed in the analysis of the case. More complicated syndrome names may be formed by combining this regime of syndrome differentiation with other regimes, e.g., "liver-gallbladder damp-heat syndrome".

Proposed Standard Nomenclature

disease-cause syndrome differentiation 病因辨證 [bìng yīn biàn zhèng][1]

disease-cause pattern identification 病因辨證 [bìng yīn biàn zhèng][1]

external wind syndrome 外風證 [wài fēng zhèng][2]

external cold syndrome 外寒證 [wài hán zhèng][2]

external dryness syndrome 外燥證 [wài zào zhèng][2]

warm-dryness syndrome 溫燥證 [wēn zào zhèng][3]

cool-dryness syndrome 涼燥證 [liáng zào zhèng][3]

dryness-heat syndrome 燥熱證 [zào rè zhèng][3]

cold-dryness syndrome 寒燥證 [hán zào zhèng][3]

wind-heat syndrome 風熱證 [fēng rè zhèng][4]

wind-heat exterior syndrome 風熱表證 [fēng rè biǎo zhèng]

wind-cold exterior syndrome 風寒表證 [fēng hán biǎo zhèng]

damp syndrome 濕證 [shī zhèng]

wind-damp syndrome 風濕證 [fēng shī zhèng][4]

damp-heat syndrome 濕熱（蘊結）證 [shī rè (yùn jié) zhèng][4]

summer heat syndrome 暑證 [shǔ zhèng]; 暑熱（內鬱）證 [shǔ rè (nèi yù) zhèng][4]

syndrome of down-pouring damp-heat 濕熱下注證 [shī rè xià zhù zhèng]

summer damp syndrome 暑濕（內蘊）證 [shǔ shī (nèi yùn) zhèng][4]

heat-toxin syndrome 熱毒（熾盛）證 [rè dú (chì shèng) zhèng][4]

fire-toxin syndrome 火毒（熾盛）證 [huǒ dú (chì shèng) zhèng][4]

excess-fire syndrome 實火證 [shí huǒ zhèng]

phlegm-damp syndrome 痰濕證 [tán shī zhèng][4]

cold-phlegm syndrome 寒痰證 [hán tán zhèng][4]

damp-phlegm syndrome 濕痰證 [shī tán zhèng][4]

heat-phlegm syndrome 熱痰證 [rè tán zhèng][4]

wind-phlegm syndrome 風痰證 [fēng tán zhèng][4]

pus-toxin syndrome 膿毒（蘊積）證 [nóng dú (yùn jī) zhèng]

food accumulation syndrome 食積證 [shí jī zhèng][5]

worm accumulation syndrome 蟲積證 [chóng jī zhèng][6]

Discussion

1. The term 病因辨證 [bìng yīn biàn zhèng] has been rendered in different ways. Besides lengthy explanatory translations, the following are succinct: "etiological differentiation of syndromes", "syndrome differentiation of etiology", "disease cause pattern identification", "identification according to the etiology" and "etiological analysis and differentiation". In this scheme, the word "etiology" is not used, in order to avoid confusion with the Western medical concept. The causal factor determined in syndrome differentiation may change at different stages of the same disease. This is alien to Western etiology.

2. The terms "external wind syndrome [pattern]" (外風證[wài fēng zhèng]), "external cold syndrome [pattern]" (外寒證 [wài fēng zhèng]), and "external dryness syndrome [pattern]" (外燥證 [wài zào zhèng]) are all general terms for syndromes caused by exogenous pathogenic wind, cold and dryness respectively. About the English equivalents, cf. the related terms on page 55－59. It should be noted that they are different from the corresponding exterior syndromes. "External cold syndrome" refers to a syndrome caused by cold pathogens from without, while "exterior cold syndrome" refers to a syndrome with the exterior portion of the body affected by cold.

3. External dryness syndrome may show heat symptoms in addition to manifestation of dryness. In this case, the syndrome is called warm-dryness or dryness-heat. Strictly speaking, the two terms have some minor difference. "Warm-dryness syndrome" refers to a syndrome occurring in a seasonal (autumnal) febrile disease caused by dryness pathogens with heat property. On the other hand, "dryness-heat" refers to the condition in which dryness pathogens turn into heat, giving rise to heat symptoms in addition to dryness. Practically, the two conditions can hardly be differentiated, and so they are taken as synonyms in the State Standard Terminology of Traditional Chinese Medical Diagnosis and Treatment, P.R. China, 1997. In this scheme, both are collected because of their common use.

"Cool-dryness syndrome" and "cold-dryness syndrome" are also synonyms.

4. For the names of syndromes caused by combined pathogens, cf. the discussion on page 62－63.

In these terms some additional words are often used to describe the pathogenesis, for example, 蘊結 [yùn jié] in 濕熱蘊結證 [shī rè yùn jié zhèng], 內鬱 [nèi yù] in 暑熱內鬱證 [shǔ rè nèi yù zhèng] and 內蘊 [nèi yùn] in 暑濕內蘊證[shǔ shī nèi yùn zhèng]. In the State Standard Terminology of Traditional Chinese Medical Diagnosis and Treatment, P.R. China, these additional words are specially labeled as omittable. Omission of these words facilitates the standardization of the terms in Chinese. In this scheme, therefore, only the abbreviated terms are proposed in the standard nomenclature.

5. Most authors render 食積證 [shí jī zhèng] as dyspepsia or indigestion. This seems too Westernized, and does not completely conform to the original Chinese medical concept. Both dyspepsia and indigestion refer to impaired function of digestion, but 食積 [shí jī] is usually an excess condition due to improper diet or overfeeding. Some other renderings such as "food retention" and "food accumulation" may be more appropriate.

6. Many authors use "intestinal parasitosis" or even "enterositosis" as the equivalent of 蟲積證 [chóng jī zhèng]. This term as a syndrome name emphasizes the symptoms caused by intestinal parasites, but not merely the presence of parasites in the intestines. Other authors render this term as "worm accumulation" or "worm stagnation". This seems closer to the original Chinese concept.

ZANG-FU ORGAN SYNDROME DIFFERENTIATION (ORGAN PATTERN IDENTIFICATION)

Zang-fu organ syndrome differentiation, or organ syndrome differentiation for short, is not limited to determination of the organ in which a disease is located. It should be made on the basis of the nature (cold, heat, deficiency or excess) and cause of the syndrome. The nomenclature of the syndrome names in terms of *zang-fu* organs usually includes the following elements: (1) the organ mainly affected, (2) the nature of the syndrome, and (3) the etiological factor that affects the diseased organ, particularly in excess syndromes of the organ. According to deficiency or excess, organ syndromes can generally classified into three categories: deficiency syndromes, excess syndromes, and complex deficiency-excess syndromes. In deficiency syndromes, the terminological structure in Chinese is: organ name + vital substance or activity (yin, yang, *qi*, blood, fluid or essence) + deficiency (or other words indicating functional insufficiency) + syndrome (or pattern). To turn them into English, a literal translation is usually acceptable. But there are two issues that need discussion. One is whether a hyphen should be inserted between the organ name and the vital substance or activity. According to punctuation rules, a hyphen is used when forming attributive compounds from two or more proper names. Many authors, particularly those who capitalize organ names and the vital substance or activity, add such a hyphen. The other issue is about the word "syndrome" or "pattern". In syndrome names that only contain the disease cause, the word "syndrome" or "pattern" should not be omitted, otherwise they will be regarded as the names of etiological factors. For the syndrome names used in organ syndrome differentiation, omission of the word "syndrome" or "pattern" will not lead to such misunderstanding. In reality, the original Chinese nomenclature in the past did not contain the character 證 [zhèng] as a rule. This can be demonstrated by the *Grand Dictionary of Traditional Chinese Medicine*, 1995, the most authoritative dictionary of Chinese medicine, jointly compiled by thirteen TCM universities and colleges. In this dictionary almost none of the syndrome names related to *zang-fu* organs end with 證 [zhèng], for example, 心氣虛 [xīn qì xū] but not 心氣虛證 [xīn qì xū zhèng] and 心火上炎 [xīn huǒ shàng yán] but not 心火上炎證 [xīn huǒ shàng yán zhèng]. In the recent publications of Chinese medicine translated or directly written in English, for the syndrome names related to *zang-fu* organs the word syndrome or pattern is not used in most instances. Only since the promulgation of the State Standard of the P.R. of China on Clinical Terminology of Traditional Chinese Medical Diagnosis and Treatment — Syndromes in 1997, are all the syndrome names including those related to *zang-fu* organs required to end with the character 證 [zhèng]. In Chinese, the addition of 證 [zhèng] can distinguish the term from the corresponding term used in pathogenesis.

In excess syndromes, there are two common patterns of terminological structure in Chinese. One is: pathogenic factor + verb (often with the meaning of "invade", "attack", "assail", "disturb", "embarrass", "harass", "torment", "obstruct", "block", "accumulate in", and so on) + organ name + syndrome (or pattern). The other pattern is organ name + pathogenic factor + verb (intransitive, often with the meaning of existing in excess) + syndrome (or pattern). When rendering the Chinese term into English, a big problem is how to treat the verb indicating the action of the etiological factor on the organ. In the past, many Chinese medical professionals especially the authors of medical books were also *literati*. They used literary language to form medical terms and write theses. They paid great attention to the elegance of the writing style and often tried to avoid duplication of the same character in different terms. Take affliction of the lungs by various pathogens as an example. The pathogens such as wind-cold, wind-heat, cool-dryness, and warm-dryness may cause lung disorders, which are called 風寒束肺證 [fēng hán shù fèi zhèng], 風熱犯肺證 [fēng rè fàn fèi zhèng], 涼燥襲肺證 [liáng zào xí fèi zhèng], and 溫燥傷肺證 [wēn zào shāng fèi zhèng] in Chinese. In the State Standard TCM Terminology, 風寒束肺證 [fēng hán shù fèi zhèng] is also called 風寒襲肺證 [fēng hán xí fèi zhèng], 涼燥襲肺證 [liáng zào xí fèi zhèng] is synonymous with 燥寒犯肺證 [zào hán fàn fèi zhèng], and 溫燥傷肺證 [wēn zào shāng fèi zhèng] is the same as 溫燥襲肺證 [wēn zào xí fèi zhèng], and in the national textbook 風寒束肺證 [fēng hán shù fèi zhèng] is also replaced by 風寒犯肺證 [fēng hán fàn fèi zhèng]. From the above examples we can see that the characters 束 [shù], 襲 [xí], 傷 [shāng] and 犯 [fàn] can replace each other. We certainly cannot say that these characters have no differences in meaning, but the differences are merely of literary significance. That is why modern Chinese medical professionals are trying to unify and standardize syndrome names. The verbs used in the second pattern of excess syndrome names present a similar problem. For example, 壅盛 [yōng shèng], 亢盛 [kàng shèng] and 熾盛 [chì shèng] are used in different syndrome names. There is really no need to render 肺熱壅盛證 [fèi rè yōng shèng zhèng] and 肺熱熾盛證 [fèi rè chì shèng zhèng] in English as two different terms, because in the State Standard TCM Terminology they are taken as one single term with two different expressions. In addition, the State Standard TCM Terminology also attaches 肺實熱證 [fèi shí rè zhèng] as a synonym. This gives another clue to its standard nomenclature in English, as from the scientific perspective, 實熱 [shí rè] is better than such flowery wordings as 熱壅盛 [rè yōng shèng] or 熱熾盛 [rè chì shèng].

As for the addition of character 證 [zhèng], since Chinese characters have no suffix to indicate different uses or show inflectional endings, the only way to do so is by adding more characters. For the standard English terms, however, it is not always necessary to add the word "syndrome" or "pattern" to the terms. A grammatical change may also work.

Proposed Standard Nomenclature

zang-fu organ syndrome differentiation 臟腑辨證 [zàng fǔ biàn zhèng][1]

syndrome differentiation [pattern identification] of lung diseases [disorders] 肺病辨證 [fèi bìng biàn zhèng][2]

syndrome differentiation [pattern identification] of stomach-intestine diseases [disorders] 胃腸病辨證 [wèi chàng bìng biàn zhèng][2]

syndrome differentiation [pattern identification] of kidney and bladder diseases [disorders] 腎與膀胱病辨證 [shèn yǔ páng guāng bìng biàn zhèng][2]

organ pattern identification 臟腑辨證 [zàng fǔ biàn zhèng][1]

syndrome differentiation [pattern identification] of heart diseases [disorders] 心病辨證 [xīn bìng biàn zhèng][2]

syndrome differentiation [pattern identification] of spleen diseases [disorders] 脾病辨證 [pí bìng biàn zhèng][2]

syndrome differentiation [pattern identification] of liver-gall-bladder diseases [disorders] 肝膽病辨證 [gān dǎn bìng biàn zhèng][2]

Discussion

Although 病 [bìng] in Chinese medicine is generally equivalent to "disease", it is usually based on functional disorders rather than morpho-pathological change, so quite a number of authors prefer using the word "disorder".

Syndromes of the Heart

Proposed Standard Nomenclature

heart-*qi* deficiency (syndrome [pattern]) 心氣虛證 [xīn qì xū zhèng][1]

heart-yin deficiency (syndrome [pattern]) 心陰虛證 [xīn yīn xū zhèng][1]

heart-yang collapse (syndrome [pattern]) 心陽虛脫證 [xīn yáng xū tuō zhèng][2]

heart-vessel obstruction (syndrome 心脈痹阻證 [xīn mài bì zǔ zhèng][3]

heart-blood deficiency (syndrome [pattern]) 心血虛證 [xīn xuè xū zhèng][1]

heart-yang deficiency (syndrome [pattern]) 心陽虛證 [xīn yáng xū zhèng][1]

heart-blood stasis (syndrome [pattern]) 心血瘀阻證 [xīn xuè yū zǔ zhèng][3]

blazing heart fire (syndrome [pattern]) 心火熾[亢]盛證 [xīn

up-flaring heart fire (syndrome [pattern]) 心火上炎證 [xīn huǒ shàng yán zhèng][4]

phlegmatic mental confusion (syndrome [pattern]) 痰迷[蒙]心竅[神]證 [tán mí [méng] xīn qiào [shén] zhèng][4]

huǒ chì[kàng] shèng zhèng][4]

phlegm-fire (mental) agitation (syndrome [pattern]) 痰火擾神[心]證 [tán huǒ rǎo shén [xīn] zhèng][4]

Discussion

1. The major divergence in the English names of these syndromes lies in the reflection of the concept 虛 [xū]. As discussed above, "deficiency" is the best choice when 虛 [xū] is used to nominate a syndrome. Another divergence is the use of the hyphen. For example, some authors render 心氣虛證 [xīn qì xū zhèng] as "heart *qi* deficiency (syndrome [pattern])", but some others prefer "heart-*qi* deficiency (syndrome [pattern]"). According to punctuation, hyphen is used when forming attributive coumpounds from two or more proper names. So, "heart-*qi* deficiency" is reasonable, but in the term "deficiency of heart *qi*" no hyphenation is needed because "heart *qi*" is not an attributive in this phrase.

Many authors capitalize some Chinese medical terms as if they are proper names when they may cause confusion with Western concepts. In this scheme, no such a rule is established simply because too many words with an initial capital letter may seemingly break up the sentence. No objection is made if a limited number of Chinese medical terms are capitalized as proper names.

2. In this term 虛 [xū] and 脫 [tuō] are not two independent words; they form one single concept. When Western medicine was introduced to China, Chinese medical professionals rendered "collapse" as 虛脫 [xū tuō] for the two terms in different languages were identically defined and described. Now, there is no reason why we should not do the reverse, i.e., rendering 虛脫 [xū tuō] as "collapse".

3. In some books 心血瘀阻證 [xīn xuè yū zǔ zhèng] and 心脈痹阻證 [xīn mài bì zǔ zhèng] are regarded as one term, but they actually refer to two different conditions. So, it is better to give two independent English equivalents.

4. The corresponding pathogenetic terms are "heart fire blazing (心火熾[亢]盛 [xīn huǒ chì [kàng] shèng])", "heart fire flaring up (心火上

炎 [xīn huǒ shàng yán])", "phlegm-fire agitating the mind [heart] 痰火擾神[心] [tán huǒ rǎo shén [xīn]]" and "phlegm confusing the mind (痰迷[蒙]心竅[神] [tán mí [méng] xīn qiào [shén]]).

Syndromes of the Liver and Gallbladder

Proposed Standard Nomenclature

liver-blood deficiency (syndrome [pattern]) 肝血虛證 [gān xuè xū zhèng][1]

liver-*qi* stagnation (syndrome [pattern]) 肝鬱(氣滯)證 [gān yù (qì zhì) zhèng][2]

up-flaring liver fire (syndrome [pattern]) 肝火上炎證 [gān huǒ shàng yán zhèng][2]

liver-gallbladder damp-heat (syndrome [pattern]) 肝膽濕熱證 [gān dǎn shī rè zhèng][2]

internal stirring of liver wind (syndrome [pattern]) 肝風內動證 [gān fēng nèi dòng zhèng][2]

wind (syndrome [pattern]) due to extreme heat 熱極生風證 [rè jí shēng fēng zhèng][2]

wind (syndrome [pattern]) due to blood deficiency 血虛動風證 [xuè xū dòng fēng zhèng][2]

liver-yin deficiency (syndrome [pattern]) 肝陰虛證 [gān yīn xū zhèng][1]

blazing liver fire (syndrome [pattern]) 肝火熾盛證 [gān huǒ chì shèng zhèng][2]

hyperactive liver yang (syndrome [pattern]) 肝陽上亢證 [gān yáng shàng kàng zhèng][2]

(syndrome [pattern] of) cold stagnation in liver meridian 寒滯肝脈證 [hán zhì gān mài zhèng][2]

(syndrome [pattern] of) liver-yang transformation into wind 肝陽化風證[gān yáng huà fēng zhèng][2]

wind (syndrome [pattern]) due to yin deficiency 陰虛動風證 [yīn xū dòng fēng zhèng][2]

gallbladder-*qi* deficiency (syndrome [pattern]) 膽氣虛證 [dǎn qì xū zhèng][1]

Discussion

1. 肝血虛證 [gān xuè xū zhèng] and 肝陰虛證 [gān yīn xū zhèng] are rendered into English according to the general rules of nominating deficiency syndromes of *zang-fu* organs.

2. The corresponding pathogenetic terms are "stagnation of liver *qi* 肝鬱氣滯 [gān yù qì zhì zhèng]", "liver fire blazing 肝火熾盛 [gān huǒ chì shèng]", "liver fire flaring up 肝火上炎 [gān huǒ shàng yán]", "hyperactivity of liver yang 肝陽上亢 [gān yáng shàng kàng]", "liver wind stirring internally 肝風內動 [gān fēng nèi dòng]", "liver yang

transforming into wind 肝陽化風 [gān yáng huà fēng]", "extreme heat producing wind 熱極生風 [rè jí shēng fēng]", "yin deficiency stirring wind 陰虛動風 [yīn xū dòng fēng]", "blood deficiency stirring wind 血虛動風 [xuè xū dòng fēng]", "damp-heat in the liver and gallbladder 肝膽濕熱 [gān dǎn shī rè zhèng]", and "stagnation of cold in the liver meridian 寒滯肝脈 [hán zhì gān mài]".

Syndromes of the Spleen

Proposed Standard Nomenclature

spleen-*qi* deficiency (syndrome [pattern]) 脾氣虛證 [pí qì xū zhèng][1]

spleen-yin deficiency (syndrome [pattern]) 脾陰虛證 [pí yīn xū zhèng][1]

(syndrome [pattern] of) spleen failure in controlling blood 脾不統血證 [pí bù tǒng xuè zhèng][3]

(syndrome [pattern] of) cold-damp disturbance of the spleen 寒濕困脾證 [hán shī kùn pí zhèng][4]

spleen-stomach damp-heat (syndrome [pattern]) 脾胃濕熱證 [pí wèi shī rè zhèng]; 中焦濕熱證 [zhōng jiāo shī rè zhèng][4]

spleen-stomach deficiency-cold (syndrome [pattern]) 脾胃虛寒證 [pí wèi xū hán zhèng][5]

spleen-yang deficiency (syndrome [pattern]) 脾陽虛證 [pí yáng xū zhèng][1]

spleen-*qi* sinking (syndrome [pattern]) 脾氣下陷證 [pí qì xià xiàn zhèng]; 脾虛氣陷證 [pí xū qì xiàn zhèng][2]

(syndrome [pattern] of) spleen insufficiency with damp retention 脾虛濕困證 [pí xū shī kùn zhèng][4]

(syndrome [pattern] of) accumulationof damp-heat in the spleen 濕熱蘊脾證 [shī rè yùn pí zhèng][4]

spleen-stomach yang deficiency (syndrome [pattern]) 脾胃陽虛證 [pí wèi yáng xū zhèng][5]

Discussion

1. The wording follows the nomenclature of deficiency syndromes of *zang-fu* organs.

2. The renderings of 下陷 [xià xiàn] include "collapse", "fall", "descending", and "sinking".

3. The corresponding pathogenetic term is "spleen failing to control blood (脾不統血 [pí bù tǒng xuè])".

4. The main pathogen that affects the spleen is damp. "Harass", "en-

cumber", "disturb", and "burden" are used by different authors to express 困 [kùn]; and "accumulate" or "retain" for 蘊 [yùn].

5. Yang-deficiency and deficiency-cold are synonyms.

Syndromes of the Stomach and Intestines

Proposed Standard Nomenclature

stomach-*qi* deficiency (syndrome [pattern]) 胃氣虛證 [wèi qì xū zhèng][1]

stomach-yin deficiency (syndrome [pattern]) 胃陰虛證 [wèi yīn xū zhèng][1]

(syndrome [pattern] of) cold stagnation in stomach and intestines 寒滯胃腸證 [hán zhì wèi cháng zhèng][2]

(syndrome [pattern] of) food stagnation in stomach and intestines 食滯胃腸證 [shí zhì wèi cháng zhèng][2]

(syndrome [pattern] of) damp-heat in intestine 腸道濕熱證 [cháng dào shī rè zhèng][2]

(syndrome [pattern] of) heat binding in large intestine 大腸熱結證 [dà cháng rè jié zhèng][2]

(syndrome [pattern] of) fluid deficiency in large intestine 大腸液虧證 [dà cháng yè kuī zhèng][2]

stomach-yang deficiency (syndrome [pattern]) 胃陽虛證 [wèi yáng xū zhèng][1]

(syndrome [pattern] of) cold invasion of stomach 寒邪犯胃證 [hán xié fàn wèi zhèng][2]

(syndrome [pattern] of) retained fluid in stomach and intestines 飲留胃腸證 [yǐn liú wèi cháng zhèng][2]

stomach fire (syndrome [pattern]) 胃火[熱](熾盛)證 [wèi huǒ [rè] (chì shèng) zhèng][3]

(syndrome [pattern] of) *qi* stagnation in stomach and intestines 胃腸氣滯證 [wèi cháng qì zhì zhèng][2]

(syndrome [pattern] of) excess-heat in small intestine 小腸實熱證 [xiǎo cháng shí rè zhèng][2]

(syndrome [pattern] of) worm accumulation in intestine 蟲積腸道證 [chóng jī cháng dào zhèng][2]

Discussion

1. Naming of deficiency syndromes follows the general rule of nomenclature.

2. Please see the previous discussion on the related etiological and pathogenetic terms

3. Various expressions of intense heat in the stomach can be collectively called "stomach fire".

Syndromes of the Lung

Proposed Standard Nomenclature

lung *qi* deficiency (syndrome [pattern]) 肺氣虛證 [fèi qì xū zhèng][1]

(syndrome [pattern] of) wind-cold restraining of the lung 風寒束肺證 [fēng hán shù fèi zhèng][2]

(syndrome [pattern] of) wind-heat invasion of the lung 風熱犯肺證 [fēng rè fàn fèi zhèng][3]

(syndrome [pattern] of) lung-yin deficiency with dryness 陰虛肺燥證 [yīn xū fèi zào zhèng]

(syndrome [pattern] of) phlegm-heat accumulation in the lung 痰熱壅肺證 [tán rè yōng fèi zhèng]

(syndrome [pattern] of) cold-phlegm obstruction of the lung 寒痰阻肺證 [hán tán zǔ fèi zhèng][4]

wind-water syndrome [pattern]風水(相搏)證 [fēng shuǐ xiāng bó zhèng]

lung yin deficiency (syndrome [pattern]) 肺陰虛證 [fèi yīn xū zhèng][1]

(syndrome [pattern] of) wind-cold attack on the lung 風寒襲肺證 [fēng hán xí fèi zhèng][2]

(syndrome [pattern] of) dryness invasion of the lung 燥邪犯肺證 [zào xié fàn fèi zhèng]

intense lung heat syndrome [pattern] 肺熱熾盛證[fèi rè chì shèng zhèng]

(syndrome [pattern] of) phlegm-heat obstruction of the lung 痰熱閉肺證 [tán rè bì fèi zhèng]

(syndrome [pattern] of) phlegm-damp obstruction of the lung 痰濕阻肺證 [tán shī zǔ fèi zhèng][4]

(syndrome [pattern] of) retained fluid in the chest 飲停胸脅證 [yǐn tíng xiōng xié zhèng]

Discussion

1. Deficiency syndromes [patterns] are named in accordance with the general rule of nomenclature.

2. Both "(syndrome [pattern] of) wind-cold restraining of lung 風寒束肺證 [fēng hán shù fèi zhèng]" and "(syndrome [pattern] of) wind-cold attack on the lung 風寒襲肺證 [fēng hán xí fèi zhèng]" may be simplified as "wind-cold (syndrome [pattern]) of the lung".

3. "(Syndrome [pattern] of) wind-heat invasion of the lung 風熱犯肺證 [fēng hán fàn fèi zhèng]" may be simplified as "wind-heat (syndrome [pattern]) of the lung".

4. "(Syndrome [pattern] of) phlegm-damp obstruction of the lung 痰濕阻肺證 [tán shī zǔ fèi zhèng]" may be simplified as "phlegm-damp (syndrome [pattern]) of the lung" and "(syndrome [pattern] of) cold-phlegm

obstruction of the lung 寒痰阻肺證 [hán tán zǔ fèi zhèng]" as "cold-phlegm (syndrome [pattern]) of the lung".

Syndromes of the Kidney and Bladder

Proposed Standard Nomenclature

kidney-*qi* deficiency (syndrome [pattern]) 腎氣虛證 [shèn qì xū zhèng][1]

(syndrome [pattern] of) kidney insufficiency with edema 腎虛水泛證 [shèn xū shuǐ fàn zhèng][2]

kidney-*qi* insecurity (syndrome [pattern]) 腎氣不固證 [shèn qì bù gù zhèng][3]

bladder heat retention (syndrome [pattern]) 熱結膀胱證 [rè jié páng guāng zhèng][3]

kidney-yang deficiency (syndrome [pattern]) 腎陽虛證 [shèn yáng xū zhèng][1]

kidney-yin deficiency (syndrome [pattern]) 腎陰虛證 [shèn yīn xū zhèng][1]

kidney essence deficiency (syndrome [pattern]) 腎精虧虛證 [shèn jīng kuī xū zhèng][1]

bladder damp-heat (syndrome [pattern]) 膀胱濕熱證 [páng guāng shī rè zhèng]

bladder deficiency-cold (syndrome [pattern]) 膀胱虛寒證 [páng guāng xū hán zhèng]

Discussion

1. Deficiency syndromes [patterns] are named in accordance of general rule of nomenclature.

2. Most authors render 水泛 [shuǐ fàn] as "edema" and "water flood (or flooding of water)". For pathogenesis "flooding" is selected, and for a syndrome [pattern] "edema" seems better.

3. For the terms 不固 [bù gù] and 熱結 [rè jié], cf. pages 78 and 83.

Organ Combination Syndromes

Proposed Standard Nomenclature

heart-kidney disharmony (syndrome [pattern]) 心腎不交證 [xīn shèn bù jiāo zhèng]

heart-lung *qi* deficiency (syndrome [pattern]) 心肺氣虛證 [xīn fèi qì

heart-kidney yang deficiency (syndrome [pattern]) 心腎陽虛證 [xīn shèn yáng xū zhèng]

heart-spleen *qi*-blood deficiency (syndrome [pattern]) 心脾氣血

xū zhèng]

heart-liver blood deficiency (syndrome [pattern]) 心肝血虛證 [xīn gān xuè xū zhèng]

lung-kidney *qi* deficiency (syndrome [pattern]) 肺腎氣虛證 [fèi shèn qì xū zhèng]

lung-kidney yang deficiency (syndrome [pattern]) 肺腎陽虛證 [fèi shèn yáng xū zhèng]

(syndrome [pattern] of) liver-*qi* invasion of the stomach 肝氣犯胃證 [gān qì fàn wèi zhèng]

(syndrome [pattern] of) liver-*qi* invasion of the spleen 肝氣犯脾證 [gān qì fàn pí zhèng]

liver-spleen disharmony (syndrome [pattern]) 肝脾不和證 [gān pí bù hé zhèng]

liver-kidney yin deficiency (syndrome [pattern]) 肝腎陰虛證 [gān shèn yīn xū zhèng]

兩虛證 [xīn pí qì xuè liǎng xū zhèng]

spleen-lung *qi* deficiency (syndrome [pattern]) 脾肺氣虛證 [pí fèi qì xū zhèng]

lung-kidney yin deficiency (syndrome [pattern]) 肺腎陰虛證 [fèi shèn yīn xū zhèng]

(syndrome [pattern] of) liver fire invasion of the lung 肝火犯肺證 [gān huǒ fàn fèi zhèng]

liver-stomach disharmony (syndrome [pattern]) 肝胃不和證 [gān wèi bù hé zhèng]\

(syndrome [pattern] of) liver stagnation and spleen insufficiency 肝鬱脾虛證 [gān yù pí xū zhèng]

spleen-kidney yang deficiency (syndrome [pattern]) 脾腎陽虛證 [pí shèn yáng xū zhèng]

Discussion

Most of the terms are combination of two related terms.

MERIDIAN SYNDROME DIFFERENTIATION (MERIDIAN PATTERN IDENTIFICATION)

Proposed Standard Nomenclature

(syndrome [pattern] of) thoroughfare-conception vessel disharmony 衝任失調證 [chōng rèn shī tiáo zhèng]

(syndrome [pattern] of) thoroughfare-conception vessel insecurity 衝任不固證 [chōng rèn bù gù zhèng]

belt vessel syndrome 帶脈病證 [dài mài bìng zhèng]

yin-heel vessel syndrome 陰蹺脈病證 [yīn qiāo mài bìng zhèng]

yang-heel vessel syndrome 陽蹺脈病證 [yáng qiāo mài bìng zhèng]

yin-link vessel syndrome 陰維脈病證 [yīn wéi mài bìng zhèng]
yang-link vessel syndrome 陽維脈病證 [yáng wéi mài bìng zhèng]

DISEASE NAMES

In traditional Chinese medicine, the term 病 [bìng] (disease) was not well defined. Only in recent decades, has the concept of disease been made clear, and a formal list of disease names promulgated by the State Administration of Traditional Chinese Medicine.* Since the document bears English equivalents of disease names, most English names collected in this scheme are cited from that document with or without modification. On the other hand, terms newly developed from modern Western medicine are generally excluded from this scheme, particularly those exactly identical with the Chinese terms of Western medicine. For example, most disease names in Chinese orthopedics have undergone such a change, and the traditional names are now obsolete.

A crucial issue that has to be seriously considered is the reversibility of the medical terms in English and in Chinese if they are considered as equivalents. Since modern Western medicine was first introduced to China about a century ago, a complete set of disease names was established. Most of them are still in use at present. It should be noted that, so far as the disease names are concerned, there are a lot of things in common between the two systems of medicine. But naming a disease and understanding the disease are different matters. The latter may differ greatly between the two systems of medicine, but the former may be the same, particularly when they are designated according to the symptoms or signs. For example, if a patient is suffering from pain in the abdomen, tenesmus and deposits frequent stools containing blood and mucus, the disease is called dysentery in Western medicine, and 痢 (疾) [lì (jí)] in traditional Chinese medicine. Therefore, dysentery is translated 痢疾

---

*中華人民共和國中醫藥行業標準 ── 中醫病證診斷療效標準，國家中醫藥管理局發佈，1994. (Professional Standard of Traditional Chinese Medicine, P.R. China ── Criteria of Diagnosis and Therapeutic Effect of Diseases and Syndromes in Traditional Chinese Medicine, promulgated by State Administration of Traditional Chinese Medicine, 1994)

[lì jí] as a Chinese term of Western medicine. From the terminological perspective, "dysentery" as an English name in Western medicine, 痢疾 [lì jí] as a Chinese name in Western medicine and 痢疾 [lì jí] as a Chinese name in traditional Chinese medicine should be natural equivalents, because they refer to the same disease. Regarding the causative agents of this disease, the microbiological understanding in Western medicine, and naive understanding based on natural philosophy in traditional Chinese medicine are different, but this does not interfere with the general designation of the disease name with no involvement of the causative agent. So, "dysentery" and 痢疾 [lì jí] are natural and reversible equivalents.

It is not at all infrequent that a disease has multiple names in both traditional Chinese and modern Western medicine. For standardization, the disease names in Western medicine are selected from the World Health Organization's *Classification of Diseases,* 10th edition (ICD-10) with Chinese translation, 1998, and the Chinese disease names of traditional Chinese medicine are selected from *Professional Standard of Traditional Chinese Medicine, P.R. China* — *Criteria of Diagnosis and Therapeutic Effect of Diseases and Syndromes in Traditional Chinese Medicine*, promulgated by the State Administration of Traditional Chinese Medicine, 1994 (abbreviated as *TCM Professional Standard*), with minor modifications in accordance with recent editions of national Chinese textbooks.

In accordance with the above-mentioned rules, the discussion in this section is often simplified. For example, 遺精 [yí jīng] is rendered in several ways by different authors. It is extremely difficult to select the proposed standard from "emission", "seminal emission", "nocturnal emission", "spontaneous emission", and "spermatorrhea". However, by consulting ICD-10 this problem can be easily solved, for "spermatorrhea" (N50.8) is the only formal name.

The crucial issue for determining a disease name is its definition. As in Western medicine, the knowledge about each individual disease has also undergone changes in China. For example, before 1820, 霍亂 [huò luàn] was defined as any disease characterized by sudden and drastic vomiting and diarrhea. To render this term into English is a difficult task, because it includes a variety of diseases. Afterwards, the disease gradually became confined to the category of pestilence. Now, this disease is defined as an acute diarrheal disease caused by *vibrio cholera*. Traditional Chinese medicine should not be taken as an interesting antique. Its real value lies at its practical use in the health service at present. Therefore, the obsolete concepts are excluded from this scheme.

Lastly, it should be noted that this scheme of disease names is an English-Chinese vocabulary, but not a Chinese-English vocabulary. In other words, from the following lists one can find out the

(All the TCM terms labeled with ※ are exactly identical with those of ICD-10 both in English and in Chinese.)

INTERNAL DISEASES

Proposed Standard Nomenclature

common cold 感冒 [gǎn mào][1]

externally contracted fever 外感發熱 [wài gǎn fā rè][2]

pulmonary tuberculosis 肺癆[fèi láo][4]

asthma 哮病 [xiào bìng][5]

dysphagia 噎膈 [yē gé][7]

vomiting 嘔吐 [ǒu tù]※

hematemesis 吐血 [tù xuè][9]

diarrhea 泄瀉 [xiè xiè][11]

ascites 水臌 [shuǐ gǔ][12]

purpura 紫癜 [zǐ diàn]※

cholera 霍亂 [huò luàn]※

angina pectoris 胸痹心痛 [xiōng bì xīn tòng][13]

depression 鬱病 [yù bìng][15]

depressive psychosis 癲病 [diān bìng][16]

headache 頭痛 [tóu tòng]※

vertigo 眩暈 [xuàn yūn]※

tremor 顫震 [chàn zhèn][18]

flaccidity 萎病 [wěi bìng][20]

edema 水腫 [shuǐ zhǒng]※

urolithic stranguria 石淋 [shī lín][22]

heat stranguria 熱淋 [rè lín][22]

ischuria 癃閉 [lóng bì][23]

cough 咳嗽 [ké sòu]※

fever 發熱 [fā rè]※

lung abscess 肺癰 [fèi yōng][3]

hemoptysis 咯血 [kǎ xuè]※

dyspnea 喘病 [chuǎn bìng][5]

pleural effusion 懸飲 [xuán yǐn][6]

gastralgia 胃脘痛 [wèi wǎn tòng][8]

hematochezia 便血 [biàn xuè][10]

dysentery 痢疾 [lì jí]※

jaundice 黃疸 [huáng dǎn]※

tympanites 氣臌 [qì gǔ][12]

constipation 便秘 [biàn bì]※

heat stroke 中暑 [zhòng shǔ]※

malaria 瘧疾 [nüè jí]※

palpitation 心悸 [xīn jì]※

insomnia 不寐 [bù mèi][14]

epilepsy 癲癇 [diān xián]※

manic psychosis 狂病 [kuáng bìng][16]

intermittent headache 頭風 [tóu fēng][17]

apoplexy 中風 [zhòng fēng][19]

diabetes 消渴 [xiāo kě][21]

retention of urine 癃閉 [lóng bì][23]

spermatorrhea 遺精 [yí jīng]※

impotence 陽萎 [yáng wěi][※]   rheumatic arthritis 風濕痹 [fēng
rheumatoid arthritis 尫痹 [wāng bì][24]   shī bì][24]
osteoarthrosis 骨痹 [gǔ bì][24]   polymyositis and dermatomyositis
gout 痛風 [tòng fēng][※]   肌痹 [jī bì][24]

Discussion

1. Strictly speaking, "cold" (J00 in ICD-10) and 感冒 [gǎn mào] are equivalents. As the word "cold" is so frequently used as a pathogenic factor and also as a basic property of morbid conditions or syndromes, it is better to use the term "common cold" (also J00 in ICD-10).

2. Since the proposed standard term for 外感 [wài gǎn] is "external contraction", 外感發熱 [wài gǎn fā rè] is undoubtedly "externally contracted fever". It is a general term for various fevers caused by infection and other external factors.

3. The character 癰 [yōng] refers to any acute suppurative inflammation leading to abscess formation. When it occurs in the lung, it is called 肺癰 [fèi yōng], namely "lung abscess".

4. 癆 [láo] refers to consumptive disease, and 肺癆 [fèi láo] is pulmonary tuberculosis.

5. Both 喘 [chuǎn] and 哮 [xiào] refer to difficult or labored breathing. The former is marked by short quick breaths, and the latter is accompanied by wheezing.

6. 飲 [yǐn] as a disease name refers to retention of fluid. Literally, 懸飲 [xuán yǐn] means "suspended retention of fluid".

7. 噎膈 [yē gé] means difficulty in swallowing or inability to swallow due to esophageal obstruction.

8. 胃脘痛 [wèi wǎn tòng] is "pain in the stomach cavity".

9. 吐血 [tù xuè] means "vomiting of blood".

10. 便血 [biàn xuè] means "passage of blood in the feces".

11. Both 泄 [xiè] and 瀉 [xiè] mean "diarrhea", but the former is mild diarrhea, and the latter severe diarrhea with passage of watery stools. The two characters are put together as one term, generally signifying diarrhea.

12. 臌 [gǔ] can also be written as 鼓 [gǔ] (drum). As a medical term it means distension, especially distension of the abdomen with the appearance of a drum. When the distension of the abdomen is caused by accumulation of gas, it is called 氣臌 [qì gǔ]; when such distension is caused by accumulation of fluid, it is called 水臌 [shuǐ gǔ].

13. Angina pectoris is called 胸痹心痛 [xiōng bì xīn tòng] in traditional Chinese medicine. Literally, the Chinese original means "precordial pain with obstruction".

14. 不寐 [bù mèi] means "inability to sleep". It is often called 失眠 [shī mián], which literally means "failure to sleep". The same term is used in the Chinese terminology of Western medicine (G47.0 in ICD-10).

15. 鬱病 [yù bìng] is a traditional Chinese medical term. Its corresponding name in the Chinese terminology of Western medicine is 抑鬱 [yì yù], which comes from "depression" (F32.9 in ICD-10)

16. 癲 [diān] and 狂 [kuáng] are often put together as one single term indicating psychosis, but they are actually different. The former refers to depressive psychosis, and the latter to mania. The combined term signifies maniac-depression.

17. A chronic headache with intermittent and recurrent episodes is called 頭風 [tóu fēng], which literally means "head wind".

18. "Tremor" is called 顫震 [chàn zhèn] in traditional Chinese medicine, while the Chinese terminology of Western medicine also uses the two characters, but in the reverse order, i.e., 震顫 [zhèn chàn] (R25.1 in ICD-10)

19. According to ICD-10, both apoplexy and stroke are regarded as two formal names of the same disease. Many authors use wind-stroke as the equivalent of 中風 [zhòng fēng]. There are two possible reasons. One is that wind-stroke might be better than stroke for differentiating the condition from heat stroke; the other is that wind-stroke is exactly equivalent to the Chinese original. The problem is whether 中風 [zhòng fēng] and stroke are the same disease or two different diseases. If they refer to the same disease, it is confusing to give it different names. In ICD-10 "apoplexy" and "stroke" are interchangeable, but "apoplexy" is given priority.

20. 萎病 [wěi bìng] literally means "flaccidity disease", but it actually refers to a group of diseases characterized by muscular weakness and flaccidity.

21. Many authors render 消渴 [xiāo kě] as "wasting-thirst". Since "wasting-thirst" actually refers to diabetes, there is no reason why "diabetes" should be rejected as the equivalent of 消渴 [xiāo kě]. It is celebrated that the sweet taste of a patient's urine was first recorded in the literature of traditional Chinese medicine, much earlier than the discovery of urine sugar in Western medicine. "Diabetes mellitus" is not appropriate,

because 消渴 [xiāo kě] may include some other diseases characterized by excessive thirst. However, "diabetes" alone is a term with a much broader sense. It also includes a variety of abnormal conditions characterized by polyuria and polydipsia.

According to both the *TCM Professional Standard* and the newest edition of Chinese national textbook of traditional internal medicine, the diagnostic criteria of 消渴 [xiāo kě] include examination of fasting blood sugar and glucose tolerance test. It is also clearly stated that 消渴 [xiāo kě] refers to diabetes mellitus, but may also include diabetes insipidus.

22. The situation regarding 淋 [lín] is complicated. On the one hand, 淋 [lín] was used to designate five or seven morbid conditions characterized by difficult and painful discharge of urine drop by drop. In these conditions, "stranguria" is a proper rendering. On the other hand, the Chinese terminology of Western medicine has used this character to signify "gonorrhea". This has also been adopted by traditional Chinese medical terminology. (The term 淋病 [lín bìng] is used in both the *TCM Professional Standard* and the latest edition of Chinese national textbook of traditional external diseases). Therefore, distinction between various patterns of stranguria and gonorrhea is of great importance. In order to avoid confusion, we would be better off using the general term 淋 [lín] or 淋症 [lín zhèng]. Various patterns of stranguria can be treated individually, such "heat stranguria" for 熱淋 [rè lín], and "urolithic stranguria" for 石淋 [shī lín].

23. 癃閉 [lóng bì] is now regarded as one term, but 癃 [lóng] and 閉 [bì] differ in severity, corresponding to "retention of urine" (R33 in ICD-10) and "ischuria" (R34 in ICD-10), respectively.

24. Among various disease names 痹 [bì] is probably the most difficult character to deal with. Generally speaking, it refers to any disease characterized by obstruction of *qi* and/or blood flow in a meridian and/or collateral. Numerous diseases may have such a pathological change, so there are diverse ways of classifying 痹 [bì], e.g., classification according to internal and external in terms of zang-fu organs (a specific meridian obstruction for each organ), in terms of tissues (such as skin, muscle, bone, etc.) and in terms of the limbs and joints. Many of the terms are now obsolete. Although they may have some academic interest, they are excluded from this scheme from a practical perspective. For terms that are still in common use at present, probable equivalents in Western medicine

are given so as to avoid giving the impression that these diseases had never been known in mainstream medicine.

SURGICAL DISEASES

In the ancient classification, 外科 [wài kē] is a discipline of medicine that deals with pathological changes visible externally, and the related diseases are thus called "external diseases". According to the modern classification of Chinese medicine, however, surgical diseases and skin diseases are separated into two categories.

Proposed Standard Nomenclature

furuncle 癤 [jiē][※]

carbuncle 有頭疽 [yǒu tóu jū][1]

acute suppurative subcutaneous inflammation 疔(瘡)[dīng chuāng][3]

acute suppurative parotitis 發頤 [fā yí][6]

acute thyroiditis 癭癰 [yǐng yōng][8]

scrofula 瘰癧 [luǒ lì][※]

tuberculosis of breast 乳癆 [rǔ láo][10]

carcinoma of breast 乳岩 [rǔ ái][13]

nodule in breast 乳核 [rǔ hé][15]

hydrocele 水疝 [shuǐ shàn][16]

epididymitis and orchitis 子癰 [zǐ yōng][8]

hypertrophy of prostate 精癃 [jīng lóng][19]

bedsore 褥瘡 [rù chuāng][※]

tuberculosis of bones and joints 流痰 [liú tán][17]

gangrene of digit 脫疽 [tuō jū][22]

burns and scalds 水火燙傷 [shuǐ huǒ tàng shāng][24]

frostbite 凍傷 [dòng shāng][※]

venomous snake bite 毒蛇咬傷 [dú shé yǎo shāng][※]

acute suppurative lymphadenitis 痰毒 [tán dú][2]

acute lymphangitis 紅絲疔 [hóng sī dīng][4]

gas gangrene 爛疔 [làn dīng][5]

erysipelas 丹毒 [dān dú][※]

gravity abscess 流注 [liú zhù][7]

acute mastitis 乳癰 [rǔ yōng][8]

adenoma of thyroid 肉癭 [ròu yǐng][9]

hypertrophy of breast 乳癧 [rǔ lì][11]

lump in breast 乳癖 [rǔ pǐ][12]

thelorrhagia 乳衄 [rǔ nù][14]

acute appendicitis 腸癰 [cháng yōng][8]

tuberculosis of epididymis 子痰 [zǐ tán][17]

prostatitis 精濁 [jīng zhuó][18]

chronic ulcer of shank 臁瘡 [lián chuāng][20]

suppurative osteomyelitis 附骨疽 [fù gǔ jū][21]

superficial thrombophlebitis 青蛇毒 [qīng shé dú][23]

deep-seated thrombophlebitis 股腫 [gǔ zhǒng][25]

tetanus 破傷風 [pò shāng fēng][※]

external hemorrhoids 外痔 [wài zhì][※]

internal hemorrhoids 內痔 [nèi zhì][※]

perianal abscess 肛癰[gāng yōng][27]

anal fissure 肛裂 [gāng liè][26]

rectal polyp 息肉痔 [xī ròu zhì][28]

anal fistula 肛漏 [gāng lòu][26]

anorectal cancer 鎖肛痔 [suǒ gāng zhì][28]

rectal prolapse 脫肛 [tuō gāng][26]

fibropapilloma of anus 懸珠痔 [xuán zhū zhì][28]

eczema of anus 肛門濕瘍 [gāng mén shī yáng][29]

Discussion

1. Literally 有頭疽 [yǒu tóu jū] means deep-rooted subcutaneous inflammation with openings (for discharge of pus) and necrosis.

2. 痰毒 [tán dú] as a pathogenic factor is rendered as "phlegm-toxin" or "phlegm toxic", but as a disease name it corresponds to acute suppurative lymphadenitis.

3. Acute suppurative subcutaneous inflammation is called 疔 [dīng] or 疔瘡 [dīng chuāng] in traditional Chinese medicine. In ancient Chinese, 疔 is written as 丁 [dīng], which figuratively describes a deep-rooted inflammation covered with redness and swelling.

4. In traditional Chinese medicine, acute lymphangitis is called 紅絲疔 [hóng sī dīng], which literally means "red-thread sore".

5. 爛 [làn] means "festering".

6. In traditional Chinese medicine acute suppurative parotitis is called 發頤 [fā yí], "eruption of swelling at the cheek".

7. 流注 [liú zhù] refers to an abscess in which the pus migrates to the lower portion of the body, so it is equivalent to gravity abscess.

8. 癰 [yōng] is not always equivalent to carbuncle, but may refer to any acute localized suppurative inflammation. Acute thyroiditis, particularly acute suppurative thyroiditis corresponds to 癭癰 [yǐng yōng], in which 癭 [yǐng] is an enlarged thyroid gland; acute mastitis corresponds to 乳癰 [rǔ yōng]; acute appendicitis corresponds to 腸癰 [cháng yōng].

9. Literally, 肉癭 [ròu yǐng] means "fleshy goiter".

10. 癆 [láo] is the traditional Chinese name for tuberculosis.

11. In the designation of subcutaneous nodes, the small ones are called 瘰 [luǒ], and the big ones are called 癧 [lì]. Therefore, 乳癧 [rǔ lì] refers to excessive development tof the breast.

12. 癖 [pǐ] means "aggregation", and so 乳癖 [rǔ pǐ] is "aggregation in the breast".

13. 岩 [ái] is the ancient character for 癌 [ái] (carcinoma) and is still used in traditional Chinese medicine.

14. 乳衄 [rǔ nù] is hemorrhage from the nipple.

15. 核 [hé] is equivalent to "nodule".

16. 疝 [shàn] has multiple meanings. The commonest meaning is painful swelling of the scrotum. Thus, 水疝 [shuǐ shàn] is fluid accumulation in the scrotum.

17. Besides 瘰 [láo], the character 痰 [tán] sometimes also refers to tuberculosis, especially a localized tuberculous lesion with abscess formation. Hence, tuberculosis of epididymis is called 子痰 [zǐ tán] (phlegm around the testis); tuberculosis of bones and joints is called 流痰 [liú tán] ("flowing phlegm") for the formation of wandering abscess.

18. 精濁 [jīng zhuó] is so called for the spontaneous discharge of seminal fluid from the urethral orifice.

19. 癃 [lóng] refers to difficulty in urination and retention of urine.

20. 臁瘡 [lián chuāng] literally means "shank sore".

21. 附骨疽 [fù gǔ jū] literally means "suppurative lesion attached to bone".

22. 脫疽 [tuō jū] is gangrene of the extremities that may cause loss of a finger or toe.

23. 青蛇毒 [qīng shé dú] ("dark-striped toxicosis") is characterized by redness, swelling and tenderness along a superficial vein with palpable cord.

24. The character 燙 [tàng] is composed of two basic structural parts: 氵 (water) and 火 (fire). So, in traditional Chinese medicine 燙傷 [tàng shāng] is not limited to scalds but also includes burns.

25. 股腫 [gǔ zhǒng] refers to blood stagnation with thrombus formation in a deep-seated vein of the thigh.

26. The traditional medical terms 肛裂 [gāng liè] (anal fissure), 肛漏 [gāng lòu] (anal fistula), and 脫肛 [tuō gāng] (anal prolapse) are basically the same as the Western medical terms in Chinese, though the latter uses the full terms formally, i.e., 肛門裂隙 [gāng mén liè xì], 肛門瘻 [gāng mén lòu], and 肛門脫出 [gāng mén tuō chū].

27. The character 癰 [yōng] refers to any acute localized suppurative inflammation.

28. In traditional Chinese medicine, the character 痔 [zhì] does not only refer to hemorrhoids, but is also a general name for any anorectal disease. Hence, fibropapilloma of the anus is called 懸珠痔 [xuán zhū

zhì], which literally means "suspended pearl at the anus", rectal polyp is called 息肉痔 [xī ròu zhì], which literally means "a fleshy mass growing at the anus", and anorectal cancer is called 鎖肛痔 [suǒ gāng zhì], which refers to "a mass that locks the anus".

29. Literally, 濕瘍 [shī yáng] means "damp sore".

GYNECOLOGICAL AND OBSTETRICAL DISEASES

Proposed Standard Nomenclature

frequent menstruation 月經先期 [yuè jīng xiān qī][1]

infrequent menstruation 月經後期 [yuè jīng hòu qī][1]

hypomenorrhea 月經過少 [yuè jīng guò shǎo][※]

amenorrhea 閉經 [bì jīng][※]

headache during menstruation 經行頭痛 [jīng xíng tóu tòng][3]

general aching during menstruation 經行身痛 [jīng xíng shēn tòng][3]

distension and pain of breasts during menstruation 經行乳房脹痛 [jīng xíng rǔ fáng zhāng tòng][3]

menopause syndrome 絕經前後諸證 [jué jīng qián hòu zhū zhèng][4]

threatened abortion 胎動不安 [tāi dòng bù ān][7]

habitual abortion 滑胎 [huá tāi][8]

retention of urine during pregnancy 轉胞 [zhuǎn bāo][10]

prolonged lochiorrhea 產後惡露不絕 [chǎn hòu è lù bù jué][11]

agalactia 產後缺乳 [chǎn hòu quē rǔ][11]

galactorrhea 產後乳汁自出 [chǎn hòu rǔ zhī zì chū][11]

irregular menstrual cycle 月經先後無定期 [yuè jīng xiān hòu wú dìng qī][1]

hypermenorrhea 月經過多 [yuè jīng guò duō][※]

dysmenorrhea 痛經 [tòng jīng][※]

metrorrhagia and metrostaxis 崩漏 [bēng lòu][2]

fever during menstruation 經行發熱 [jīng xíng fā rè][3]

diarrhea during menstruation 經行泄瀉 [jīng xíng xiè xiè][3]

hematemesis and/or epistaxis during menstruation 經行吐衄 [jīng xíng tǔ nù][3]

oral aphtha during menstruation 經行口糜 [jīng xíng kǒu mí][3]

leukorrheal disease 帶下病 [dài xià bìng][5]

hyperemesis gravidarum 妊娠惡阻 [rèn shēn ě zǔ][6]

gestational edema 子腫 [zǐ zhǒng][9]

stranguria during pregnancy 子淋 [zǐ lín][9]

postpartum hemorrhage 產後血崩 [chǎn hòu xuè bēng][11]

puerperal constipation 產後大便難 [chǎn hòu dà biàn nán][11]

uterine prolapse 陰挺 [yīn tǐng][12]   female infertility 不孕 [bù yùn][13]

Discussion

1. In Chinese medicine the abnormal menstrual cycles are described as prolonged, shortened or irregular, while in Western medicine they are described as frequent menstruation (N92.0), infrequent menstruation (N91.5), and irregular menstrual cycle (N92.6). Literal translation of the Chinese as "advanced menstruation" and "delayed menstruation" causes misunderstanding that the first appearance of menstruation is precocious or delayed beyond the sixteenth year.

2. Both 崩 [bēng] and 漏 [lòu] refer to abnormal uterine bleeding.

3. All these terms are common complaints during menstruation. They are regarded as diseases in Chinese medicine. For making diagnosis, other diseases, particularly other organic diseases, should be ruled out.

4. Menopause syndrome is called 絕經前後諸證 [jué jīng qiān hòu zhū zhèng] in traditional Chinese medicine, and 絕經綜合徵 [jué jīng zōng hé zhēng] in the Chinese terminology of Western medicine (N95.1).

5. leukorrheal disease 帶下病 [dài xià bìng]

6. In the term 惡阻 [ě zǔ], the character 惡 [ě] is an abbreviation of 惡心 [ě xīn] ("nausea"), and 阻 [zǔ] ("obstruction") means severe vomiting as if the stomach were obstructed.

7. 胎動不安 [tāi dòng bù ān] means "stirring fetus", indicating threatened abortion.

8. Habitual abortion is called 滑胎 [huá tāi] in traditional Chinese medicine, literally meaning "sliding fetus".

9. In the terms 子腫 [zǐ zhǒng] and 子淋 [zǐ lín], 子 [zǐ] refers to the fetus, and so the former term means edema caused by the fetus, and the latter, stranguria caused by the fetus.

10. Literally, 轉胞 [zhuǎn bāo] means "shifted bladder", which explains difficulty in urination with retention of urine resulting from pressure on the bladder in the late stage of pregnancy.

11. All the disease names preceded by 產後 [chǎn hòu] (postpartum) belong to the category of 產後病 [chǎn hòu bìng] (postpartum diseases). 血崩 [xuè bēng] refers to massive uterine bleeding; 惡露不絕 [è lù bù jué] means persistent discharge of lochia following delivery; 大便難 [dà biàn nán] literally means "difficulty in defecation"; 缺乳 [quē rǔ] is lack of secretion of milk; 乳汁自出 [rǔ zhī zì chū] is spontaneous flow of

milk from the nipple.

12. Uterine prolapse is called 陰挺 [yīn tǐng] in traditional Chinese medicine, which literally means "vaginal protrusion".

13. 不孕 [bù yùn] means "inability to conceive".

PEDIATRIC DISEASES

Proposed Standard Nomenclature

common cold 感冒 [gǎn mào][1]

asthma 哮喘 [xiào chuǎn][*]

diarrhea 泄瀉 [xiè xiè][2]

infantile malnutrition 疳症 [gān zhèng][3]

rubella 風痧 [fēng shā][4]

varicella 水痘 [shuǐ dòu][*]

whooping cough 頓咳 [dùn ké][6]

summer unacclimation 疰夏 [zhù xià][8]

infantile convulsion 驚風 [jīng fēng][9]

neonatal jaundice 胎黃 [tāi huáng][11]

roseola infantum 奶麻 [nǎi má][13]

cough 咳嗽 [ké sòu][*]

thrush 鵝口瘡 [é kǒu chuāng][*]

anorexia 厭食 [yàn shí][*]

edema 水腫 [shuǐ zhǒng][*]

measles 麻疹 [má zhěn][*]

scarlatina 丹痧 [dān shā][4]

mumps 痄腮 [zhà sāi][5]

fulminant dysentery 疫毒痢 [yì dú lì][7]

epilepsy 癲癇 [diān xián][*]

enuresis 遺尿 [yí niào][*]

indigestion 食積 [shí jī][10]

infantile eczema 奶癬 [nǎi xuǎn][12]

hydrocephalus 解顱 [jiě lú][14]

Discussion

1. cf. Discussion 1 of Internal Diseases.

2. cf. Discussion 11 of Internal Diseases.

3. 疳 [gān] refers to malnutrition, especially in children.

4. 痧 [shā] (rash) refers to any of various eruptive diseases, 風痧 [fēng shā] ("wind rash") refers to rubella, and 丹痧 [dān shā] ("red rash") refers to scarlatina.

5. 痄腮 [zhà sāi] is a disease characterized by swelling of the cheek. It is also called 蛤蟆瘟 [há má wēn] ("toad-head epidemic"), showing that it is an epidemic contagious disease with the cheeks swollen like a toad's head.

6. 頓咳 [dùn ké] literally means "bouts of coughing".

7. Fulminant dysentery is called 疫毒痢 [yì dú lì] in traditional Chinese medicine, literally meaning "pestilential toxic dysentery".

8. 疰 [zhù] meant chronic consumptive diseases, including pulmonary tuberculosis, in ancient times. 疰夏 [zhù xià] is a children's disease characterized by lassitude and anorexia in summer and spontaneous recovery in autumn.

9. 驚風 [jīng fēng] is also called 小兒驚風 [xiǎo ér jīng fēng], equivalent to infantile convulsion. But the Western medical term infantile convulsion is not translated into Chinese as such, and 驚風 [jīng fēng] is replaced by 驚厥 [jīng jué] (R56.8 in ICD-10). Therefore, in Chinese, although 驚風 [jīng fēng] and 驚厥 [jīng jué] refer to the same diseased condition, the former is a traditional Chinese medical term, while the latter is a Western medical term.

10. 食積 [shí jī] literally means retention of (undigested) food.

11. Neonatal jaundice is called 胎黄 [tāi huáng] (fetal jaundice) in traditional Chinese medicine because it is believed that jaundice of the newborn results from stagnant heat or damp-heat affection at the fetal stage.

12. Infantile eczema is called 奶癬 [nǎi xuǎn] in traditional Chinese medicine, literally meaning pruritic skin lesion of breast-fed babies.

13. 奶麻 [nǎi má] literally means "infant's rash".

14. Hydrocephalus is called 解顱 [jiě lú] in traditional Chinese medicine, literally meaning non-closure of skull sutures.

EYE DISEASES

Proposed Standard Nomenclature

hordeolum 針眼 [zhēn yǎn][1]

blepharitis marginalis 瞼弦赤爛 [jiǎn xián chì làn][3]

vesicular dermatitis of eyelid 風赤瘡痍 [fēng chì chuāng yí][5]

trichiasis 倒睫(拳毛) [dǎo jié (quán máo)][※]

pterygium 胬肉攀睛 [nǔ ròu pān jīng][7]

puffiness of eyelid 胞虚如球 [bāo xū rú qiú][9]

blepharospasm 胞輪振跳 [bāo lún

chalazion 胞生痰核 [bāo shēng tán hé][2]

erysipelas of eyelid 眼丹 [yǎn dān][4]

trachoma 沙眼 [shā yǎn][※]

frequent nictitation 目劄 [mù dá][6]

severe inflammatory edema of eyelid 胞腫如桃 [bāo zhǒng rú táo][8]

ptosis of eyelid 上胞下垂 [shàng bāo xià chuí][10]

epiphora 冷淚症 [lěng lèi zhèng][12]

acute catarrhal conjunctivitis 暴風

zhèn tiào][11]

acute dacryocystitis 漏睛瘡 [lòu jīng chuāng][13]

epidemic keratoconjunctivitis 天行赤眼 [tiān xíng chì yǎn][15]

xerosis conjunctiva 神水將枯 [shén shuǐ jiāng kū][17]

herpetic keratitis 聚星障 [jù xīng zhàng][19]

interstitial keratitis 混睛障 [hún jīng zhàng][19]

panus totalis 血翳包睛 [xuè yì bāo jīng][20]

fascicular keratitis 風輪赤豆 [fēng lún chì dòu][22]

hypopyon 黃液上冲 [huáng yè shàng chōng][24]

acute glaucoma 綠風內障 [lù fēng nèi zhàng][26]

chronic glaucoma 青風內障 [qīng fēng nèi zhàng][26]

traumatic cataract 驚震內障 [jīng zhèn nèi zhàng][26]

blurred vision 視瞻昏渺 [shì zhān hūn miǎo][28]

myopia 近視 [jìn shì][※]

strabismus 目偏視 [mù piān shì][30]

optic atrophy 青盲 [qīng máng][31]

nystagmus 轆轤轉關 [lù lú zhuàn guān][33]

客熱 [bào fēng kè rè][14]

vernal conjunctivitis 時復症 [shí fù zhèng][16]

phlyctenular conjunctivitis 金疳 [jīn gān][18]

episcleritis 火疳 [huǒ gān][18]

serpent corneal ulcer 凝脂障 [níng zhī zhàng][19]

keratohelcosis 花翳白陷 [huā yì bái xiàn][20]

corneal opacity 宿翳 [sù yì][20]

keratomalacia 疳積上目 [gān jī shàng mù][21]

iridocyclitis 瞳神緊小 [tóng shén jǐn xiǎo][23]

vitreous hemorrhage 血灌瞳神 [xuè guàn tóng shén][25]

senile cataract 圓翳內障 [yuán yì nèi zhàng][26]

vitreous opacity 雲霧移睛 [yún wù yí jīng][27]

metamorphopsia 視直如曲 [shì zhí rú qū][29]

hyperopia 遠視 [yuǎn shì][※]

sudden visual loss 暴盲 [bào máng][32]

exophthalmos 鶻眼凝睛 [gǔ yǎn níng jīng][34]

Discussion

　　1. 針眼 [zhēn yǎn] is a small furuncle on the edge of the eyelid, and is equivalent to sty in English.

　　2. Literally, 胞生痰核 [bāo shēng tán hé] means "phlegm node of the eyelid".

　　3. 瞼弦赤爛 [jiǎn xián chì làn] is an eye disease characterized by redness, swelling and ulceration of the margin of the eyelid.

　　4. 丹 [dān] as a disease name refers to any acute redness and hotness

(inflamation) of the skin as if painted with cinnabar.

5. 風赤瘡痍 [fēng chì chuāng yí] ("wind red sore") is characterized by redness, swelling and pain of the eyelid with vesicle formation.

6. 目剳 [mù dá] means blinking.

7. 胬肉攀睛 [nǔ ròu pān jīng] means "fleshy growth creeping over the eye".

8. 胞腫如桃 [bāo zhǒng rú táo] means swelling of the eyelid like a peach.

9. 胞虛如球 [bāo xū rú qiú] means puffiness of the eyelid like a ball.

10. 上胞下垂 [shàng bāo xià chuí] means "drooping of the upper eyelid"

11. 胞輪振跳 [bāo lún zhèn tiào] means "spasmodic winking"

12. 冷淚症 [lěng lèi zhèng] is a morbid condition characterized by excessive secretion of tears without hotness, redness and pain in the eye.

13. 漏睛瘡 [lòu jīng chuāng] is an eye disease characterized by sudden onset of redness and swelling of the lacriminal sac followed by pustulosis.

14. Acute catarrhal conjunctivitis is called 暴風客熱 [bào fēng kè rè] in traditional Chinese medicine, literally meaning "sudden onset of wind with invading heat".

15. 天行赤眼 [tiān xíng chì yǎn] means "pidemic red eye".

16. Vernal conjunctivitis is called 時復症 [shí fù zhèng] ("seasonal recurrence disease") in traditional Chinese medicine.

17. Xerosis conjunctiva is called 神水將枯 [shén shuǐ jiāng kū], which means "drying up of eye water".

18. The character 疳 [gān] has two major meanings: one is malnutrition with emaciation, and the other, any of the superficial ulcers with concave necrosis but not much pus discharge. 金疳 [jīn gān] and 火疳 [huǒ gān] belong to the latter. Phlyctenular conjunctivitis is called 金疳 [jīn gān] ("metal ulcerative eye"), because traditional Chinese medicine believes that the formation of small vesicles or ulcers on the white of the eye is caused by heat in the lung meridian that pertains to metal. Episcleritis is called 火疳 [huǒ gān] ("fire ulcerative eye") in traditional Chinese medicine because the red granule bulging from the deep layer of the white of the eye results from pathogenic fire.

19. In traditional Chinese ophthalmology, 障 [zhàng] ("screen" or "hindrance") is any pathological change of the eye that impairs vision.

聚星障 [jù xīng zhàng] ("star-clustered screen of the eye") is an eye disease characterized by ulceration of the dark of the eye with the appearance of a cluster of stars, corresponding to herpetic keratitis in Western medicine.

凝脂障 [níng zhī zhàng] ("congealed-fat screen of the eye") is characterized by a creeping suppurative ulcer of the dark of the eye with the appearance of congealed lard, and it is called serpent corneal ulcer in Western medicine.

混睛障 [hún jīng zhàng] ("murky screen of the eye") is characterized by a grayish screen covering the dark of the eye, which becomes hazzy with a ground-glass appearance, and so it is equivalent to interstitial keratitis in Western medicine.

20. 翳 [yì] is opacity of the dark of the eye, i.e., corneal opacity. Thus, 宿翳 [sù yì] ("old corneal opacity") refers to cicatrix cornea, 花翳白陷 [huā yì bái xiàn] ("flowery white pitted opacity") refers to keratohelcosis, and 血翳包睛 [xuè yì bāo jīng] ("vascularized opacity covering the eye") refers to panus totalis in Western medicine.

21. 疳積上目 [gān jī shàng mù] literally means malnutrition involving the eye.

22. 風輪 [fēng lún] ("wind-orbiculus") is another name for the dark of the eye. 風輪赤豆 [fēng lún chì dòu] ("wind-orbiculus red bean") is an eye disease characterized by formation of a band of blood vessels on the cornea like a red bean. It is called fascicular keratitis in Western medicine.

23. Iridocyclitis is called 瞳神緊小 [tóng shén jǐn xiǎo] (pupilary contraction) in traditional Chinese medicine, for a highly contracted pupil is usually the chief manifestation.

24. 黃液 [huáng yè] ("yellow liquid") is a metaphorical way of saying pus. 黃液上沖 [huáng yè shàng chōng] ("upward surging of pus") refers to accumulation of pus in the eye, i.e., hypopyon.

25. Literally, 血灌瞳神 [xuè guàn tóng shén] means "blood pouring into the pupil".

26. 內障 [nèi zhàng] ("internal screen") refers to diseases of the lens and posterior to the lens that impair vision. Acute angle-closure glaucoma is called 綠風內障 [lù fēng nèi zhàng] ("green-wind internal screen") for the greenish color of the pupil, 青風內障 [qīng fēng nèi zhàng] ("blue-wind internal screen") for the bluish color of the pupil, senile cataract is called 圓翳內障 [yuán yì nèi zhàng] ("round internal

screen") for the round shape of the opaque lens, and traumatic cataract is called 驚震內障 [jīng zhèn nèi zhàng] ("internal screen secondary to trauma").

27. Vitreous opacity is called 雲霧移睛 [yún wù yí jīng] in traditional Chinese medicine, which literally means "cloud moving in the eye".

28. 視瞻昏渺 [shì zhān hūn miǎo] ("blurred vision") is a symptom in which vision is impaired while no abnormal change of the eye can be found from without.

29. 視直如曲 [shì zhí rú qū] is a disturbance of vision that distorts objects.

30. strabismus is called 目偏視 [mù piān shì] in traditional Chinese medicine, which means "deviation of the eye".

31. 青盲 [qīng máng] is characterized by loss of vision with no abnormal appearance of the eye.

32. 暴盲 [bào máng] ("sudden blindness") is actually a symptom that may be caused by various eye diseases such as acute inflammation of the optic nerve and occlusion of central retinal artery or vein.

33. 轆轤轉關 [lù lú zhuàn guān] literally means "windlass winding".

34. 鶻眼凝睛 [gǔ yǎn níng jīng] literally means "dove-like fixed eye".

EAR, NOSE AND THROAT DISEASES

Proposed Standard Nomenclature

catarrhal otitis media 耳脹 [ěr zhàng][1]

suppurative otitis media 膿耳 [nóng ěr][1]

sudden hearing loss 暴聾 [bào lóng][2]

chronic deafness 久聾 [jiǔ lóng][2]

coryza 傷風鼻塞 [shāng fēng bí sāi][4]

Ménière's disease 耳眩暈 [ěr xuán yùn][3]

chronic rhinitis 鼻窒 [bí zhì][5]

atrophic rhinitis 鼻槁 [bí gǎo][5]

nosebleed 鼻衄 [bí nù][7]

sinusitis 鼻淵 [bí yuān][6]

acute pharyngitis 急喉痹 [jí hóu bì][8]

chronic pharyngitis 慢喉痹 [màn hóu bì][8]

acute laryngitis 急喉瘖 [jí hóu yīn][8]

chronic laryngitis 慢喉瘖 [màn hóu yīn][8]

acute tonsillitis 乳蛾 [rǔ é][9]

globus hystericus 梅核氣 [méi hé qì][11]

peritonsillar abscess 喉關癰 [hóu guān yōng][10]

aphtha 口瘡 [kǒu chuāng][12]   periodontal diseases 牙宣 [yá xuān][13]

Discussion

1. 耳脹 [ěr zhàng] is also called 耳脹痛 [ěr zhàng tòng], "distension and pain in the ear", and refers to catarrhal otitis media in Western medicine. 膿耳 [nóng ěr], which means "suppuration in the ear", refers to suppurative otitis media.

2. 聾 [lóng] and deafness (ICD-10 H91.9) are natural equivalents.

3. 耳眩暈 [ěr xuán yùn] is literally equivalent to otogenic vertigo, but most authors in China believe that it refers to Ménière's disease, i.e., labrinthine vertigo (ICD-10 H81.0).

4. 傷風鼻塞 [shāng fēng bí sāi] is common cold with snuffles, referring to coryza (acute rhinitis).

5. Chronic rhinitis is called 鼻窒 [bí zhì] (obstructed nose), and atrophic rhinitis, 鼻槁 [bí gǎo] ("withered nose") in traditional Chinese medicine.

6. The character 淵 [yuān] is a deep pool, and 鼻淵 [bí yuān] literally means that the nasal discharge comes from a deep source.

7. At present, 鼻衄 [bí nù] is more commonly called 鼻出血 [bí chū xuè] as the Chinese term used in both traditional Chinese medicine and Western medicine.

8. In Chinese medicine 喉 [hóu] is an abbreviation for 咽喉 [yān hóu] (throat) that includes the pharynx and larynx. Pharyngitis is chiefly manifested by pain, and so is called 喉痹 [hóu bì]. Laryngitis is chiefly manifested by hoarseness, and so is called 喉喑 [hóu yīn].

9. Acute tonsilitis is called 乳蛾 [rǔ é] or 蛾子 [é zi] ("moth") in traditional Chinese medicine, for the inflammed tonsil looks like a moth.

10. 喉關 [hóu guān] refers to the isthmus of the fauces.

11. 梅核氣 [méi hé qì] ("plum-stone sensation") is a disease characterized by subjective sensation of choking with a lump in the throat that can neither be swallowed nor ejected.

12. 口瘡 [kǒu chuāng] literally means "oral sore".

13. Periodontal diseases are generally called 牙宣 [yá xuān] (exposure of teeth), for one of the prominent features of these diseases is exposure of the roots of teeth. In addition, 牙宣 [yá xuān] is also manifested by swelling or atrophy of the tissues surrounding the teeth.

SKIN DISEASES

Proposed Standard Nomenclature

impetigo 黃水瘡 [huáng shuǐ chuāng][1]

favus 肥瘡 [féi chuāng][2]

tinea circinata 圓癬 [yuán xuǎn][3]

tinea blanca 白禿瘡 [bái tū chuāng][3]

tinea manuum 鵝掌風 [é zhǎng fēng][3]

tinea pedis 腳濕氣 [jiǎo shī qì][3]

herpes zoster 蛇串瘡 [shé chuàn chuāng][4]

scabies 疥瘡 [ji chuāng][※]

herpes simplex 熱瘡[rè chuāng][4]

wart 疣目 [yóu mù][5]

verruca plana 扁瘊 [biǎn hóu][5]

molluscum contagiosum 鼠乳 [shǔ rǔ][6]

clavus 雞眼 [jī yǎn][※]

callus 胼胝 [pián zhī][※]

eczema 濕瘡 [shī chuāng][7]

urticaria 隱疹 [yǐn zhěn][8]

dermatitis medicamentosa 藥毒 [yào dú][9]

Pemphigus 天皰瘡 [tiān pào chuāng][※]

lupus erythematosus 紅蝴蝶瘡 [hóng hú dié chuāng][10]

erythema multiforme 貓眼瘡 [māo yǎn chuāng][11]

erythema nodosum 瓜藤纏 [guā téng chán][12]

pityriasis rosea 風熱瘡 [fēng rè chuāng][13]

scleroderma 皮痹 [pí bì][14]

psoriasis 白疕 [bái bǐ][15]

neurodermatitis 牛皮癬[niú pí xuǎn][16]

lichen planus 紫癜風 [zǐ diàn fēng][17]

vitiligo 白駁[癜]風 [bái bó fēng][18]

chloasma 黧黑斑 [lí hēi bān][20]

seborrhoic dermatitis 面游风 [miàn yóu fēng][19]

rosacea 酒齇鼻 [jiǔ zhā bí][※]

keloid 蟹足腫 [xiè zú zhǒng][22]

acne 粉刺 [fěn cì][21]

Discussion

1. 黃水瘡 [huáng shuǐ chuāng] ("yelow-water sore") is a skin disease characterized by vesicles and pustules with yellowish watery discharge. It is known as impetigo.in Western medicine.

2. 肥瘡 [féi chuāng] ("fat sore") is a skin disease of the scalp, characterized by yellow scabs and hair loss at the affected area. It is known as favus in Western medicine.

3. Various kinds of tinea are designated in Chinese medicine by describing the appearance of lesions. 圓癬 [yuán xuǎn] is ringworm with the skin lesion round in shape. 鵝掌風 [é zhǎng fēng] is ringworm of the palms with itching and thickening of the skin like the feet of a goose. 腳濕氣 [jiǎo shī qì] is ringworm of the foot with exudation. 白禿瘡 [bái tū

chuāng] literally means "white bald sore".

4. Herpes zoster and herpes simplex are called 蛇串瘡 [shé chuàn chuāng] (snake-like string sore) and 熱瘡 [rè chuāng] ("heat sore") respectively. The former is designated in accordance with the appearance of the lesions, and the latter is designated by pathogenesis.

5. Both 疣 [yóu] and 瘊 [hóu] refer to wart. 疣目 [yóu mù] is "lobulated wart" and 扁瘊 [biǎn hóu] is "flat wart".

6. Molluscum contagiosum is called 鼠乳 [shǔ rǔ] ("mouse nipple") in traditional Chinese medicine for its appearance and white caseous discharge on squeezing.

7. Eczema is called 濕瘡 [shī chuāng] ("damp sore") in traditional Chinese medicine for its oozing vesicular lesions.

8. Urticaria is called 隱疹 [yǐn zhěn] (dormant papule) in traditional Chinese medicine, for it is latent between eruptions.

9. 藥毒 [yào dú] is also called 藥疹 [yào zhěn], i.e., skin lesion caused by medication.

10. Lupus erythematosus is called 紅蝴蝶瘡 [hóng hú dié chuāng] ("red butterfly sore") in traditional Chinese medicine, for the "butterfly" distribution of malar rash.

11. Erythema multiforme is called 貓眼瘡 [māo yǎn chuāng] ("cat's eye sore") in traditional Chinese medicine, for the characteristic lesion consists of a central papule with concentric rings resembling a cat's eye.

12. Erythema nodosum is called 瓜藤纏 [guā téng chán] (vine twining) in traditional Chinese medicine, for the skin lesions are most commonly located around the shins as if twined by a vine.

13. Pityriasis rosea is called 風熱瘡 [fēng rè chuāng] ("wind-heat sore") in traditional Chinese medicine, for it is a wind-heat contraction.

14. 皮痹 [pí bì] is characterized by chronic hardening and thickening of the skin, corresponding to scleroderma in Western medicine.

15. 白疕 [bái bǐ] is a skin disease characterized by circumscribed patches covered with white scales, corresponding to psoriasis in Western medicine.

16. Neurodermatitis is called 牛皮癬 [niú pí xuǎn] ("oxhide lichen") in traditional Chinese medicine, because the affected skin is thickened and hardened, giving the appearance of the skin of an ox's neck.

17. 紫癜風 [zǐ diàn fēng] ("purple wind-patch") is a pruritic skin disease characterized by an eruption of umbilicated, flat-topped papules, corresponding to lichen planus in Western medicine.

18. Vitiligo is called 白駁風 [bái bó fēng] in traditional Chinese medicine, but is more commonly called 白癜風 [bái diàn fēng] ("white wind-patch") at present.

19. 面遊風 [miàn yóu fēng] ("wandering wind of the face") is a pruritic skin disease, commonly located on the face, characterized by dry, moist or greasy scaling, and yellow crusted patches. It corresponds to seborrhoic dermatitis in Western medicine.

20. Literally, 黧黑斑 [lí hēi bān] means "blackish spots".

21. Acne corresponds to 粉刺 [fěn cì] in traditional Chinese medicine, but in the Chinese terminology of modern Western medicine, 痤瘡 [cuò chuāng] refers to acne, and 粉刺 [fěn cì] to comedo

22. Keloid is called 蟹足腫 [xiè zú zhǒng] (crab's leg swelling) in traditional Chinese medicine, for its crab-legged shape.

THERAPEUTICS

TERMS OF TREATMENT PRINCIPLES

In traditional Chinese medicine, treatment principles are usually classified into 治則 [zhì zé] and 治法 [zhì fǎ], which are often rendered literally as "treatment principle" and "treatment method" respectively. The term "treatment" is easy to understand, but the term "treatment method" may cause confusion. In English the word "method" refers to an established way of doing something or the means by which something is done. Therefore, when we say "treatment method", we first think of whether the patient is to be treated with herbal medication, acupuncture, surgical operation or some other method. In Chinese, however, the character 法 [fǎ] primarily means "law" or "rule". The difference between 法 [fǎ] and 則 [zé] is not always clear, and the two characters are often used in combination, forming a compound word 法則 [fǎ zé]. In the word 方法 [fāng fǎ], the character 法 [fǎ] means "method", but in the word 法則 [fǎ zé], the character 法 [fǎ] means "rule".

This issue can be further clarified with the following examples. 祛邪 [qū xié] (to eliminate pathogenic factors) is 治則 [zhì zé], while 清熱 [qīng rè] (to clear heat) is 治法 [zhì fǎ]. The only difference is that "eliminating pathogenic factors" is a general expression, and "clearing heat" is somewhat specific. If the former is called "treatment principle", one can hardly imagine that the latter should be called "treatment method". In Chinese medical publications written (but not translated) by Westerners the term "treatment method" is no more used in these cases, and "clearing heat" is also regarded as a treatment principle. This does not mean that the Chinese term 治法 [zhì fǎ] is irrational. In fact, its equivalent is "rule of treatment" rather than "method of treatment". Both 治則 [zhì zé] and 治法 [zhì fǎ] are guiding rules for treatment, the former being the guiding rule in general and the latter, the somewhat specific guiding rule.

In the standard nomenclature, there is no need to stick to the existing translation of Chinese terms. Since the two terms 治法 [zhì fǎ] and 治則 [zhì zé] can be combined into 治療法則 [zhì liáo fǎ zé], it is better to use the combined term instead of two separate ones. Jeremy Ross and other authors have tried this in their writings with success.

GENERAL TREATMENT PRINCIPLES

Chinese medicine has the following special features in terms of its concept of disease: Firstly, disease is regarded as a struggling process of the health *qi* against pathogenic factors. Therefore, the therapeutic principle should decide whether the treatment is aimed at strengthening the health *qi* or eliminating the pathogenic factors, or both. Secondly, from the holistic perspective, disease is considered as disharmony between different parts of the body and between the parts of the body and the whole, and so the basic principle of treatment is to restore the normal harmony. Thirdly, also from the holistic perspective, the patients and their diseases are always under the influence of the environment, and so the treatment should be suited to the environment, particularly to the time and place.

Proposed Standard Nomenclature

treatment principle 治療法則 [zhì liáo fǎ zé]

treatment based on pattern identification 辨證施[論]治 [biàn zhèng shī [lùn] zhì][1]

treating the secondary 治標 [zhì biāo][2]

same treatment for different diseases 異病同治 [yì bìng tóng zhì][3]

paradoxical treatment 反治 [fǎn zhì][4]

strengthen the healthy and dispel the pathogenic 扶正祛邪 [fú zhèng qū xié][6]

suiting (treatment) to place 因地制宜 [yīn dì zhì yí][7]

treatment based on syndrome differentiation 辨證施[論]治 [biàn zhèng shī [lùn] zhì][1]

treating the primary 治本 [zhì běn][2]

different treatments for same disease 同病異治 [tóng bìng yì zhì][3]

routine treatment 正治 [zhèng zhì][4]

preventive treatment 治未病 [zhì wèi bìng][5]

suiting (treatment) to person 因人制宜 [yīn rén zhì yí][7]

suiting (treatment) to time 因時制宜 [yīn shí zhì yí][7]

Discussion

1. 辨證施[論]治 [biàn zhèng shī [lùn] zhì] is a very important term in Chinese medicine. Grammatically it is composed of two verb-object word groups, 辨證 [biàn zhèng] and 施[論]治 [shī [lùn] zhì], without any connecting "functional character" to show the relationship between them. They may be coordinate, or the one may be subordinated to the other. Therefore, the whole term can be explained in different ways when it is used on different occasions.

When the term 辨證施[論]治 [biàn zhèng shī [lùn] zhì] is used as a subheading under the discussion of diseases in the textbooks and monographs, the verb-object word groups are usually coordinate. Generally, there are descriptions of the major clinical manifestations, analysis of the manifestations, treatment principle, exemplified formulae with possible modifications, and even discussion on the ingredients of the formulae. In such cases, the corresponding English subheading is "syndrome differentiation [pattern identification] and treatment".

On the other hand, 辨證施[論]治 [biàn zhèng shī [lùn] zhì] is the basic principle of treatment, reflecting one of the most unique features of Chinese medicine. In this context, the expressions in recent publications include "selection of treatment based on differential diagnosis", "therapy with syndrome differentiation", "planning treatment according to diagnosis", "treatment based on differential diagnosis", "determining treatment by patterns identified", "syndrome differentiation treatment", "treatment based on pattern discrimination", etc. From the above expressions, "treatment based on syndrome differentiation" or "treatment based on pattern identification" are selected as the proposed standard.

2. The first principle of Chinese medical treatment is 治病必求於本 [zhì bìng bì qiú yú běn], which has been rendered in various ways, such as "searching for the primary cause of disease in treatment", "to treat disease one should find its cause", "treatment should focus on the principal cause of a disease", "to treat disease, it is necessary to seek the root", "treatment must aim at the cause of the disease", "treatment must search for the primary cause of the disease", "to treat a disease one should find its root or cause" and "treating a disease by treating its primary cause". It is apparently a statement in a complete sentence rather than a technical term. None of the renderings can be regarded as a term. Nevertheless, 本 [běn] and 治本 [zhì běn] as well as their contrasts 標 [biāo] and 治標 [zhì biāo] are technical terms with unique features

of Chinese medicine. The equivalents of 本 [běn] versus 標 [biāo] suggested by different authors are "root" versus "tip", "root" versus "appearance", "radical" versus "symptomatic", "fundamental (aspect)" versus "incidental (aspect)", "cause" versus "effect", etc. The wide diversity comes from the multiple implications of the Chinese original. In terms of healthy *qi* and pathogenic *qi*, 本 [běn] refers to healthy *qi*, while 標 [biāo] refers to pathogenic *qi*; in terms of cause and manifestations, 本 [běn] refers to the cause of a disease, while 標 [biāo] refers to the manifestations or symptoms. In terms of primary and secondary diseases, 本 [běn] refers to the primary disease, while 標 [biāo] refers to secondary diseases or complications. Therefore, it is extremely difficult to find a single pair of English words that meet all the requirements. The phrase "root versus tip" is seemingly the briefest, but it corresponds to 本末 [běn mò] rather than 標本 [biāo běn]. "Radical treatment" versus "symptomatic treatment" is easy to understand, but too Westernized. Furthermore, 治標 [zhì biāo] is not limited to the treatment of symptoms; it also includes the treatment of secondary diseases and complications. Two pairs of wordings appearing in recent publications — "fundamental" vs "incidental", and "primary" vs "secondary" are probably applicable. Since the word "incidental" may imply something unimportant, "primary" vs "secondary" is thus selected.

3. In Chinese medicine different treatment principles are often applied to patients with the same disease, while the same treatment principle is often applied to patients with different diseases. This is called 同病異治 [tóng bìng yì zhì] and 異病同治 [yì bìng tóng zhì]. The English expressions "different treatments for same disease" and "same treatment for different diseases" seem appropriate, though there are other expressions such as "treat the disease with different principles [therapies or methods]" and "treat different diseases with the same principle [therapy or method]".

4. The characters 正 [zhèng] and 反 [fǎn] mean "straight [regular or ordinary]" and "opposite [contrary or reverse]", rspectively. Most authors express 正治 [zhèng zhì] as "routine treatment", which is generally acceptable. However, for 反治 [fǎn zhì], "contrary treatment" is obscure, and "treatment contrary to routine" is too wordy. Some authors prefer "paradoxical treatment". Since the word "paradoxical" means "seemingly absurd or contradictory but actually true", it is a suitable word to express the Chinese concept. For example, in Chinese

medicine the routine treatment of cold syndromes is the use of drugs hot in nature, but in exceptional cases, particularly when there is pseudo-cold manifestation, drugs cold in nature should be used. Such treatment of cold with cold is said to be 反治 [fǎn zhì], contrary to the routine treatment.

5. In Chinese medicine 治未病 [zhì wèi bìng] has dual meanings. It includes a treatment to prevent the occurrence of disease, and also an early treatment of a disease to prevent the occurrence of complications. Therefore, "preventive treatment" is more appropriate than simply "prevention".

6. A disease is always considered as a process of struggle between healthy (normal) *qi* and pathogenic (evil) *qi*, and their growth and decline determine the occurrence, development and outcome of the disease. Therefore, the basic principle of treatment is to strengthen healthy (normal) *qi*, and/or to dispel pathogenic (evil) *qi*. In Chinese this is called 扶正祛邪 [fú zhèng qū xié], which is rendered in various ways by different authors, e.g., "strengthening the body's resistance to eliminate pathogenic factors", "strengthening healthy *qi* to eliminate pathogens", "reinforcing the body's resistance to eliminate pathogens", "supporting healthy energy to eliminate evils", "strengthening body resistance to eliminate pathogens", "strengthening body resistance to eliminate pathogenic factors", "supporting healthy-*qi* to eliminate pathogenic factors", "reinforcing body resistance to eliminate pathogens", "supporting upright *qi* and expelling pathogenic factors", "strengthening the patient's resistance and dispelling pathogenic factors", "strengthening the body resistance and removing pathogenic factors", "supporting right and dispelling evil", etc. Again, the major divergence comes from the omission of the "functional character" between the two phrases 扶正 [fú zhèng] and 祛邪 [qū xié]. In reality, under this heading there may be several different patterns of treatment principles related to strengthening healthy *qi* and dispelling pathogenic factors: (1) separate application, as "strengthening healthy *qi*" (扶正 [fú zhèng]) alone or "dispelling pathogenic factors" (祛邪 [qū xié]) alone; (2) concurrent application, with one as primary and the other as secondary, i.e., "strengthening healthy *qi* and dispelling pathogenic factors in addition" (扶正兼祛邪 [fú zhèng jiān qū xié]) or "dispelling pathogenic factors while strengthening healthy *qi* in addition" (祛邪兼扶正 [qū xié jiān fú zhèng]); (3) sequential application, as one followed by the other, i.e., "strengthening healthy *qi* followed by dispelling pathogenic factors"

(扶正後祛邪 [fú zhèng hòu qū xié]) or "dispelling pathogenic factors followed by strengthening healthy *qi*" (祛邪後扶正 [qū xié hòu fú zhèng]). The last two terms can also be expressed as "reinforcement followed by attack" (先補後攻 [xiān bǔ hòu gōng]) and "attack followed by reinforcement" (先攻後補 [xiān gōng hòu bǔ]), respectively. Based on the above discussion, it is better to express this concept in the most general way, i.e., "strengthening healthy *qi* and dispelling pathogenic factors".

7. Individualization is another prominent feature of Chinese medical treatment. According to the holistic perspective, with correspondence between a person and the universe, one of the basic principles of treatment is that the treatment should be suited to the patient's constitution, sex, age and other features, to the geographical circumstances, and to seasonal and climatic factors, which are called "suiting the person" (因人制宜 [yīn rén zhì yí]), "suiting the place" 因地制宜 [yīn dì zhì yí], and "suiting the time" (因時制宜 [yīn shí zhì yí]), respectively. There are other English expressions, such as "treatment chosen according to the variability of climate, locality and physique of the individual", "treat a disease according to the individual, the environment and the season", "treatment in accordance with the physique of the individual, with regard to local and seasonal conditions", "treating a disease according to the seasons, the environment and the individual", "treating the disease according to the individual's condition, to the environment and to the climate", "act(ion) according to the person, place and time", etc. Almost all these expressions are concerned with treatment, but the original Chinese terms are common idioms applicable to designing any measures other than medical treatment.

SPECIFIC TREATMENT PRINCIPLES

Most terms regarding specific treatment principles are verb-object word groups. The basic form of such a word group is usually composed of a transitive verb and its object, i.e., a two-character phrase, but customarily two or more word groups are combined to form the term. For example, "strengthen the spleen (健脾 [jiàn pí])" and "resolve damp (化濕 [huà shī])" are often used in combination as 健脾化濕 [jiàn pí huà shī]. In the compound terms, the functional character (equivalent to a preposition or conjunction in English) between the two basic terms is often omitted, and different explanations may be given. Thus, 健脾化濕 [jiàn pí huà shī] may be understood as "strengthen the spleen and resolve damp simultaneously", "strengthen the spleen primarily and resolve damp secondarily", "strengthen the spleen first and then resolve damp", and "strengthen the spleen to resolve damp". It is hard to say which one is definitely right or wrong. In fact, one can use the term in any of the senses as one wishes. So, in order to avoid this kind of uncertainty, only the basic terms of treatment principles are given in this scheme. Various arrangements and combinations of the basic terms with necessary insertion of conjunctions or prepositions may be made by the users themselves.

In Chinese medicine, the terms for expressing the treatment principles are also used for describing the actions of medicines and acupuncture points. For example, "strengthen the spleen" (健脾 [jiàn pí])" is a treatment principle, and it is also one of the pharmacological effects of ginseng and an action of the acupoint zusanli (ST36). In this scheme, the verb form is used for these purposes, but whenever the term is used as attributive the present participle form may be adopted, such as "spleen-strengthening".

The characters used as verbs in these terms can be listed in the following table. For each of these characters there are usually several renderings suggested by different authors. Selection of one or two equivalents will be very helpful for standardizing the related terms.

Because of the rich and colorful vocabulary of Chinese language, many characters are used with subtle differences in meaning; when they are used mainly for rhetoric purposes, the differences are negligible. For example, one can hardly make any definite distinction among 補益氣血 [bǔ yì qì xuè], 氣血雙補 [qì xuè shuāng bǔ], 益氣養血 [yì qì yǎng xuè] and 補氣養血 [bǔ qì yǎng xuè]. They have the same meaning, and are selected in accordance with the context. The Chinese pay attention to parallelism in composition. If the preceding phrase is a double-character verb + double-character object, 補益氣血 [bǔ yì qì xuè] is a preferable choice. If the preceding phrase is a combination of two word groups, each containing a single-character verb + single-character object, it is usually followed by 益氣養血 [yì qì yǎng xuè] or 補氣養血 [bǔ qì yǎng xuè]. The habitual variation of word-formation in Chinese is not necessarily reflected in the English expression; on the contrary, only one uniform phrase pattern should be adopted in the standard terminology.

In the above examples, also from the rhetorical perspective, some characters are added. Deletion of these characters does not at all change the real meaning of the phrase. There is actually no difference between 補氣血 [bǔ qì xuè] and 補益氣血 [bǔ yì qì xuè] or 氣血雙補 [qì xuè shuāng bǔ]. In the latter two terms, the characters 益 [yì] and 雙 [shuāng] are rhetorically necessary but explanatorily negligible. Therefore, all the expressions including 益氣養血 [yì qì yǎng xuè] and 補氣養血 [bǔ qì yǎng xuè] can be rendered as "tonify *qi* and blood" or "*qi*-blood tonifying".

For standardizing the terms of this category, the key words are the verbs used in these terms. In Chinese, synonyms are often used. They may have the same meaning, but may also differ in meaning subtly. Before the discussion of each term, it is better to have a general review of the various renderings of the verbs appearing in recent publications. They are listed in the following table.

Specific characters commonly used in therapeutic principles

Chinese character		Translations by different authors	Standard term recommended
解	表	release, relieve, resolve, flush (the exterior); relieve, resolve (exterior syndrome); induce diaphoresis	release (the exterior)
	肌	release (muscles), resolve (flesh)	release (muscles)
	毒	resolve, relieve (toxicity), eliminate (toxin), detoxicate	relieve (toxicity)
	痙	relieve (spasm)	relieve (spasm)
發	表	release, effuse, vent (the exterior)	release (the exterior)
	汗	induce, promote (sweating); effuse, induce (sweat); induce, cause (diaphoresis)	promote (sweating)
疏	風	dispel, course, dissipate, expel, disperse (wind)	disperse (wind)
	肝	soothe, clear, course (the liver) disperse, spread (liver *qi*)	soothe (the liver)
散	風、寒	disperse, dispel, expel (cold)	disperse (wind, cold)
	結、瘀	dissipate, disperse (nodulation or accumulation, stasis)	dissipate (nodulation, stasis)

宣	肺	diffuse, clear, ventilate (the lung); disseminate ventilate, release, mobilize (lung-*qi*); restore the dispersing and descending (of lung-*qi*); facilitate the flow (of lung-*qi*); promote the dispersing function (of the lung); open the inhibited (lung-*qi*); release stagnated (lung-*qi*)	disseminate (lung *qi*)
祛	風、寒 暑、痰 濕	dispel, expel, eliminate (wind, cold, summer heat, phlegm, damp)	dispel (wind, cold, summer heat, phlegm, damp)
	瘀	dispel, eliminate, remove (blood stasis)	dispel (stasis)
去	腐	remove, eliminate (putridity or necrotic tissue)	eliminate (putridity)
逐	寒、瘀 水、飲	expel, dispel, eliminate, remove (cold, stasis, water, fluid)	expel (cold, stasis, water, fluid)
除	痞、熱	relieve (stuffiness, fever)	relieve
	濕、痰	eliminate, disperse, remove, expel, relieve (dampness, phlegm)	eliminate (dampness, phlegm)
熄	風	calm, check, extinguish, inhibit, stop (wind)	extinguish (wind)
清	熱	clear, clear up, clear away, eliminate, remove, purge (heat)	clear (heat)
	火	clear, clear away, purge, quench (fire)	clear (fire)
	暑	clear, clear away (summer heat)	clear (summer heat)
	裏、營 心、肝 肺、胃 腸、膽	clear, clear away, remove, purge, eliminate, quench (the interior, nutrient, heart, liver, lung, stomach, intestine, or gallbladder)	clear (the interior, nutrient, heart, liver, lung, stomach, intestine, or gallbladder)
涼	血、營 膈	cool, remove heat from (the blood, nutrient, diaphragm)	cool (the blood, nutrient, diaphragm)
瀉	火	purge, drain, reduce (fire)	purge (fire)
	心、肝 脾、肺 腎	purge, discharge (the heart, liver, spleen, lung, kidney)	purge (the heart, liver, spleen, lung, kidney)

下	乳	promote, encourage, induce, stimulate (lactation)	stimulate (lactation)
降	氣	send down, direct downward, redirect downward, downbear, descend (*qi*), restore the descending of (*qi*), depress upward-reverse flow of (*qi*)	send (*qi*) downward
升	陽	elevate, raise, lift, upbear, activate, invigorate (yang)	raise (yang)
提	膿	draw out (pus)	draw out (pus)
化	痰、濕 濁、瘀	resolve, dissipate, eliminate, remove, transform (damp, phlegm, turbidity or stasis)	resolve (damp, phlegm, turbidity or stasis)
燥	濕	dry, eliminate (dampness)	dry (dampness)
滲	濕	drain, percolate, excrete, remove, eliminate, leach out (dampness)	drain (dampness)
排	膿	drain, discharge, evacuate, expel (pus)	expel (pus)
止	痛、癢 咳、嘔 呃、瀉 渴	stop, alleviate, relieve, arrest (a symptom or suffering, such as pain, itching, cough, vomiting, hiccups, diarrhea, thirst)	stop, relieve (pain, itching, cough, vomiting, hiccups, diarrhea, thirst)
	汗	stop, check, suppress, inhibit (sweating or perspiration)	stop, check (sweating)
	血	stop, arrest (bleeding or hemorrhage)	stop (bleeding)
	帶	arrest, stop, check, cure (vaginal discharge, leukorrhea, or leukorrhagia)	arrest (vaginal discharge)
	遺	arrest (enuresis)	arrest (enuresis)
平	肝	calm, pacify, check (the liver)	pacify (the liver)
	喘	relieve, arrest (asthma)	relieve (asthms)
潛	陽	anchor, check, suppress, subdue, restrain, pacify (yang)	subdue (yang)
熄	風	check, subdue, calm, extinguish (wind)	extinguish (wind)
安	神	calm, tranquilize, quiet (the mind)	calm (the mind)
	蛔	quiet (roundworm), relieve (ascaris colic)	quiet (ascaris)

	胎	prevent (abortion), prevent (miscarriage), quiet (the fetus)	prevent (abortion)
寧	心	calm, tranquilize (the mind) quite (the heart)	calm (the mind)
定	志	stabilize (the mind) calm (the emotional strain)	stabilize (the mind)
寬	中、胸	soothe (the middle, the chest), loosen (the center, the chest)	soothe (the middle, chest)
疏	肝	soothe, course, clear (the liver); spread (liver *qi*)	soothe (the liver)
	風	disperse, dissipate, dispel, expel, course (wind)	disperse (wind)
和	胃、絡	harmonize (the stomach, meridian)	harmonize (the stomach, meridian, nutrient, blood)
	營、血	harmonize, regulate, enrich (the nutrient, blood)	
理	氣	regulate, rectify, regulate the flow of, normalize the flow of (*qi*)	regulate (*qi*)
溫	陽	warm (yang)	warm (yang)
	中、裏 經、臟 腑	dispel cold from, warm (the middle, interior, meridian, kidney, spleen, stomach, etc.)	warm (the middle, interior, meridian, kidney, spleen, stomach, etc.)
補	陰、陽 火、氣 精、血 心、肝 脾、肺 腎、中	benefit, invigorate, nourish, recuperate, reinforce, replenish, supplement, tonify (yin, yang, fire, *qi*, essence, blood, heart, liver, spleen, lung, kidney, middle energizer, etc.)	tonify or reinforce (yin, yang, fire, *qi*, essence, blood, heart, liver, spleen, lung, kidney, middle energizer, etc.)
益	氣	aid, augment, benefit, boost, enhance, invigorate, nourish, reinforce, replenish, supplement, tonify	replenish (*qi*)
	精	boost, nourish, replenish, tonify (the essence)	replenish (essence)
	肺、胃 腎	benefit, boost, reinforce, nourish, replenish, tonify (the lung, stomach, kidney)	tonify (the lung, stomach, kidney)
滋	陰、肝 腎	nourish, enrich (yin, liver, kidney)	nourish (yin, liver, kidney)

養	血、陰 心、胃	nourish, replenish, enrich (blood, yin, heart, stomach)	nourish (blood, yin, heart, stomach)
健	脾、胃	invigorate, strengthen, fortify, reinforce, activate, improve the function of , promote the function of (the spleen or stomach)	invigorate (the spleen or stomach)
壯	陽	invigorate, promote, strengthen, support, fortify, tonify (yang)	strengthen
扶	正	support, reinforce, strengthen, assist (healthy *qi*, right, or body resistance)	support (healthy *qi*)
助	陽	support, assist (yang)	support (yang)
生	肌	generate; regenerate (flesh) promote (granulation or tissue regeneration)	regenerate (flesh or tissue)
	津	promote (secretion, salivation, or fluid production) improve (secretion) produce (salivation) engender (liquid)	promote (fluid production)
醒	脾	enliven, activate, arouse invigorate (the spleen)	enliven (the spleen)
開	胃	improve, increase, induce, whet, promote, stimulate (appetite) open, promote the function of (the stomach)	promote (appetite)
	音	recover (yang)restore, ease-up (voice)	restore (yang)restore (voice)
	竅	induce, promote (resuscitation) open (the orifices)	induce (resuscitation)
回	陽	recuperate, restore, revive, return (yang)	restore (yang)
	乳	stop, terminate (lactation or milk secretion)	stop (lactation)
行	氣	activate, promote the flow of, promote the circulation of , conduct, move (*qi*)	move (*qi*)
通	陽	activate, invigorate, free, warm, unblock, promote the flow of, ensure the flow of (yang)	unblock (yang)

	腑	free, relax, clear (the bowels, hollow viscera)	free (the bowels)
	絡	dredge, unblock, remove obstruction from (collaterals)	unblock (collateral)
	經	free, clear, dredge, remove obstruction of, dispel obstruction of (the meridian)	unblock (meridian)
		promote, free, induce, stimulate, restore (menstruation)	promote (menstruation)
	乳	promote (lactation), free (milk)	promote (lactation)
	淋	treat, free, unblock, relieve (stranguria)	relieve (stranguria)
	竅	free, open (the orifices)	free (the orfices)
明	目	improve, promote (vision, acuity of vision, visual acuity) brighten (the eyes)	improve (vision)
利	濕	drain, disinhibit, eliminate, expel, remove, excrete, clear away (damp or dampness)	drain (dampness)
	水、尿	induce, promote (diuresis or urination), disinhibit (water)	promote (urination)
	咽	relieve (sore throat) benefit, strengthen (the throat)	relieve (sore throat)
	膽	benefit, normalize, promote (the gallbladder or the function of the gallbladder)	promote (bile flow)
消	食	promote, improve (digestion) remove (food stagnancy) disperse (food accumulation)	promote (digestion)
	腫	alleviate, reduce (edema) disperse (swelling)	alleviate (edema or swelling)
	痰	eliminate, disperse, resolve (phlegm)	resolve (phlegm)
	痞	remove, eliminate, disintegrate (mass) disperse (glomus)	disperse (mass)
	癥	eliminate, disperse (abdominal mass)	disperse (abdominal mass)
退	黃、熱	cure, relieve (fever, jaundice)	relieve (fever, jaundice)

固	本	consolidate, enhance, secure, strengthen (the origin, root, constitution or body resistance)	strengthen (the body resistance)
	表	consolidate, secure, strengthen (the exterior or superficies)	strengthen (the superficies)
	脫	restore from (collapse) stem (desertion)	restore from (collapse)
	經	arrest (uterine bleeding) cure, treat (metrorrhagia), secure (the menses)	arrest (uterine bleeding)
澀	腸	astringe, bind up (the intestines)	astringe (the intestines)
	精	Arrest, astringe, treat, control (seminal emission); bind up, astringe, preserve (essence or semen)	astringe (essence or semen)
潤	燥、肺 腸、膚	moisten, emolliate (dryness, lung, intestine, skin)	moisten

Lengthy explanatory translations that disrupt the basic form of technical terms are not collected in this table because they cannot be regarded and used as terms, no matter how completely they express the original Chinese medical concept. For example, "set the *qi* in motion"; and "let the *qi* circulate" are not listed in the table as equivalents of 行氣 [xíng qì]. Similarly, "warm the kidney to reinforce its vital function" cannot be taken as an equivalent for 溫腎(陽) [wēn shèn (yáng)].

I. Exterior-releasing (Diaphoresis) 解表 (汗法)

Releasing the exterior is a general term for dispelling pathogenic factors from the exterior of the body, a common principle for treating exterior syndromes. As this therapeutic principle is often implemented by inducing sweating, it is also called diaphoresis. Under this heading, the following terms are commonly encountered.

Proposed Standard Nomenclature

release the exterior 解表 [jiě biǎo][1]   exterior-releasing therapy 解表法

release muscles 解肌 [jiě jī][2]   [jiě biǎo fǎ][1]

diaphoresis 汗法 [hàn fǎ][3]   induce sweating 發汗 [fā hàn][3]
dispel wind 祛風 [qū fēng][4]   disperse wind 疏風 [shū fēng][5]
disperse cold 散寒 [sàn hán][6]   promote (skin) eruption 透疹 (tòu zhěn)[7]

Discussion

1. A variety of translations have been used for expressing 解表 [jiě biǎo]. The translation "relieve the exterior syndrome" is correct, but explanatory, and "expel (or dispel) pathogenic factors from the exterior of the body" is totally explanatory and too lengthy. A group of expressions are related to diaphoresis, e.g., to induce diaphoresis. This is not exact, because besides diaphoresis there are other ways to relieve exterior syndromes. Some authors abbreviate the term "relieve the exterior syndrome" to "relieve the exterior". The abbreviated form seems to coincide with the original Chinese term, but there is a problem in collocation, as the object of "relieve" is usually a pain, distress or suffering. Two other verbs are used in this case: "resolve" and "release". In comparison, the latter is more appropriate, and has been easily and smoothly used in Dan Bensky's and Giovanni Maciocia's books.

2. 解肌 [jiě jī] is a general term for dispelling pathogenic factors from the superficial muscles. For similar reasons as stated above, "release muscles" is an appropriate choice.

3. For 發汗 [fā hàn] many authors prefer using the word "diaphoresis", and 發汗藥 [fā hàn yào] "diaphoretics". Undoubtedly, these terms can be well accepted for the terms in Chinese and in English are generally recognized equivalents in the reverse manner in Western medicine. Furthermore, in order to make the terminology parallel to the related terms, a verb-object phrase is also preferred. Among various but basically similar expressions, "induce sweating" is selected as the proposed standard.

4. Both the terms "dispel wind" 祛風 [qū fēng] and "disperse wind" 疏風 [shū fēng] are used as the treatment principle of external wind contraction, but they have some minor differences. The latter is only used for removing pathogens from the body surface, while the former is effective for expelling pathogens not only from the body surface, but also from the meridians, muscles and joints. In some Chinese books 祛風 [qū fēng] may also be a therapeutic principle of endogenous wind,

but in the State Standard Terminology it is only indicated for treating exogenous wind. As the English equivalent of 祛 [qū], most authors use "dispel" or "eliminate".

5. 疏風 [shū fēng] is a treatment principle for relieving exterior syndromes caused by external wind. It is an abbreviation for 疏散風邪 [shū sàn fēng xié], and so it is also called 散風 [sàn fēng]. The characters 疏 [shū] and 散 [sàn] are only used for getting rid of external wind, not endogenous wind, for it may be misunderstood as spreading the pathogenic wind throughout the body. For endogenous wind, the ordinary treatment is called 熄風 [xī fēng] ("extinguish wind")

The character 疏 [shū] has several translations: "dispel", "dissipate", "expel", "disperse", "course", etc. Most authors use the word "disperse", which means scatter and disappear, which best conforms to the original Chinese concept.

6. The characters 疏 [shū] and 散 [sàn] are synonymous, but the treatment of exterior cold is customarily called 散寒 [sàn hàn]. In this scheme, either 疏 [shū] or 散 [sàn] is rendered as "disperse", and so "disperse cold" is taken as the proposed standard equivalent of 散寒 [sàn hàn].

It should be noted that "dispersing cold" can also be applied to the treatment of interior cold syndromes, particularly when there is direct attack of external cold to the interior.

7. 透疹 [tòu zhěn] is a special therapeutic principle in the treatment of measles and some other eruptive infectious diseases when the skin eruption is impaired or inadequate. It is believed that the pathogens can be expelled from the body through the eruption, so that complications can be prevented. Most authors use the term "promote (skin) eruption", but some use other terms such as "let out skin eruptions", "outthrust papules", "expose exanthema", "vent rashes". By comparison with papules, exanthema and rashes, the word eruption or skin eruption may be more appropriate. Firstly, it is not confined to papule. The rashes in measles are usually maculopapular. Secondly, it refers not only to the skin lesions, but particularly to the process of rash appearance, for this therapeutic principle is indicated in treating 疹出不暢 [zhěn chū bù chàng] (impaired eruption).

II. Heat-clearing 清熱 (清法)

"Heat-clearing", abbreviated as "clearing", is a general term indicating the basic principle of treating various heat syndromes. Since fire is intense heat, clearing therapy also includes fire-clearing. In practical use, the terminology often contains the site where the heat or fire is located. For example, "clear the heart" (清心 [qīng xīn]) means "clear the heart of fire", and is also called "clear heart fire" (清心火 [qīng xīn huǒ]). In this scheme, only the briefer expression is adopted in order to keep consistency with the Chinese version of *Clinical Terminology of Traditional Chinese Medical Diagnosis and Treatment — Therapeutic Methods* promulgated by the State Technology Supervision Bureau, P.R. China in 1997. Similarly, "clear the lung" (清肺 [qīng fèi]) means "clear away heat or fire from the lung", and "clear the stomach" (清胃 [qīng wèi]) means "clear stomach heat or fire", etc. Treatment of heat in the blood is an exception. It is called 清血分熱 [qīng xuè fèn rè] or 涼血 [liáng xuè], but not 清血 [qīng xuè], and so the proposed standard terminology is "cool the blood" or "blood-cooling".

Proposed Standard Nomenclature

clear heat 清熱 [qīng rè][1]

(heat- or fire-)clearing therapy 清法 [qīng fǎ][2]

clear the lung 清肺 [qīng fèi][1]

clear the intestines 清腸 [qīng cháng][1]

clear the nutrient 清營 [qīng yíng][1,5]

purge the lung 瀉肺 [xiè fèi][4]

cool the blood 涼血 [liáng xuè][5]

clear fire 清火 [qīng huǒ][1]

clear the heart 清心 [qīng xīn][1]

clear the stomach 清胃 [qīng wèi][1]

clear the liver 清肝 [qīng gān][1]

clear the gallbladder 清膽 [qīng dǎn][1]

clear the *qi* 清氣 [qīng qì]

purge fire 瀉火 [xiè huǒ][3]

purge the liver 瀉肝 [xiè gān][4]

Discussion

1. 清熱 [qīng rè] is an important therapy for treating interior heat. As its equivalent, the term "clear heat" has already been accepted by most authors. Some other expressions such as "remove heat" and "eliminate heat" are not recommended, because they are too general, and 清熱 [qīng rè] has its specific implication. It is believed in Chinese medicine that heat in the exterior is usually removed by dispersion, but

heat in the interior should not be dispersed; it should be cleared out or purged away. A variety of technical terms are formed on the basis of "clear heat". For the terms associated with clearing heat from a certain organ or part of the body, the rule of word-building is "clear + name of the organ or site". For example, "clear the lung of heat" of "clear heat from the lung" is expressed as "clear the lung". Some authors prefer the term "clear lung heat", for its correspondence with "清肺熱 [qīng fèi rè]". In this scheme of nomenclature "clear the lung" is recommended because it is most succinct, and in the Chinese State Standard only the term 清肺 [qīng fèi] is used. In addition, fire is considered as intense heat, and so 清肺熱 [qīng fèi rè] and 清肺火 [qīng fèi huǒ] may be mixed up, but they actually refer to the same thing. Sticking to the Chinese terminology, there would be two proposed standard terms "clear lung heat" and "clear lung fire", while "clear the lung" is applicable in either case. Similarly, "clear the heart" means "clear heat or fire from the heart" or "clear the heart of heat or fire", "clear the liver" means "clear heat or fire from the liver" or "clear the liver of heat or fire", and so forth. "Clear the nutrient" means "clear the nutrient system of heat" or "clear away heat from the nutrient system.". But for removing heat from the blood, the word "clear" is not applicable.

2. "Clearing therapy" (清 [qīng fǎ]) includes "heat-clearing" (清熱 [qīng rè]) and "fire-clearing" 清火 ([qīng huǒ]).

3. "Purge fire" (瀉火 [xiè huǒ]) is a treatment similar to "clear heat" but more drastic since fire is more intense than heat. In addition, purgatives are often used to clear the fire, and so the term "purge the fire" is advocated by most authors.

4. A number of technical terms are derived from 'purge fire" in a similar way to "clear heat". For example, "purge the liver" actually means "purge the liver of fire" or "purge the liver fire". 清 [qīng] and 瀉 [xiè] are often used in combination when a double-charactered verb is necessary for word-building in Chinese, e.g., 清瀉肝膽 [qīng xiè gān dǎn]. In this case, "purge the liver and gallbladder" is an appropriate term. There is no need to say "clear and purge the liver and gallbladder" because "purge" already has the meaning of clear or clean, and in Chinese the addition of the character 清 [qīng] is purely for rhetorical purposes.

5. Most authors render 涼血 [liáng xuè] as "cool the blood". The definition of this term is clear-cut, i.e., to remove pathogenic heat from the blood. It is not called 清血 [qīng xuè] However, the treatment to remove

pathogenic heat from the nutrient is called "clear the nutrient". In Chinese medicine, nutrient and blood are closely associated, and heat invading the nutrient often involves the blood. For rhetorical reasons, if the term "clear the nutrient" is given to the removal of pathogenic heat from the nutrient system, it is better not to use the term "clear the blood" in order to avoid such a repetition as "clear the nutrient and clear the blood" 清營清血 [qīng yíng qīng xuè], and hence "cool the blood" 涼血 [liáng xuè].

III. Dampness-dispelling 祛濕

Dampness-dispelling is a general term collectively indicating various treatments for dampness. It includes resolving dampness with aromatics, draining dampness through diuresis, and drying dampness by means of desiccating agents.

Proposed Standard Nomenclature

dispel damp(ness) 祛濕 [qū shī][1]

resolve damp(ness) 化濕 [huà shī][2]

promote urination 利水[尿] [lì shuǐ [niào][4]

dry dampness 燥濕 [zào shī][5]

damp-dispelling therapy 祛濕法 [qū shī][1]

drain damp(ness) 利濕 [lì shī][3] 滲濕 [shèn shī][3]

diuresis 利水[尿] [lì shuǐ [niào][4]

eliminate damp(ness) 除濕 [chú shī][6]

Discussion

1. The general term indicating treatment for getting rid of dampness is 祛濕 [qū shī]. It is rendered as "dispel damp(ness)" by most authors.

2. 化濕 [huà shī] is treatment for dispelling dampness, especially that lodging in the upper energizer or exterior portion of the body by using aromatics. The Chinese character 化 [huà] has many different meanings when it is used as a verb in medicine. It means (1) change (變化 [biàn huà]) or transform (轉化 [zhuǎn huà]), (2) digest (消化 [xiāo huà]), and (3) dissolve (融化 [róng huà]) or cause to vanish (化滅 [huà miè]). Therefore, for the term 化濕 [huà shī] various translations have appeared in recent publications, such as "dissolve damp", "eliminate damp", "remove damp", "transform damp", and "resolve damp". Among these translations, "eliminate damp" and "remove damp" are too general,

and cannot exactly reflect the original meaning. The word "transform" is quite frequently used for the translation of the word 化 [huà], probably because it is suitable for expressing pathological terms such as 化火 [huà huǒ], 化風 [huà fēng], 化熱 [huà rè] and 化燥 [huà zào], which mean transform into fire, wind, heat and dryness, respectively. But 化濕 [huà shī] as a treatment principle has a different meaning from a pathological change, and it can never be understood as transform something into damp. Rendering it as "transform damp" will naturally lead to the question "into what?" "Resolve damp" may be the most appropriate translation, because "resolve" used in medicine means "to cause to disperse or to be absorbed without the formation of pus" (*The New International Webster's Comprehensive Dictionary of the English Language*, 1996 edition). This is also what 化痰 [huà tán] means. Many authors prefer "resolve damp" and "resolve phlegm" for these terms.

3. To remove dampness by promoting urination is called 利水滲濕 [lì shuǐ shèn shī], or 滲濕 [shèn shī] for short, in which the character 滲 is rendered as "drain", "percolate", "leach out", "remove", "eliminate" or "excrete" by different authors. Among these words, "drain" best reflects the Chinese concept. 利濕 [lì shī] is synonymous with 滲濕 [shèn shī], and so it is unnecessary to propose another standard term.

4. 利水 [lì shuǐ], same as 利尿 [lì niào], is usually expressed as "induce diuresis" or "promote urination". Some authors suggest "disinhibit water", which is difficult to understand.

5. Most authors render 燥濕 [zào shī] as "dry dampness", while a few others render it as "eliminate dampness". The word "dessicate" suggested by some authors seems to be too serious, as it means to remove all the moisture.

6. In the Chinese language, 祛 [qū] and 除 [chú] are synonymous, and often used in combination as 祛除 [qū chú]. Customarily, 祛濕 [qū shī] and 除濕 [chú shī] have some minor differences in use. The former is a general term including all kinds of dampness-relieving treatment, while the latter usually refers to treatment of dampness involving the meridians or in morbid conditions with liquid discharge. Most authors render 除濕 [chú shī] as "eliminate dampness", while others render it as "remove dampness".

IV. (Dryness-)Moistening 潤燥

Moistening is a general term indicating the treatment of dryness. It includes the treatment of endogenous dryness due to consumption of body fluid and that of exogenous dryness in external contractions.

Proposed Standard Nomenclature

produce fluid 生津 [shēng jīn][1]

moistening therapy 潤(燥)法 [rùn zào fǎ][3]

moistening the intestines; 潤腸 [rùn cháng][4]

increase fluid 增液 [zēng yè][2]

moisten dryness 潤燥 [rùn zào][3]

moisten the lung 潤肺 [rùn fèi][4]

moisten the skin 潤膚 [rùn fū][4]

Discussion

1. The rational way to cure internal dryness is to promote the production of body fluid. This is called 生津 [shēng jīn], and in English expressed as "engender liquid", "produce fluid", "increase fluid", or "promote fluid production". Since the character 津 [jīn] in its narrow sense means saliva, some authors render 生津 [shēng jīn] as "promote salivation". This is not recommended.

2. There are several ways to express 增液 [zēng yè] if 液 [yè] is rendered as "fluid": "increase fluid", "produce fluid", "increase the production of fluid", and "promote the production of fluid", among which "increase fluid" as well as "fluid-increasing" is direct to the point.

3. Most authors render 潤燥 [rùn zào] as "moisten dryness", though the expression may not be so idiomatic. In many instances, the word "moisten" or "moistening" is clear enough.

4. In these terms, most authors use the word "moisten". Some other suggestions such as "wet", "moisturize" and "lubricate" are not widely accepted.

V. Purgation 瀉下(下法)

Purgation refers to a variety of treatment characterized by vigorous evacuation of the bowels. In Chinese medicine, purgation is not only used for relieving intestinal stagnancy, but also for removing heat, fire, toxins, and even retained fluid or water.

Proposed Standard Nomenclature

purge; purgation 瀉下 [xiè xià][1]

purgative therapy 下法 [xià fǎ][1]

cold purgation 寒下 [hán xià][2]

laxation 緩下 [huǎn xià][3]

expel water 逐水 [zhú shuǐ]

purgation 下法 [xià fǎ][1]

warm purgation 溫下 [wēn xià][2]

drastic purgation 峻下 [jùn xià][3]

lubricant laxation 潤下 [rùn xià][3]

hydragogue 逐水 [zhú shu][4]

Discussion

1. Some authors always want to designate Chinese medical terms with words different from those of Western medicine. It is true that the Chinese and Western systems of medicine have their own characteristic features that should not be mixed up. However, this does not mean that they have nothing in common. "Purgation" in Western medicine and 瀉下 [xiè xià] in Chinese medicine refer to the same action. Even the drugs used for this purpose are often identical, such as rhubarb, aloe, senna leaf and sodium sulfate. Therefore, it is unnecessary to express the concept 瀉下 [xiè xià] with a word other than "purgation".

2. The character 下 [xià] in the terms 溫下 [wēn xià] and 寒下 [hán xià] is an abbreviation of 瀉下 [xiè xià]. If we agree that purgation or catharsis is equivalent to 瀉下 [xiè xià], there is no need for a special rendering of 下 [xià].

3. The drastic act of purging the bowels is called 峻下 [jùn xià], and the mild act of evacuating the bowels is called 緩下 [huǎn xià]. The latter is consistent with "laxation", and 緩下劑 [huǎn xià jì], laxative. There is really no need for creation of new English terms.

4. Literally, 逐水 [zhú shuǐ] means "expelling water". It basically conforms to hydragogue. However, while hydragogue refers to producing watery discharge from the bowels, the Chinese term stresses the discharge of water rather than watery discharge.

VI. Harmonization 和法，和解法

Harmonization is a therapy for adjusting the functions of the human body for restoring normal correlation between the internal organs or between *qi* and blood, or eliminating the pathogenic factors from the part between the exterior and interior of the body, also known as harmonizing therapy.

Proposed Standard Nomenclature

harmonization 和法 [hé fǎ][1]

harmonize the exterior and interior 和解表裏 [hé jiě biǎo lǐ][2]

check malaria 截瘧 [jié nüè][2]

harmonize the spleen and stomach 調和脾胃 [tiáo hé pí wèi][3]

harmonize the liver and spleen 調和肝脾 [tiáo hé gān pí][3]

harmonize the nutrient 和營 [hé yíng][3]

harmonize qi and blood 調和氣血 [tiáo hé qì xuè][3]

harmonize 和解 [hé jiě]; 調和 [tiáo hé][1]

harmonize the lesser yang 和解少陽 [hé jiě shào yáng][2]

harmonize the stomach 和胃 [hé wèi][3]

harmonize the liver and stomach 調和肝胃 [tiáo hé gān wèi][3]

harmonize the blood 和血 [hé xuè][3]

harmonize the nutrient and defense 調和營衛 [tiáo hé yíng wèi][3]

Discussion

1. Different expressions have been suggested to express the concept of 和(法) [hé (fǎ)]: "mediation", "harmonization", "regulation", and "reconciliation". More and more authors are using the word "harmonization", probably because it has more sense of restoring the normal harmonious correlation. In the Chinese terms, 和 [hé] is an abbreviation of 和解 [hé jiě] and 調和 [tiáo hé]. Strictly speaking, the latter two terms have some minor difference: 和解 [hé jiě] means harmonize and release, and 調和 [tiáo hé] means regulate and harmonize. The former treatment is indicated in relieving external contractions, while the latter is suitable for adjusting functional activities.

2. "Harmonizing the exterior and interior" (和解表裏 [hé jiě biǎo lǐ]) is a treatment for relieving half-exterior and half-interior syndromes. It includes harmonizing the lesser yang, checking malaria, and some other treatments.

A half-exterior and half-interior syndrome is characterized by alternate chills and fever. That is why the treatment of malaria is classified in the category of exterior-interior harmonizing. The term 截瘧 [jié nüè] is rendered in various ways by different authors: "check malarial conditions", "prevent attack of malaria", "stop malaria paroxym", "interrupt malaria", etc.

In lesser yang syndrome, the pathogen exists between the exterior and the interior, and the clinical manifestation is marked by alternate chills and fever. So it should also be treated by harmonization.

3. Harmonization is an important treatment for relieving functional disorders of internal organs. In this case, the single character 和 [hé] is an abbreviation of 調和 [tiáo hé]. In Chinese terminology, whether 和 [hé] or 調和 [tiáo hé] is used depends upon the total number of characters that the term contains. For example, it is customary to say 和胃 [hé wèi] and 調和脾胃 [tiáo hé pí wèi], but not 調和胃 [tiáo hé wèi] or 和脾胃 [hé pí wèi]. In the proposed standard nomenclature, however, both the single-charactered 和 [hé] and the double-charactered 調和 [tiáo hé] is rendered as "harmonize".

In addition, 調和脾胃 [tiáo hé pí wèi] is sometimes changed to 調脾和胃 [tiáo pí hé wèi] on account of rhetorical parallelism, according to the context. This need not be considered in the proposed standard nomenclature, and both terms are expressed as "harmonize the spleen and stomach". The same rule is applied to 調和肝胃 [tiáo hé gān wèi] vs. 調肝和胃 [tiáo gān hé wèi], 調和肝脾 [tiáo hé gān pí] vs. 調肝和脾 [tiáo gān hé pí] and 調和氣血 [tiáo hé qì xuè] vs. 調氣和血 [tiáo qì hé xuè].

和血 [hé xuè] and 和營 [hé yíng] are often used to refer to a basic element of treatment principles such as "harmonize blood to regulate menstruation" (和血調經 [hé xuè tiáo jīng]), "harmonize blood to prevent abortion" (和血安胎 [hé xuè ān tāi]) and "harmonize nutrient to promote regeneration" (和營生新 [hé yíng shēng xīn])

Another term closely related to 調和 [tiáo hé] (abbreviated as 和 [hé]) is 調理 [tiáo lǐ] (abbreviated as 理 [lǐ]). Among various renderngs, most authors use "harmonize" for 調和 [tiáo hé] or 和 [hé] and "regulate" for 調理 [tiáo lǐ] or 理 [lǐ]. If the character 調 [tiáo] is used singly, it may be an abbreviation of either 調和 [tiáo hé] or 調理 [tiáo lǐ].

VII. Warming 溫法

Warming is a general term indicating the treatment of any kind of interior cold syndrome. Since it is only used in the treatment of interior cold, it is also called "interior-warming". For exterior cold, "exterior-releasing" is the proper treatment. Terminologically, the characters 溫 [wēn] and 暖 [nuǎn] are synonyms, and can be replaced with each other, e.g., 溫胃 [wēn wèi] can also be called 暖胃 [nuǎn wèi]. In the proposed nomenclature, however, only those appearing in the State Standard of Traditional

Chinese Medical Diagnosis and Treatment, 1997, are selected.

Proposed Standard Nomenclature

warming (therapy) 溫法 [wēn fǎ][1]
dispel cold 祛寒 [qū hán][2]
warm the interior 溫裏 [wēn lǐ][3]
warm the lung 溫肺 [wēn fèi]
warm the stomach 溫胃 [wēn wèi][4]
warm the middle (energizer) 溫中
    [wēn zhōng][5]
warm the meridian 溫經 [wēn jīng][6]
restore yang 回陽 [huí yáng][7]

cold-dispelling (therapy) 祛寒法
    [qū hán fǎ][2]
warm yang 溫陽 [wēn yáng]
warm the spleen 溫脾 [wēn pí][4]
warm the kidney 溫腎 [wēn
    shèn][4]
warm the liver 暖肝 [nuǎn gān][6]
warm the uterus 暖宮 [nuǎn
    gōng][6]

Discussion

1. Almost all authors use the word "warming" for 溫 [wēn] in the term 溫法 [wēn fǎ]. The divergence exists in the expression of 法 [fǎ] as "method" or "therapy", or as omitted.

2. 祛寒法 [qū hán fǎ] is another name for 溫法 [wēn fǎ].

3. Warming therapy is chiefly used for relieving interior cold syndromes caused by yang deficiency, and hence the names "interior-warming" (溫裏 [wēn lǐ]) and "yang-warming" (溫陽 [wēn yáng]). Both are general terms, and can be further divided in accordance with individual *zang-fu* organs and yang of each organ, e.g., "warm the spleen" (溫脾 [wēn pí]) and "warm the spleen yang" (溫脾陽 [wēn pí yáng]). Two terminological formulas can be thus established: one is "warm" + organ name, and the other is "warm" + organ name + yang. Of the two expressions, only the first one, i.e., "warm the spleen" is adopted in this scheme.

4. Since the standard names of *zang-fu* organs have already been approved by the WHO Scientific Group and are used by almost all authors at present, there is no question about the rendering of 溫脾 [wēn pí], 溫胃 [wēn wèi] and 溫腎 [wēn shèn] as "warm the spleen", "warm the stomach" and "warm the kidney".

On these basic terms, a variety of compound terms can be formed. Taking the kidney as an example, "warm the kidney to induce diuresis" (溫腎利水 [wēn shèn lì shuǐ]) is the treatment principle for relieving edema due to kidney yang deficiency; "warm the kidney to reduce urination" (溫腎縮尿 [wēn shèn suō niào]) is treatment of frequent micturition or enuresis by warming the kidney; "warm the kidney to stop diarrhea" (溫腎止瀉 [wēn shèn zhǐ xiè]) is a therapy of chronic diarrhea caused by kidney yang deficiency; "warm the kidney to invigorate yang" (溫腎壯陽 [wēn shèn zhuàng yáng]) refers to the treatment of sexual impotence.

5. 中 [zhōng] of the term 溫中 [wēn zhōng] comes from 中焦 [zhōng jiāo] ("the middle energizer"). Since the corresponding abbreviation in English is not widely used, "warm the middle (energizer)" is proposed as the standard term.

6. For warming the liver and uterus, the character 暖 [nuǎn] is customarily used in Chinese terminology. The probable reason is that the liver and kidney are believed to be of the same origin, and warming the liver is usually associated with warming the kidney. In Chinese rhetoric, 溫腎暖肝 [wēn shèn nuǎn gān] is apparently better than 溫腎溫肝 [wēn shèn wēn gān], So is the term 溫經暖宮 [wēn jīng nuǎn gōng]. In English the repetition can be easily avoided by rendering the terms as "warm the kidney and liver" and "warm the meridian and uterus".

7. 回陽 [huí yáng] is also called 回陽救逆 [huí yáng jiù nì] or 回陽固脫 [huí yáng gù tuō], referring to the treatment of shock or collapse. Several English expressions appear in the publications: "restore yang", "revive yang", "recuperate yang", "return yang", "recover yang", etc.

VIII. Tonification 補(益)法; Reinforcement 補法

In herbal medication, tonification (補法 [bǔ fǎ]) is one of the major principles for treating deficiency syndromes. It is so called because various kinds of tonics are used in the treatment. In acupuncture, 補法 [bǔ fǎ] is also one of the major treatment principles. In the latter case, although some authors also render it as tonification, most authors prefer the word "reinforcement", for the term involves certain manipulations but not tonics.

Proposed Standard Nomenclature

tonify 補益 [bǔ yì][1]	tonification 補法 [bǔ fǎ][1]
tonify *qi* 補氣 [bǔ qì][1]	replenish *qi* 益氣 [yì qì][1]
qi tonification 補氣 [bǔ qì][1]	*qi* replenishment 益氣 [yì qì][1]
replenish essence 益[填]精	replenish marrow 益[填]髓

[yì [tián] jīng][1]

tonify the heart 補心 [bǔ xīn][1]

heart tonification 補心 [bǔ xīn][1]

tonify the spleen 補脾 [bǔ pí][1]

spleen tonification 補脾 [bǔ pí][1]

tonify the kidney 補腎 [bǔ shèn][1]

kidney tonification 補腎 [bǔ shèn][1]

tonify heart *qi* 補益心氣 [bǔ yì xīn qì][1]

tonify middle *qi* 補益中氣 [bǔ yì zhōng qì][1]

tonify kidney *qi* 補益腎氣 [bǔ yì shèn qì][1]

tonify the spleen and kidney 補益脾腎 [bǔ yì pí shèn][1]

tonify essence and blood 補益精血 [bǔ yì jīng xuè][1]

nourish blood 養血 [yǎng xuè][1]

blood nourishment 養血 [yǎng xuè][1]

nourish the stomach 養胃 [yǎng wèi][1]

stomach nourishment 養胃 [yǎng wèi][1]

nourish yin 滋陰 [zī yīn]; 養陰 [yǎng yīn][1]

yin nourishment 滋陰 [zī yīn]; 養陰 [yǎng yīn][1]

tonify yin; yin tonification 補陰 [bǔ yīn][1]

tonify [nourish] lung yin 滋補 [養]肺陰 [zī bǔ [yǎng] fèi yīn][1]

tonify [nourish] spleen yin 滋補 [養]脾陰 [zī bǔ [yǎng] pí yīn][1]

tonify [nourish] kidney yin 滋補 [養]腎陰 [zī bǔ [yǎng] shèn yīn][1]

[yì [tián] suǐ][1]

tonify the lung 補肺 [bǔ fèi][1]

lung tonification 補肺 [bǔ fèi][1]

tonify the liver 補肝 [bǔ gān][1]

liver tonification 補肝 [bǔ gān][1]

replenish the kidney 益腎 [yì shèn][1]

kidney replenishment 益腎 [yì shèn][1]

tonify lung *qi* 補益肺氣 [bǔ yì fèi qì][1]

tonify liver *qi* 補益肝氣 [bǔ yì gān qì][1]

tonify the heart and lung 補益心肺 [bǔ yì xīn fèi][1]

tonify *qi* and blood 補益氣血 [bǔ yì qì xuè][1]

tonify blood; blood tonification 補血 [bǔ xuè][1]

nourish nutrient 養營 [yǎng yíng][1]

nourish the heart 養心 [yǎng xīn][1]

heart nourishment 養心 [yǎng xīn][1]

nourish the liver 養肝 [yǎng gān][1]

liver nourishment 養肝 [yǎng gān][1]

tonify [nourish] heart yin 滋補 [養]心陰 [zī bǔ [yǎng] xīn yīn][1]

tonify [nourish] liver yin 滋補 [養]肝陰 [zī bǔ [yǎng] gān yīn][1]

tonify [nourish] the heart and lung 滋補[養]心肺 [zī bǔ [yǎng] xīn fèi][1]

tonify [nourish] the spleen and

tonify [nourish] the liver and stomach 滋補[養]肝胃 [zī bǔ [yǎng] gān wèi][1]

tonify [nourish] the liver and kidney 滋補[養]肝腎 [zī bǔ [yǎng] gān shèn][1]

tonify [nourish] the lung and kidney 滋補[養]肺腎 [zī bǔ [yǎng] fèi shèn][1]

warm-tonify lung yang 溫補肺陽 [wēn bǔ fèi yáng][2]

warm-tonify stomach yang 溫補胃陽 [wēn bǔ wèi yáng][2]

warm-tonify kidney yang 溫補腎陽 [wēn bǔ shèn yáng][2]

warm-tonify the heart and lung; 溫補心肺 [wēn bǔ xīn fèi][2]

strengthen the spleen 健脾 [jiàn pí]

raise yang 升陽 [shēng yáng][3]

invigorate yang 壯陽 [zhuàng yáng][1]

fire supplement 補火 [bǔ huǒ][1]

regenerate fluid 生津 [shēng jīn][4]

fluid regeneration 生津 [shēng jīn][4]

regenerate muscles 生肌 [shēng jī][4]

stomach 滋補[養]脾胃 [zī bǔ [yǎng]pí wèi][1]

tonify [nourish] the heart and kidney 滋補[養]心腎 [zī bǔ [yǎng]xīn shèn][1]

tonify yang 補陽 [bǔ yáng][1]

yang tonification 補陽 [bǔ yáng][1]

warm-tonify heart yang 溫補心陽 [wēn bǔ xīn yáng][2]

warm-tonify spleen yang 溫補脾陽 [wēn bǔ pí yáng][2]

warm-tonify liver yang 溫補肝陽 [wēn bǔ gān yáng]

warm-tonify the life gate 溫補命門 [wēn bǔ mìng mén][2]

strengthen the stomach 健胃 [jiàn wèi]

strengthen bones 健骨 [jiàn gǔ]

strengthen muscles 強筋 [qiáng jīn]

support yang 扶陽 [fú yáng]; 助陽 [zhù yáng]

supplement fire 補火 [bǔ huǒ][1]

regenerate blood 生血 [shēng [shēng xuè][4]

blood regeneration 生血 [shēng xuè][4]

muscle regeneration 生肌 [shēng jī][4]

Discussion

1. Tonification is a general principle for treating various deficiency syndromes by using tonics; it is one of the eight principal therapeutic methods. The words "tonify" and "tonification" can not be found in an English dictionary. They come from the word "tonic" and so are often used in herbal medicine, but in acupuncture many authors also use this word, though more authors prefer the word "reinforcement". In herbal medicine tonic, tonify, and tonification form a series of related words, among which "tonic" is adjective and also a noun referring to tonic agents,

"tonify" is the verb indicating the tonic action, and "tonification" refers directly to the tonic action. Since they coincide with the Chinese term 補 [bǔ] in every respect, many American and European authors including Dan Bensky, Andrew Gamble, Giovanni Maciocia, Gérard Guillaume, Mach Chieu prefer this word.

Of course, different ways of rendering this concept exist, such as "replenish", "invigorate", "nourish", "reinforce", "strengthen" and "supplement". In Chinese medicine, quite a few synonyms of 補 [bǔ] are commonly used, so most of the above words are of use in expressing the Chinese concepts. For example, "replenish", "invigorate", "nourish", "strengthen" and "invigorate" are equivalent to "益""養""健" and "壯" respectively.

Strictly speaking, the concept of 補 [bǔ] reflects one of the crucial features of Chinese medicine. It does not mean direct supplement of what is deficient. There is no blood transfusion for blood deficiency, no parenteral fluid therapy for fluid deficiency, no vitamin supplement for vitamin deficiency, no oxygen inhalation for oxygen deficiency, etc. In general, the word "supplement" is somewhat different from the Chinese concept of 補 [bǔ], and so it is not recommended.

In Chinese medicine, physiological substances and activities include yin, yang, *qi*, blood, essence, fluid, etc. Tonification 補法 [bǔ fǎ] or 補益 [bǔ yì] is suitable for treating deficiency of any physiological substance or activity. It should be noted that the original term is simply 補 [bǔ], and the character 益 [yì] is added in order to make a double-character term. Although the two characters can be replaced with each other, e.g., 補氣 [bǔ qì] is also called 益氣 [yì qì], they have some minor difference. 補 [bǔ] as a treatment principle can cover all kinds of deficiency conditions, but 益 [yì] cannot. The former can be applied to treating deficiency conditions of any cause, while the latter is usually indicated in the treatment of deficiency conditions caused by consumption. Therefore, 補法 [bǔ fǎ] cannot be called 益法 [yì fǎ].

As for the English equivalent of 益 [yì], various words have been suggested by different authors: "aid", "benefit", invigorate", "reinforce", "replenish", "supplement" and "tonify". Most authors prefer "replenish", probably because it has the meaning of filling something again after is has been consumed.

When 補 [bǔ] and 益 [yì] are used as one word, it is unnecessary to make a distinction between the two characters. For example, 補益心肺

[bǔ yì xīn fèi] can be simply regarded as 補心肺 [bǔ xīn fèi], and rendered as "tonify the heart and lung". Sometimes the term can be rearranged as 補心益肺 [bǔ xīn yì fèi]. In either case, "tonify and replenish the heart and lung" or "tonify the heart and replenish the lung" are wordy expressions. However, this is not always true for all the terms of the kind. In most instances 補脾益肺 [bǔ pí yì fèi] means "tonify the spleen to replenish the lung" (a treatment likened to "earth engenders metal"). Therefore, in this scheme only the elementary terms of treatment priniciples are included. The readers themselves can make the combinations at their own wishes. Many Chinese terms can be expressed in different ways, for example, 補益心氣 [bǔ yì xīn qì] vs 補心益氣 [bǔ xīn yì qì], 補益肺氣 [bǔ yì fèi qì] vs 補肺益氣 [bǔ fèi yì qì], and 補益中氣 [bǔ yì zhōng qì] vs 補中益氣 [bǔ zhōng yì qì]. Only the former terms of these pairs are regarded as elementary, while the latter ones are not adopted because of their ambiguity.

For tonifying or replenishing yin and blood, besides 補 [bǔ], the characters 滋 [zī] and 養 [yǎng] are frequently encountered, forming such expressions as 補養 [bǔ yǎng], 滋養 [zī yǎng], and 滋補 [zī bǔ]. According to the majority opinion, the word "nourish" is selected for 滋 [zī] and 養 [yǎng], either used singly or in combination.

2. 溫補 [wēn bǔ] is different from 補益 [bǔ yì], 補養 [bǔ yǎng] and 滋補 [zī bǔ]. The latter terms are used to express the treatment of deficiency conditions, while the former refers to a combined treatment of deficiency-cold. So, it should not be rendered simply as "warming" or "tonification".

3. There are a couple of ways to express the character 升 in the term 升陽 [shēng yáng], such as "elevate" and "lift". But the word "raise" suggested by Dan Bensky seems to be more appropriate. 升陽 [shēng yáng] is also called 升陽舉陷 [shēng yáng jǔ xiàn], in which 陷 [xiàn] means something sunken. To cause a sunken thing to rise, "raise" is probably the most suitable word.

4. Various words are used to express the concept of 生 [shēng] in treatment principles. "Engender", "generate", "produce", and "grow" may all bear the meaning of 生 [shēng] as a common word, but in medical treatment 生 [shēng] actually refers to generating or producing (fluid, blood or muscles) anew or again. So, "regenerate" or "regeneration" seem the best words.

IX. Qi Regulation 理氣法

Regulation of *qi* is a general principle for treating disordered flow of *qi*. The major problems of *qi* flow are *qi* stagnation and *qi* counterflow. Hence, *qi* regulation includes moving *qi* to relieve stagnation, and sending *qi* downward to treat abnormal upward flow of *qi*. As for raising sunken *qi*, it belongs to the category of tonification.

Proposed Standard Nomenclature

qi regulation 理氣法 [lǐ qì fǎ][1]

regulate *qi* 理氣 [lǐ qì][1]

move *qi* 行氣 [xíng qì][2]

soothe the liver 疏[舒]肝 [shū gān][3]

send *qi* downward 降氣 [jiàng qì][5]

disseminate lung *qi* 宣肺 [xuān fèi][7]

regulate the middle (energizer) 理中 [lǐ zhōng][1]

soothe the chest 寬胸 [kuān xiōng][4]

soothe the middle (energizer) 寬中 [kuān zhōng][4]

break up (stagnant) *qi* 破氣 [pò qì][6]

relieve depression 解鬱 [jiě yù][8]

Discussion

1. The English equivalent of 理氣 [lǐ qì] includes "regulate the flow of *qi*", "regulate the circulation of *qi*", "normalize the flow of *qi*", "rectify *qi*" and "regulate *qi*". Most authors prefer "regulate *qi*, and the word "regulate" is also used for the Chinese character "理" [lǐ] in other instances, such as "regulate the middle" (理中 [lǐ zhōng]).

2. For the term 行氣 [xíng qì], there are a number of translations, such as "promote the flow of *qi*", "promote movement of *qi*", "activate *qi*", "conduct *qi*", "set the *qi* in motion", "let the *qi* circulate". All of them seem to be indirect. Nigel Wiseman, Giovanni Maciocia and some other authors solve this problem in a direct and simple way; they use the term "move *qi*", which is exact and appropriate in their writings.

3. The term 疏[舒]肝 [shū gān] is also rendered into English in various ways: "soothe the liver", "disperse the stagnated liver-*qi*", "course the liver", "spread the liver *qi*", "relieve the liver *qi*", "clear the liver", etc. "Soothe the liver" is more frequently used than the others.

4. The character 寬 [kuān] is originally an adjective, describing a spacious room. It is the opposite of narrow. Used as a verb, it has multiple meanings, such as "broaden", "loosen", "relax", "relieve" and "comfort" in different word groups. For the terms 寬胸 [kuān xiōng] and 寬中 [kuān zhōng], the word "soothe" may be the best choice.

5. In the basic terms of treatment principles, the first word is usually a transitive verb. This is also true for the term 降氣 [jiàng qì]. None of the available equivalents of 降 [jiàng], such as "lower", "drop" and "reduce", is exactly appropriate. Some authors suggest a new word — "downbear". This is also open to question, because "bear" means "carry something while moving". As discussed previously, "send" may be better, for it means "cause something to go without going oneself".

6. In severe cases of *qi* stagnation, the treatment is often potent, not only smoothing the *qi* flow, but also breaking up the stagnation. This treatment is called 破氣 [pò qì]. The corresponding renderings include "relieve the stagnation of *qi* with potent drugs" "relieve stagnation of *qi* with drastic drugs", "dissipate stagnant *qi*", "disperse *qi*". "disintegrate aggregated and stagnated *qi*", "break up *qi* (stagnation)", "break up stagnant *qi*", "break the stagnant *qi*", and "break *qi*". The last expression is the most direct and literal, but it is difficult to understand. So some modification is necessary.

7. The character 宣 [xuān] is difficult to understand even for the Chinese. Originally, it was a noun, meaning the emperor's office building where decrees were issued. Turned into a verb, 宣 [xuān] means "decree" or "declare". Decreeing an order is for dissemination of the order, and so the meaning of this character is extended as "disseminate", "lead off", etc.

In recent publications, there are various renderings of this term, such as "clear the lung", "release stagnated lung-*qi*", "facilitate the flow of lung-*qi*", "promote the dispersing function of the lung", "ventilate the lung", "ventilate lung-*qi*", "mobilize lung *qi*", "diffuse the lung", "release lung *qi*", "activate the dispersing function of the lung", "disseminate lung *qi*", "restore the dispersing of lung-*qi*", and "move stagnant lung *qi*". All these expressions are basically correct, but "clear the lung" is often understood as "clear the lung of heat or fire", and is an appropriate equivalent of 清肺 [qīng fèi]; the words "mobilize" and "activate" seem to be too general. The terms "facilitate the flow of lung-*qi*" and "release stagnated lung-*qi*" are more consistent with the Chinese original, but are explanatory and difficult to change into the noun form.

It should be noted that 宣肺 [xuān fèi] is an abbreviation of 宣通[發]肺氣 [xuān tōng[fā] fèi qì]. So the addition of "*qi*" to the English equivalent of this term is reasonable. Among the above-listed expressions, Dan Bensky's "disseminate lung *qi*" may be the best choice.

8. 解鬱 [jiě yù] is also called 開鬱 [kāi yù] or 疏鬱理氣 [shū yù lǐ

qì]. It is a common treatment for liver *qi* depression. The term is rendered into English in different ways, such as "relieve constraint", "remove stagnation", "eliminate stagnation of *qi*", "resolve depression", "alleviate mental depression", "disperse the depressed *qi*", "relieve depression", "relieve mental depression", and "restore the normal function of a depressed liver". Among these expressions, some are apparently explanations that cannot be taken as technical terms. In Chinese medicine 鬱 [yù] refers to depression, but is not confined to mental depression. In addition, 鬱 [yù] is different from 滯 [zhì]. The latter means sluggishness in motion, possibly with detention, and is usually rendered as "stagnation", but the former refers to the state of being compelled to inaction, maybe associated with emotion. Both "constraint" and "depression" are appropriate renderings. In this scheme, "depression" is selected owing to its use by many authors and also to its emotional implication.

X. Blood Regulation 理血法

Blood regulation is a general term including various treatments of disordered blood flow. Customarily, regulation of blood flow includes relieving blood stasis and arresting hemorrhage.

Proposed Standard Nomenclature

blood regulation 理血法 [lǐ xuè fǎ]

regulate blood 理血 [lǐ xuè]

activate blood 活血 [huó xuè][1]

dispel (blood) stasis 祛瘀 [qū yū][1]

resolve (blood) stasis 化瘀 [huà yū][2]

dissipate stasis 散瘀 [sàn yū][2]

break up (blood) stasis 破血[瘀] [pò xuè [yū]][3]

expel stasis 逐瘀 [zhú yū][3]

disperse mass 消癥 [xiāo zhēng][4]

arrest bleeding 止血 [zhǐ xuè][5]

Discussion

1. 活血 [huó xuè] is a general term for various treatments for curing blood stasis. It is often used in combination with 化瘀 [huà yū] (resolve stasis) or 祛瘀 [qū yū] (dispel stasis). If herbs with drastic action are used, the treatment is often called 破血 [pò xuè]. The equivalents of 活血 [huó xuè] can be listed as follows: "invigorate blood circulation (or flow)", "activate blood circulation (or flow)", "promote blood circulation

(or flow)", "quicken the blood", "invigorate the blood" and "activate the blood". It is really difficult to make a selection, because each term has a number of advocates. The first point that can be decided is to make the term as short as possible. So, it is better to take out such words as "circulation" or "flow" from the proposed standard terms. Comparatively speaking, more authors prefer the word "activate".

2. As for 化瘀 [huà yū], some authors take the word "transform" as the equivalent of 化 [huà]. It should be noted that this character used in medicine has different meanings. Since 化熱 [huà rè] can be properly rendered as "transform into heat", some authors insist on using the word "transform" as the equivalent of 化 [huà] on every occasion. However, if we say "transform blood stasis", we must ask "transform it into what?" Besides "transform", this character has two important meanings when it is used in medicine. It means 消逝 [xiāo shì] (perish) and 消散 [xiāo sàn] ("dissipate")*. So, in this case, the majority of authors use the word "resolve". As a medical term, "resolution" means "the subsidence of a pathological state", and "resolve" means "to cause resolution of the pathological state".**

3. 破血 [pò xuè] refers to the treatment of blood stasis with drastic drugs. The literal translation of this term —"break the blood" — will lead to confusion. One cannot understand why "breaking the blood" can be a cure. In ancient literature, Zhang Yuansu (12th century) made an annotation to peach seed that it "breaks the accumulation of stagnated blood" ("破蓄血"). The annotation is more logical than the simplified term "break the blood". In addition, in Chinese 破血 [pò xuè] is usually used in combination with 逐瘀 [zhú yū], and they can be regarded as an integral whole. In Dan Bensky and Andrew Gamble's translation of Chinese Herbal Medicine — Materia Medica "break up and drive out blood stasis" is used for 破血逐瘀 [pò xuè zhú yū], and "break up blood stasis" for 破血 [pò xuè].

4. 癥 [zhēng] and 瘕 [jiǎ] refer to mass formation in the female abdomen. The former has a definite shape, fixed in location, while the latter may change from time to time. Since the former is formed in asso-

---

*簡明中醫字典 (*Concise Dictionary of Characters in Chinese Medicine*) (in Chinese), Guizhou People's Publish House, 1985, p.30 (with annotations from classical literature).

**_Merriam Webster's Medical Desk Dictionary_, Merriam-Webster Inc., Massachusetts, U.S.A. 1996, p.698.

ciation with blood stasis, its treatment belongs to the category of blood regulation.

XI. Phlegm-Dispelling 祛痰法

In Chinese medicine, phlegm is not only regarded as a pathological product, but also as a pathogenic factor. So, phlegm-dispelling therapy is not merely a symptomatic treatment, and phlegm syndromes are varieties of pathological conditions.

Proposed Standard Nomenclature

phlegm-dispelling therapy 祛痰法 [qū tán fǎ][1]

eliminate phlegm 豁痰 [huō tán]; 滌痰 [dì tán][2]

resolve phlegm 化痰 [huà tán][1]

dispel phlegm 祛痰 [qū tán][1]

resolve fluid 化飲 [huà yǐn][3]

expel fluid 逐飲 [zhú yǐn][3]

Discussion

1. "Dispel phlegm" (祛痰 [qū tán]) is a general term indicating various treatments for getting rid of phlegm. But the term "resolve phlegm" (化痰 [huà tán]) is even more frequently used, and the various ways of dispelling phlegm can be classified as "dry dampness and resolve phlegm" (燥濕化痰 [zào shī huà tán]), "clear heat and resolve phlegm" (清熱化痰 [qīng rè huà tán]), "moisten dryness and resolve phlegm" (潤燥化痰 [huà tán]), "warm-resolve cold-phlegm" (溫化寒痰 [wēn huà hán tán]), and "resolve phlegm and extinguish wind" (化痰熄風 [huà tán xī fēng]).

2. 豁 [huō] means "break" and "eliminate", and 滌 [dì] means "cleanse" and "eliminate". Both 豁痰 [huō tán] and 滌痰 [dì tán] often refer to the treatment of stubborn phlegm syndrome with mental involvement. Various renderings are suggested by different authors, such as "eliminate", "dispel", "reduce" and "resolve" phlegm for 豁痰 [huō tán], and "remove", "flush" and "wipe out" phlegm for 滌痰 [dì tán]. Since the two terms are not often used, and the difference between them is only literal and not technical, both are rendered as "eliminate phlegm" in this scheme.

3. Phlegm and retained fluid belong to the same category of pathology, and so the treatment for expelling or resolving retained fluid is grouped under the heading of phlegm-dispelling therapy.

XII. Resuscitation 開竅法

Loss of consciousness is called 神昏竅閉 [shén hūn qiào bì] which literally means "unconsciousness with the orifices closed", and the treatment is 醒神 [xǐng shén] (cause to recover consciousness) or 開竅 [kāi qiào] (open the orifices). The two therapeutic principles are actually the same, but the latter is more frequently used as a formal term.

Proposed Standard Nomenclature

open the orifices 開竅 [kāi qiǎo][1]
resuscitation 開竅法 [kāi qiǎo fǎ][1]
cooling resuscitation 涼開 [liáng kāi][3]

resuscitate with aromatics 芳香 開竅 [fāng xiāng kāi qiǎo][2]
warming resuscitation 溫開 [wēn kāi][3]

Discussion

1. Many authors use the word "resuscitate" to express the concept of 開竅 [kāi qiǎo], but some others prefer the literal translation as "open the orifices". Both are adopted in this scheme.

2. Aromatic stimulants are often used for resuscitation, and hence the term 芳香開竅 [fāng xiāng kāi qiǎo], namely, "resuscitate with aromatics".

3. Resuscitating treatment can be generally classified into two categories. One is resuscitation by using warming agents, called 溫開 [wēn kāi], and the other by using cooling agents, called 涼開 [liáng kāi].

XIII. Tranquilization 安神法

安神 [ān shén] is treatment to relieve mental tension and uneasiness, equivalent to tranquilization. The terms of this category include the relevant wordings of tranquilization.

Proposed Standard Nomenclature

tranquilize 安神 [ān shén][1]
calm the mind 安神 [ān shén]; 寧心 [níng xīn][2]
allay excitement 鎮驚 [zhèn jīng][4]

tranquilization 安神法 [ān shén fǎ][1]
stabilize the mind 定志 [dìng zhì][3]

Discussion

1. Tranquilization and 安神 [ān shēn] are appropriate equivalents, though each may have other ways of expression.

2. 安神 [ān shēn] and 寧心 [níng xīn] have the same meaning. The corresponding expressions are "calm the mind [spirit]", "quite the mind [spirit]", "allay restlessness", "tranquilize the mind", "relieve mental strain", etc.

3. For the term 定志 [dìng zhì], among the existing expressions "calm the emotional strain", "relieve emotional distress" and "stabilize the mind", the last one seems suitable, while the others are explanatory.

4. Since 驚 [jīng] as an emotional factor means "fright", some authors suggest for the English rendering of 鎮驚 [zhèn jīng] "settle fright". On the other hand, quite a few authors even regard 驚 [jīng] as an abbreviation for 驚風 [jīng fēng], i.e., convulsion, and express 鎮驚 [zhèn jīng] as "relieve convulsion". Both are open to discussion. In Chinese medicine, 熄風 [xī fēng] is the proper term for "relieve convulsion. Since 鎮驚 [zhèn jīng] is a term indicating a therapeutic principle, 驚 [jīng] is a morbid condition referrring to the response to fright (such as restlessness, palpitations and insomnia) rather than the emotional factor of fright itself. So, "settle the mind" or "allay excitement" may be more appropriate.

XIV. Astringency 固澀法

Astringency is a category of treatment that checks discharge, particularly discharge of *qi*, blood, essence or fluids. Generally, astringency is not a radical or primary treatment, and is often used in combination with tonification

Proposed Standard Nomenclature

strengthen the superficies 固表 [gù biǎo]

restore from collapse 固脫 [gù tuō]

astringe menses 固經 [gù jīng]

astringe the thoroughfare vessel 固衝 [gù chōng]

astringe the intestines 澀腸 [sè cháng]

astringe seminal discharge 澀精 [sè jīng]

astringe the lung 斂肺 [liǎn fèi]

astringe sweat 斂汗 [liǎn hàn]

Discussion

The verbs commonly used in these treatments are 固 [gù], 澀 [sè] and 斂 [liǎn]. The last two verbs are more or less specific in meaning, and can be expressed as "astringe". The verb 固 [gù] has multiple meanings, which may or may not be related to "astringe". For example, 固齒 [gù chǐ] has nothing to do with astringency. But, 固脫 [gù tuō] means to restore from collapse with astringents to arrest excessive discharge.

精 [jīng] in its broad sense refers to any kind of essence, but in the term 澀精 [sè jīng] it only refers to semen or seminal fluid. 澀精 [sè jīng] is a treatment for arresting nocturnal or spontaneous emission or spermatorrhea.

XV. Others

Proposed Standard Nomenclature

relieve spasm 解痙 [liě jìng][1]

stop [relieve] coughing 止咳 [zhǐ ké][1]

relieve [alleviate] itching 止癢 [zhǐ yǎng][1]

relieve [alleviate] pain 止痛 [zhǐ tòng][1]

stop [relieve] hiccups 止呃 [zhǐ è][1]

promote digestion 消食 [xiāo shí][3]

return fire to its source 引火 歸原 [yǐn huǒ guī yuán][4]

soothe the throat 利咽 [lì yān][2]

relieve dyspnea 平喘 [píng chuǎn]; 止喘 [zhǐ chuǎn][1]

quench thirst 止渴 [zhǐ kě][1]

stop [arrest] bleeding 止血 [zhǐ xuè][1]

stop [relieve] vomiting 止嘔 [zhǐ ǒu][1]

alleviate swelling 消腫 [xiāo zhǒng][1]

relieve stuffiness 消痞 [xiāo pǐ][1]

promote heart-kidney interaction 交通心腎 [jāio tóng xīn shèn][5]

Discussion

1. Most of the terms listed in this table indicate symptomatic relief. As therapeutic principles, they are seldom prescribed alone, but are often combined with other principles as an auxiliary treatment or as the expected effect. For example, 止痛 [zhǐ tòng] (relieve pain) may be used in combination with 行氣 [xíng qì] (move *qi*), 活血 [huó xuè] (activate blood), 溫經 [wēn jīng] (warm the meridian), etc., forming compound terms 行氣止痛 [xíng qì zhǐ tòng], 活血止痛 [huó xuè zhǐ tòng], and 溫經止痛 [wēn jīng zhǐ tòng]. To render these terms into English, we should be very careful, because in many instances, to relieve pain is the

purpose of *qi*-moving, blood-activating or meridian-warming therapy.

In these terms, such common verbs as 止 [zhǐ], 解 [liě], 消 [xiāo] are usually used. In English, each has quite a few equivalents, mostly interchangeable, e.g., "relieve", "stop", "arrest", "alleviate", "counteract", etc. Standardization is impractical. The table only shows the words that are most often used by authors, serving as a reference.

2. Many authors use the word "benefit" to translate 利 [lì]. It is true that this character has such a meaning, but as a term of treatment, "benefit" seems too general, for any therapeutic effect is beneficial. However, this character is only used in a limited number of terms with an implication of smoothing the passage. In this context, 利 [lì] would rather refers to the component character of 順利 [shùn lì] (smooth) than that of 利益 [lì yì] (benefit). Thus, 利膽 [lì dǎn] means to promote the discharge of bile. As for the throat (咽 [yān]), it is the passage through which food passes to the stomach. The passage is impeded when the throat is sore, and relief of the sore throat will smooth the passage. So, quite a few authors prefer "soothe the throat". Comparatively speaking, the latter expression is better than "benefit the throat".

3. A direct and literal translation of 消食 [xiāo shí] is "disperse food" or "remove retained food". In fact, it is an abbreviation for 消食化滯 [xiāo shí huà zhì], closely related to the modern Chinese term 消化 [xiāo huà] (digestion). Therefore, it is easier to understand by using the word "digestion".

4. 引火歸原 [yǐn huǒ guī yuán] is a special treatment of up-floating kidney fire. The English expressions used by various authors are largely identical, with minor differences, e.g., "conduct the fire back to its origin", "direct fire to return to its source", "guide the fire to its original place", "let the fire go back to its origin", and "return fire to its source".

5. 交通心腎 [jiāo tóng xīn shèn] is a special treatment of incoordination of the heart and kidney. Variations of the English expressions lie in the term 交通 [jiāo tóng]. This term is widely used in modern Chinese with the meaning of "communication" and "traffic", but it appeared in the *Canon of Medicine* two thousand years ago*. Nelson Wu and Andrew Wu rendered this word as "intercrossing" in their translation of this classical work. For the term 交通心腎 [jiāo tóng xīn shèn], Nigel Wiseman pro-

---

* 素問・四氣調神大論篇第二 (*Plain Questions*: Chapter II. On Preserving Health in Accordance with the Four Seasons)

posed "promote heart-kidney interaction". The words "intercrossing" and "interaction" more precisely reflect the Chinese original than the words "balance" and "coordination".

PHARMACEUTIC TERMS

The Chinese expression 中藥 [zhōng yào] is a very common medical term, but its implications may vary greatly according to the context. Sometimes it refers to prepared drugs, and sometimes it refers to medicinals or medicinal materials. In a broad sense, it refers to all kinds of medicinals and prepared drugs in Chinese medicine, but when it is used in contrast with 草藥 [cǎo yào], it only refers to those recorded in Chinese materia medica, while the latter is called herbal drugs, referring to those not yet collected in the materia medica. It should be noted that the character 草 does not always mean "grass" or "herb". It also has the meaning of "preliminary" or "unofficial". For example, 草稿 [cǎo gǎo] is a preliminary draft, and 草圖 [cǎo tú], a sketch. Therefore, 草藥 [cǎo yào] refers to herbal drugs that have not yet been officially recognized, and are usually used in folk medicine. The term 中草藥 [zhōng cǎo yào] is even more vaguely defined. It is a collective name for 中藥 [zhōng yào] and 草藥 [cǎo yào], including officially recognized Chinese drugs and the drugs used in folk medicine as well.

Because the majority of Chinese medicinals are of botanical source, the books that recorded them were called 本草 [běn cǎo]. This term is composed of two characters: 本 [běn] means "origin" or "source"*, and 草 [cǎo] means "herbs" or "herbal medicinals". Traditionally, 本草 [běn cǎo] was rendered as "materia medica", but recently a new term has been developed — "herbology". However, the most appropriate designation of that branch of health sciences dealing with the preparation, dispensing and proper utilization of Chinese drugs is "Chinese pharmaceutics (中藥學 [zhōng yào xué])".

---

*The use of the character 本 in the sense of "origin" or "source" is frequently encountered in ancient Chinese medical classics. For example, in the *Canon of Medicine* there are 本輸 [běn shù] and 本病論 [běn bìng lùn] as chapter topics. They can be rendered into English as "On the Origin of Acupoints" and "Study on the Source of Disease".

Since these terms reflect various concepts and a clear-cut differentiation between them is often difficult to make, in the proposed standard nomenclature, a careful selection of the concepts is even more important than selection of the corresponding terms.

Proposed Standard Nomenclature

Chinese pharmaceutics 中藥學 [zhōng yào xué]

materia medica 本草 [běn cǎo]

Chinese drugs 中藥 [zhōng yào]

Chinese medicinals 中藥 [zhōng yào]

medicinal herbs 草藥 [cǎo yào]

herbal drugs 草藥 [cǎo yào]

medicinal substance 藥材 [yào cái]

medicinal material 藥材 [yào cái]

CHINESE MEDICINALS AND FORMULAE

The standard English and Latin names of officially recognized Chinese medicinals and formulae have already been formulated in the *Pharmacopieia of the People's Republic of China* (English edition, 1997).

DRUG PROCESSING

The terms for drug processing in Chinese pharmaceutics are chiefly verbs, i.e., words or phrases indicating actions. The corresponding nouns are also useful, but they are often derived from the verbs. For example, when a noun is needed the verb form "process (the drug)" can be turned to "(drug) processing", and "calcine" to "calcination".

Proposed Standard Nomenclature

(drug) processing 炮製 [páo zhì][1]

process 炮製 [páo zhì][1]

wash 洗 [xǐ][2]

macerate 泡 [pào][2]

refine with water 水飛 [shuǐ feī][3]

calcine 煅 [duàn][4]

carbonize 制炭 [zhì tàn][5]

bake 烘焙 [hōng bèi][6]

roast (with liquid adjuvant) 炙 [zhì][7]

roast (in ashes) 煨 [wèi][7]

stir-bake without adjuvant 清炒 [qīng chǎo][9]

stir-bake 炒 [chǎo][8]

stir-bake to just dry 微炒 [wēi chǎo][9]

stir-bake with adjuvant 加輔料炒 [jiā fǔ liào chǎo][9]

stir-bake to cracking 炒爆 [chǎo

stir-bake to yellow 炒黄 [chǎo huáng][9]

stir-bake to brown 炒焦 [chǎo jiāo][9]

stir-bake to charcoal 炒炭 [chǎo tàn][9]

steam 蒸 [zhēng][10]

stew 熬 [áo][10]

simmer in a bath 燉 [dùn][10]

blanch (in water) 潬 [dàn][11]

boil 煮 [zhǔ][10]

burn with original property retained 燒存性 [shāo cún xìng][12]

quench 淬 [cuì][11]

make into frost 制霜 [zhì shuāng][13]

Discussion

1. The word "processing" is used for 炮製 [páo zhì] by most authors, and hence is the proposed standard. Some others use the word "preparation", or a literal translation — "roast and broil".

2. There is no dispute about the terms "wash 洗 [xǐ]" and "macerate 泡 [pào]". They are common words.

3. Two expressions are often used for 水飛 [shuǐ feī]: "refining with water" and "grinding in water". The actual process is not limited to grinding, but is to retrieve the fine powder from the water suspension of the ground substance. So the first expression is better, and the second one is equivalent to 水磨 [shuǐ mò].

4. Most authors use the word calcine to express 煆 [duàn]. Some render it as "charring". The latter is not appropriate because 煆 [duàn] is the process of burning a drug on a fire to make it crispy, but not necessarily to make it black.

5. 制炭 [zhì tàn] means "to convert into charcoal".

6. Strictly speaking, 烘 [hōng] and 焙 [bèi] are not exactly the same. The former means "to dry by a fire", and the latter, "to bake".

7. Both 煨 [wèi] and 炙 [zhì] can be rendered as "roast" in English. The difference is that when we say 煨 [wèi], we mean that the medicinals are roasted in ashes or cinders. So some authors render it as "roast in ashes", "roast in hot ashes" or "roast in fresh cinders". Since there may be other sources of heat, it is better to delete the additional words and simply render the term as "roast" as the proposed standard nomenclature. When we say 炙 [zhì], we mean that during the roasting process some liquid adjuvant is added to and infiltrated into the medicinal materials.

8. Quite a number of authors render 炒 [chǎo] as "stir-fry". This is probably influenced by Chinese cookery, in which stir-frying is one of the most important cooking procedures, and it is called 炒 [chǎo] in Chinese.

Strictly speaking, the character 炒 [chǎo] simply means "stir while heating". In Chinese cooking, when one is engaged in the process of 炒, one cooks the vegetables, meat, etc. in very hot oil for a short time while stirring them. And so this process is called stir-fry in English. However, stir-fry and 炒 are not always consistent with each other. In drug processing, no oil is added while the medicinals are heated and stirred. Therefore, "stir-bake" is more exact to express the concept of 炒 [chǎo].

9. Under the heading of stir-bake there are a number of modifications, e.g., stir-bake without adjuvant 清炒 [qīng chǎo], stir-bake with adjuvant 加輔料炒 [jiā fǔ liào chǎo], stir-bake to just dry 微炒 [wēi chǎo], stir-bake to cracking 炒爆 [chǎo bào], stir-bake to yellow 炒黄 [chǎo huáng], stir-bake to brown 炒焦 [chǎo jiāo] and stir-bake to charcoal 炒炭 [chǎo tàn]. The wordings by different authors chiefly diverge in the expression of 炒 [chǎo]. In all these terms "stir-fry" is not the appropriate word. "Parch" is not appropriate either, for it means "make something very dry and hot". In other words, it indicates the result, not the processing measure to achieve the result. In addition, by means of stir-baking the medicinals are not always made very dry and hot. It should be further emphasized that "stir-fry" is not an appropriate equivalent of 炒 [chǎo] in drug processing, and "fry" is even worse for it refers to "cook in boiling oil" with no mentioning of stirring. So, "scorch-fry" for 炒焦 [chǎo jiāo] and "char-fry" for 炒炭 [chǎo tàn] are not recommended.

10. The processing of medicinal materials includes steaming 蒸 [zhēng], simmering 燉 [dùn], stewing 熬 [áo], and boiling 煮 [zhǔ]. These are also common words used in Chinese cuisine. It is often said in Chinese medicine that food and drugs have the same source. This not only denotes that some medicinal materials cannot be strictly distinguished from foodstuffs, but also refers to the fact that the culinary art and drug-processing techniques are quite similar.

11. It is interesting to note that each of the two characters 潬 [dàn] and 淬 [cuì] has two different forms of writing: 燂 same as 潬 and 焠 same as 淬. The left component of the characters can be either fire 火 or water 氵. The former stresses that heat should be applied, and the latter stresses that water should be used. The English word "blanch" is exactly equivalent to 燂 or 潬, and "quench" to 焠 or 淬. In the processes of blanching and quenching, both heat and water are necessary. Divergent views exist on the expression of 焠 or 淬. Some authors emphasize the

heat applied in the processing, and render the term as "calcination"; some emphasize the water used in the processing, and render the term as "temper mineral drugs by dipping into water". The word "quench" is selected for it means "cool a hot substance rapidly by placing it in water".

12. 燒存性 [shāo cún xìng] is the process of burning a medicinal herb till its outer part is charred while its inner part becomes yellowish-brown, so that its original property is retained. Some authors render the term as "charring with the original property retained". This might be overdone, for the medicinal is usually partially charred.

13 For the term 制霜 [zhì shuāng], there are different expressions such as "make (or prepare) drugs into frostlike powder", "frost-like powder making", "crystallizing", "powdering", "frosting", etc. In Western medicine, "frost" means "a deposit that resembles frozen dew or vapor". So the character 霜 [shuāng] and the English word "frost" have the same meaning when they are used as nouns. But as a verb, "frost" means "to cover with frost", "to damage by frost", and "to apply frosting to". The word "frosting" refers to a mixture of sugar, egg white or fat used to coat or cover a cake, or the rough surface produced on metal or glass in imitation of frost, or coarsely powdered glass. In order to avoid misunderstanding, "make into frost" or "frost making" are recommended.

PROPERTIES AND TASTES OF CHINESE DRUGS

The basic properties of drugs are classified into cold, hot, warm and cool, collectively called the "four properties [natures]". The tastes or flavors of drugs are pungent, sweet, sour, bitter, and salty, collectively called the "five tastes". Other properties include meridian tropism and direction of drug actions. The proposed standard nomenclature can be listed as follows.

Proposed Standard Nomenclature

property (of drug) 藥性 [yào xìng][1]

nature (of drug) 藥性 [yào xìng][1]

flavor (of drug) 藥味 [yào wèi][2]

taste (of drug) 藥味 [yào wèi][2]

meridian tropism 歸經 [guī jīng][3]

ascending, descending, floating and sinking 升降浮沈 [shēng jiàng fú chén][4]

toxicity 毒性 [dú xìng][5]

toxic 有毒 [yǒu dú][5]

non-toxic 無毒 [wú dú][5]

Discussion

1. For the basic properties of drugs, i.e., cold, hot, warm and cool, some designate them as natures, and some simply called them properties. Other words such as "characters", and "*qi*" have also been used, but they are not widely accepted. Both "property" and "nature" are selected as the proposed standard nomenclature. As for the words cold, hot, warm and cool, they are generally accepted, and can be used together with nature or property in different ways, e.g., cold-natured, cold-propertied, cold in nature, or cold in property.

2. For the tastes or flavors of drugs, "flavor" is more appropriate than "taste", for flavor includes taste and smell. Sweet, sour, bitter and salty are tastes, but pungent is smell. Both "taste" and "flavor" are selected as the standard nomenclature because the word "taste" is used by many authors. They prefer "taste" probably because "flavor" usually refers to pleasant taste and smell, but the taste of drug is not always so pleasant.

3. Classification of drugs according to the meridian(s) on which their therapeutic action is manifested is called 歸經 [guī jīng]. This term has been rendered into English in several different ways even if only the word "meridian" is used as an equivalent for 經 [jīng]. The character 歸 [guī] is expressed as "tropism", "distribution", "entry" or "entered" by different authors. By comparing these words, one can find that "tropism" is more appropriate than "distribution" and "entry". "Channel (meridian) distribution" is understood as the distribution of the drug or drug action to each meridian or *zang-fu* organ. It does not stress that the drug action is predisposed to a certain meridian or *zang-fu* organ. "Channel (meridian) entry" or "channel (meridian) entered" makes one misunderstand that the term stresses the meridian through which the drug enters the body.

4. The direction of the drug action is an important element of the drug's properties. The Chinese term 升降浮沉 [shēng jiàng fú chén] is used to express this concept. The four characters actually represent four different directions, namely, upward, downward, outward and inward. There are disputes about the English expressions. The key divergence lies in whether these characters are transitive or intransitive verbs. Since they are used to describe the directions of drug action, they are bound to be intransitive. But some authors believe that they are also transitive. For example, 升 [shēng] may indicate a drug action that causes something (such as *qi*) to ascend. In Chinese, 升 is both intran-

sitive and transitive, equivalent to both "rise" and "raise", but in English no corresponding word can be found. Although "ascend" and "descend" are both intransitive and transitive, when they are used as transitive verbs, their meaning is different from the Chinese original, not referring to causing something to go up or to go down, but referring to going up something or going down something (such as stairs). Thus, a new English word "upbear" was initiated for 升, and "downbear" for 降. This is a brilliant way to solve this translation problem. However, so far as the standard nomenclature is concerned, it is not necessary to find a single set of English words to match the Chinese. The words "upbear" and "downbear" are not ideal for they might be misunderstood as "cope with" (bear up) and "overcome" (bear down). One can either use "ascending, descending, floating and sinking" or "lifting, lowering, floating and sinking" in accordance with the necessity of the wording.

5. Chinese medicine puts great emphasis on the toxicity of drugs. Drugs are usually classified as highly toxic (大毒 [dà dú]), moderately toxic (常毒 [cháng dú]), slightly toxic (小毒 [xiǎo dú]) and non-toxic drugs (無毒 [wú dú]). "Toxic" and "poisonous" are synonyms, but the latter word is derived from "poison", a word often referring to a substance used for the purpose of causing death or harm.

DRUG COMBINATION

In Chinese medicine, when two or more drugs are used in combination the relationships between them should be seriously considered. There are six kinds of interactions, which, together with the administration of a single drug, are collectively called the "seven relations". When rendering them into English, first of all, one should determine the meaning of the character 相 [xiāng]. It may mean "mutual" or "each other", but in many instances it only stresses an action on somebody or something else. For these terms, rendering 相 [xiāng] as "mutual" may cause confusion. For example, 相畏 [xiāng wèi] and 相殺 [xiāng shā] describe the two aspects of one single event. In Chinese, we say pinellia tuber fears (畏 [wèi]) fresh ginger, for the latter removes the toxicity of the former, but we never say the reverse. We say fresh ginger eliminates (殺 [shā]) the toxicity of pinellia tuber, but we do not say the reverse either. The relation represented by 相使 [xiāng shǐ] is also not mutual. When two drugs are used with such a relationship, one drug should be the principal, and the other as an assistant or guide to enhance the therapeutic effect of the principal one. Take the combination of omphalia and rhubarb for example. Rhubarb is used to assist the anthelmintic effect of omphalia, but omphalia is not used for enhancing the cathartic effect of rhubarb. It is the same for 相惡 [xiāng wù]. We say ginseng is averse to radish seed, for the latter reduces the tonic action of ginseng, but we do not say radish seed is averse to ginseng. The term 相反 [xiāng fǎn] does not mean that the drugs used together have a contradictory action on each other, but indicates that the combined use of these drugs may cause or enhance the toxic or side effects. In this case, 相 [xiāng] still does not mean "mutual".

Proposed Standard Nomenclature

reinforcement 相須 [xiāng xū][1] assistance 相使 [xiāng shǐ][2]
restraint 相畏 [xiāng wèi][3] suppression 相殺 [xiāng shā][4]
aversion 相惡 [xiāng wù][5] incompability 相反 [xiāng fǎn][6]
prohibited combination 配伍禁忌 dietary prohibition 食忌 [shí jì][8]
  [pèi wǔ jìn jì][7]

Discussion

1. For the term 相須 [xiāng xū], the following expressions have appeared in recent publications: "mutual reinforcement", "mutual potentiation", "mutual need", "mutual promotion", "mutual accentuation", and "potentiation". The diversity comes from the explanation of the character 須 [xū]. Its most exact literal translation is the word "need", but many authors would rather use other words. Before discussing this issue, we had better review the definition of this term. According to the national Chinese textbook this term has the following basic elements: drugs with similar property and effect used together to enhance their efficacy.* In this sense, the words other than "need" seem to be more appropriate. They are also used in Western medicine: "accentuation" refers to "increased loudness or distinctness"; "potentiation" means "the increase of potency", particularly,

---

*"相須即性能功效相類似的藥物配合應用，可以增強原有療效。"— cited from Lei ZQ (chief ed.) Zhong Yao Xue, *Chinese Pharmaceutics* (in Chinese), the Textbook Series for Programmed Courses of the TCM Universities and Colleges, Shanghai Science and Technology Press, 1998, p.20.

the synergic action of two drugs, being greater than the sum of effects of each used alone; "promotion" is a special term used in genetics, referring to the activity of a promoter or the results of such activity; and "reinforcement" used in behavioral science refers to the presentation of a stimulus following a response that increases the frequency of subsequent responses.

2. For the term 相使 [xiāng shǐ] there are also multifarious expressions: "mutual assistance", "assistance", "mutual enhancement", "enhancement", "enhancement of effect by another medicine" and "empowering". Among these terms, "assistance" or "assisting" are recommended.

3. The available expressions for 相畏 [xiāng wèi] are "mutual restraint", "restriction", "fearing", "mutual counteraction", "counteraction", "incompatibility between drugs" and "incompatibility".

4. The English terms used for expressing 相殺 [xiāng shā] are "mutual detoxication", "mutual detoxicity", "decreasing toxicity", "neutralization", "killing", "mutual suppression" and "suppression". "Detoxication" or "detoxicating" are only partially correct, because the wording is limited to the toxic effect. In fact, the term 相殺 may cover other undesirable effects. So the word "suppression" is selected.

5. For the term 相惡 [xiāng wù] the following expressions have been used: "mutual inhibition", "inhibition", "counteraction", "aversion", "mutual antagonism", and "antagonism". The word "aversion" is most acceptable, for all the others may cause difficulty in practical use, e.g., "A 惡 B" cannot be rendered as "A inhibits B", "A counteracts on B" or "A is antagonistic to B" (the reverse being correct in all three sentences), but it can be rendered as "A is averse to B".

6. Rendering the term 相反 [xiāng fǎn] is also a problem. The word 反 [fǎn] does not simply indicate the opposite actions of drugs; it refers to the increased toxic or adverse side effects when drugs are used in combination. The available expressions include "antagonism", "antagonism between two drugs", "incompatibility", "mutual incompatibility" "incompatibility between two drugs", "clashing" and "mutual addition". The word "incompatibility" seems to be the least problematic.

7. Among the expressions appearing in recent publications are "incompatibility of drugs in a prescription", "prescription incompatibility" and "prohibited combinations". The last one seems the best, for the first one is explanatory and too lengthy as a term, and the second one may

lead to the misunderstanding that certain prescriptions should not be used together.

8. In Chinese medicine, some species of food are not allowed to be taken during a given drug treatment. This is called 服藥食忌 [fú yào shí jì] or simply 食忌 [shí jì]. Several English expressions have been suggested by different authors: "food prohibition", "dietary contraindication", "foods contraindicated", and "dietary incompatibilities". The word "contraindication" means "something (as a symptom or condition) that makes a particular treatment or procedure inadvisable" (*Merriam Webster's Medical Desk Dictionary*, 1996, p. 162). "Dietary contraindication" may lead to the misunderstanding that if one has taken a certain kind of food, one should not receive that treatment. The original Chinese term has the reverse implication, i.e., if one is receiving that treatment, one should not take certain kinds of food. The term "dietary incompatibilities" does not cause such misunderstanding, and "dietary prohibition" may be more appropriate to express this concept.

PREPARATIONS

The forms of prepared drugs are multifarious. Some of them are common among Western drugs, but some are unique to Chinese medicine, hence the names.

Proposed Standard Nomenclature

preparation 劑型 [jì xíng][1]

bolus 丸 [wán][2]

honeyed pill [bolus] 蜜丸 [mì wán][2]

minute pill 微丸 [wēi wán][2]

powder 散 [sǎn][3]

ointment 軟膏 [ruǎn gāo][4]

cream 乳膏 [rǔ gāo][4]

distillate 露 [lù][5]

lozenge 錠 [dìng][6]

decoction 湯劑 [tāng jì][8]

(medicinal) tea 茶 [chá][9]

gelatin 膠 [jiāo][10]

decocting slices 飲片 [yǐn piàn][12]

pill 丸 [wán][2]

watered pill 水丸 [shuǐ wán][2]

pasted pill 糊丸 [hú wán][2]

concentrated pill 濃縮丸 [nóng suō wán][2]

soft extract 煎膏 [jiān gāo][4]

adhesive plaster 膏藥 [gāo yào][4]

pastil 錠 [dìng][6]

medicinal wine 藥酒 [yào jiǔ][7]

cold decoction 飲 [yǐn][8]

glue 膠 [jiāo][10]

tablet 片 [piàn][11]

granules 沖劑 [chōng jì][11]

Discussion

1. Many authors render 劑型 [jì xíng] as "dosage form" or "dose pattern". This reflects a misunderstanding of the character 劑 [jì] as an abbreviation of 劑量 [jì liàng] (dosage). In fact, 劑 [jì] in this term refers to 藥劑 [yào jì] (prepared drug), and this term means "form of preparation", so rendering it simply as "preparation" is clear enough.

2. 丸 [wán] (pill or bolus) is a solid globular mass, coated or uncoated, made of finely powdered drugs with a suitable excipient or binder. A small medicated mass to be swallowed is a "pill", and a large pill to be chewed and then swallowed is a "bolus". A pill with water used as the binder is called 水丸 [shuǐ wán] (watered pill), and with rice-paste or flour-paste used as the binder is called 糊丸 [hú wán] (pasted pill). A bolus is often made with honey as the binder, and is called 蜜丸 [mì wán] (honeyed bolus), but it may also be small (honeyed pill). In a concentrated pill (濃縮丸 [nóng suō wán]), part of the medicament is made into extract, used as the binder. A very small globular medicated mass with a diameter less than 2.5 mm is called 微丸 [wēi wán] (minute pill).

3. It is generally agreed that 散 [sǎn] and "powder" are equivalents, though some authors prefer "medicinal powder" or "medicine in powder form".

4. 膏 [gāo] is a general term for soft extract, ointment and adhesive plaster. Soft extract is called 煎膏 [jiān gāo], which literally means "extract made by concentrating a decoction". Ointment, an unguent for application to the skin, is called 軟膏 [ruǎn gāo]. Cream, ointment with an emulsifying base, is called 乳膏 [rǔ gāo], and adhesive plaster, a medicated dressing that consists of a film (as of cloth or paper) spread with a medicated substance is called 膏藥 [gāo yào].

5. It is generally agreed that "distillate" and 露 [lù] are exact equivalents.

6. 錠 [dìng], pastil and lozenge refer to the same preparation.

7. There are various combinations of 藥 [yào] (medicated, medicinal, and medical) and 酒 [jiǔ] (wine, and liquor) to express 藥酒 [yào jiǔ].

8. Both 湯劑 [tāng jì] and 飲 [yǐn] are "decoction", but the latter is often taken cold.

9. 茶 [chá] is indisputably rendered as "tea". Actually, the word "tea" has at least four meanings: (1) the plant *Camellia sinensis*, (2) dried leaves of *Camellia sinensis*, (3) a decoction of infusion of these

leaves, and (4) any decoction or infusion. Here, the term 茶 [chá] is the abbreviation of 茶劑 [chá jì], i.e., a preparation of crushed medicinal made into the form of brick tea for infusion or decoction. Some authors render it as "herb tea", and some others prefer "medicinal tea".

10. Two words are commonly used to express 膠 [jiāo]: glue and gelatin, both being exact. Strictly speaking, gelatin is more purified than glue.

11. 片 [piàn] and 冲劑 [chōng jì] are not traditional preparations. They are newly developed, corresponding to "tablet" and "granules" respectively. Some authors use "soluble granules" to further specify 冲劑 [chōng jì].

12. 飲片 [yǐn piàn] is rendered in different ways: "medicinal pieces", "decocting pieces", "medical herb in pieces", and "pieces of herbal medicine". Comparatively speaking, "decocting pieces" fits the Chinese original better.

DECOCTION METHODS

Decoction is one of the most common form of drug preparation. The following terms related to decoction-making need standardization.

Proposed Standard Nomenclature

slow fire 文火 [wén huǒ][1]

decoct first 先煎 [xiān jiān][2]

decoct with wrapping 包煎 [bāo jiān][3]

decoct alone 單煎 [dān jiān][4]

dissolve 溶化 [róng huà][5]

fierce fire 武火 [wǔ huǒ][1]

decoct later 後下 [hòu xià][2]

wrap-decoct 包煎 [bāo jiān][3]

decoct separately 另煎 [lìng jiān][4]

melt 烊化 [yáng huà][5]

Discussion

1. The terms 文火 [wén huǒ] and 武火 [wǔ huǒ] are common words in daily use, particularly for cooking. Each term has a number of English expressions: "civil fire", "low fire", "soft fire", "gentle fire", "slow fire", and "mild fire" for 文火, and "martial fire", "high fire", "fierce fire", "strong fire", "quick fire", and "intense fire" for 武火. The use of 文 and 武 in the Chinese original is metaphorical. As standard nomenclature,

straightforward expressions are preferred, and so "low fire" and "high fire" are selected.

2. The terms 先煎 [xiān jiān] and 後下 [hòu xià] are usually rendered as "decoct first" or "(be) decocted first" and "decoct later" or "(be) decocted later", but the latter might be somewhat misleading. "Decoct later" may be misunderstood as "add the ingredients to be decocted following those decocted first". The actual procedure is as follows: decoct some ingredient(s) first, then add the main portions of the ingredients to continue decocting, and finally add some ingredient(s) when the decoction process is close to the end. The term 後下 [hòu xià] refers to the third part but not the second part of the procedure. So, the wordings "add at end", "end addition" or "add near end" are appropriate. Comparatively speaking, "add near end" is probably the best, because a short period of decocting after the addition is still necessary.

3. Various expressions are used for the procedure 包煎 [bāo jiān]: "decoction of a wrapped drug", "decoct a drug wrapped", "decocting in wrapped condition", "wrap-boiling", "medicines wrapped during decocting", "decocting with wrappings", "decocted in packet", and "decocted in gauze". In these expressions the words "packet" and "gauze" are not appropriate, because they are associated with the wrapping material. Among these terms "wrap-boiling" is the most succinct. In order to keep consistency with other related terms such as "decoct first", it is better to use "wrap-decoct".

4. The terms 另煎 [lìng jiān] and 單煎 [dān jiān] are synonymous. There is not much disagreement on their English equivalents except the word order: "decoct separately", "separate decocting" and "separately decocted". In order to keep consistency with other related terms, "decoct separately" is selected for 另煎 [lìng jiān], and "decoct alone" for 單煎 [dān jiān].

5. Most authors use the word "dissolve" for 溶化 [róng huà] and "melt" for 烊化 [yáng huà].

METHOD OF TAKING MEDICINES

Athough most Chinese medicines are taken orally, different methods of oral administration are required for different medicines to achieve the desired effects.

Proposed Standard Nomenclature

take infused 冲服 [chōng fú][1]

take mixed 調服 [tiáo fú][2]

swallow 吞服 [tūn fú][3]

take with fluid 送服 [sòng fú][4]

melt in the mouth 噙化 [qín huà][5]

take between meals 食遠服 [shí yuǎn fú][6]

take on an empty stomach 空腹服 [kōng fù fú][7]

take in one single dose 頓服 [dùn fú][8]

take frequently 頻服 [pín fú][9]

take warm 溫服 [wēn fú][10]

take hot 熱服 [rè fú][10]

take cold 冷服 [lěng fú][10]

Discussion

1. There are many expressions for the term 冲服 [chōng fú]: "take the drug following its infusion", "take medicine after infusion", "take soon after being infused", "take after pouring liquid on it", "take after mixing with decoction", "take medicine after mixing with water, wine, etc.", "take with decoction", "take medicine with water", "take with the strained decoction" and "take drenched [mixed with a large amount of water]". All these expressions are basically correct, but most of them are too lengthy. Since the liquid used for infusion can be flexibly changed, the addition of such words as "water", "wine", "decoction" and "strained decoction" is unnecessary. The most succinct form is "take drenched", but the word "drench" means "make something completely wet" and an additional explanation is needed for increasing the amount of water. The word "infuse" means "pouring liquid on", and so the term can be rendered as "take infused".

2. 調服 [tiáo fú] is rendered in the following ways: "take after mixing with liquid", "take after mixing with decoction", "take mixed (with liquid)", "take mixed medicine", etc.

3. Some authors render 吞服 [tūn fú] as "take by swallowing". The most direct expression is probably "swallow" or "be swallowed".

4. 送服 [sòng fú] is often rendered as "take with water", but besides water, other liquids can be used.

5. 噙化 [qín huà] is to hold a pill or pastil in the mouth and let it melt.

6. 食遠服 [shí yuǎn fú] means that the medicine should be taken at a long interval before and after meals, i.e., midway between meals.

7. 空腹服 [kōng fù fú] is not exactly the same as "take before meal".

8. There are quite a few expressions for 頓服 [dùn fú]: "take at a draught", "take medicine at a draft", "take totally at one time", "take a dose all at once", and "take in one single dose". Comparatively speaking, the last one is the most precise and non-misleading.

9. The English expressions suggested by different authors for 頻服 [pín fú] include: "take in frequent small doses", "take medicine in multiple doses", "take frequently", "take in several small doses", "take in small doses at short intervals" and "take in divided doses"

10. There is not much disagreement on the English expressions for 溫服 [wēn fú] 熱服 [rè fú], and 冷服 [lěng fú]. Most authors use "take warm", "take hot" and "take cold", respectively, though some make the expressions more detailed, such as "take medicine warm", "decoction to be taken warm" for 溫服, and so forth.

CLASSIFICATION OF DRUGS [MEDICINALS]

In Chinese medical history, there were several different ways to classify medicinals: classification chiefly according to toxicity, e.g., classification into three grades: non-toxic, not very toxic, and toxic; classification according to substances, such as plants, animals, minerals, etc.; and classification according to the therapeutic effects. Nowadays, the last approach is generally adopted. Thus the related terms should be closely consistent with those used to designate the treatment principles.

Proposed Standard Nomenclature

exterior-releasing drug [medicinal] 解表藥 [jiě biǎo yào][1]

diaphoretic exterior-releasing drug [medicinal] 發汗解表藥 [fā hàn jiě biǎo yào]

wind-cold-dispersing drug [medicinal] 發散風寒藥 [fā sàn fēng hán yào]

wind-heat-dispersing drug [medicinal] 發散風熱藥 [fā sàn fēng rè yào]

pungent-warm exterior-releasing drug [medicinal] 辛溫解表藥 [xīn wēn jiě biǎo yào]

pungent-cool exterior-releasing drug [medicinal] 辛涼解表藥 [xīn liáng jiě biǎo yào]

heat-clearing drug [medicinal] 清熱藥 [qīng rè yào]

heat-clearing and fire-purging drug [medicinal] 清熱瀉火藥 [qīng rè xiè huǒ yào]

heat-clearing and blood-cooling drug [medicinal] 清熱涼血藥 [qīng rè liáng xuè yào]

heat-clearing and dampness-drying

heat-clearing and toxicity-relieving drug [medicinal] 清熱解毒藥 [qīng rè jiě dú yào]

purgative (drug [medicinal]) 瀉下藥 [xiè xià yào]

offensive purgative (drug [medicinal]) 攻下藥 [gōng xià yào]

laxative (drug [medicinal]) 潤下藥 [rùn xià yào]

wind-damp-dispelling drug [medicinal] 祛風濕藥 [qù fēng shī yào]

wind-damp-dispelling and heat-clearing drug [medicinal] 祛風濕清熱藥 [qù fēng shī qīng rè yào]

damp-resolving drug [medicinal] 化濕藥 [huà shī yào]

diuretic (drug [medicinal] 利尿藥 [lì niào yào]

damp-draining diuretic (drug [medicinal]) 利水滲濕藥 [lì shuǐ shèn shī yào]

edema-alleviating diuretic (drug [medicinal]) 利水消腫藥 [lì shuǐ xiāo zhǒng yào]

stranguria-relieving drug [medicinal] 通淋藥 [tōng lín yào]

bile-draining anti-icteric (drug [medicinal]) 利膽退黃藥 [lì dǎn tuì huáng

interior-warming drug [medicinal] 溫裏藥 [wēn lǐ yào]

qi-regulating drug [medicinal] 理氣藥 [lǐ qì yào]

digestant (drug [medicinal]) 消食藥 [xiāo shí yào]

worm-expelling drug [medicinal] 驅蟲藥 [qū chóng yào]

drug [medicinal] 清熱燥濕藥 [qīng rè zào shī yào]

deficiency-heat-clearing drug [medicinal] 清虛熱藥 [qīng xū rè yào]

warm purgative (drug [medicinal]) 溫下藥 [wēn xià yào]

drastic hydragogue 峻下逐水藥 [jùn xià zhú shuǐ yào]

wind-damp-dispelling and cold-dispersing drug [medicinal] 祛風濕散寒藥 [qù fēng shīsàn hán yào]

wind-damp-dispelling and tendon-bone-strengthening drug [medicinal] 祛風濕強筋骨藥 [qù fēng shī qiáng jīn gǔ yào]

fragrant damp-resolving drug [medicinal] 芳香化濕藥 [fāng xiāng huà shī yào]

damp-draining drug [medicinal] 利濕藥 [lì shī yào]

stranguria-relieving diuretic (drug [medicinal]) 利尿通淋藥 [lì niào tōng lín yào]

damp-draining anti-icteric (drug [medicinal]) 利濕退黃藥 [lì shī tuì huáng yào]

bile-draining drug [medicinal] 利膽藥 [lì dǎn yào]

diuretic hydragogue (drug [medicinal]) 利尿逐水藥 [lì niào zhú shuǐ yào]

cold-expelling drug [medicinal] 祛寒藥 [qù hán yào]

qi-moving drug [medicinal] 行氣藥 [xíng qì yào]

digestant and evacuant drug [medicinal] 消導藥 [xiāo dǎo yào]

anthelmintic 驅蟲藥 [qū chóng yào]

hemostatic (drug [medicinal]) 止血

blood-regulating drug [medicinal] 理血藥 [lǐ xuè yào]

stasis-resolving hemostatic (drug [medicinal]) 化瘀止血藥 [huà yū zhǐ xuè yào]

meridian-warming hemostatic (drug [medicinal]) 溫經止血藥 [wēn jīng zhǐ xuè yào]

stasis-resolving drug [medicinal] 化瘀藥 [huà yū yào]

blood-activating and stasis-dispelling drug [medicinal] 活血祛瘀藥 [huó xuè qù yū yào]

blood-activating and menstruation-regulating drug [medicinal] 活血調經藥 [huó xuè tiáo jīng yào]

blood-breaking and mass-eliminating ing drug [medicinal] 破血消癥藥 [pò xuè xiāo zhēng yào]

warming phlegm-resolving drug [medicinal] 溫化寒痰藥 [wēn huà hán tán yào]

antitussive (drug [medicinal]) 止咳藥 [zhǐ ké yào]

tranquilizing drug [medicinal] 安神藥 [ān shén yào]

heart-nourishing tranquilizing drug [medicinal] 養心安神藥 [yǎng xīn ān shén yào]

liver-pacifying and yang-suppressing drug [medicinal] 平肝抑陽藥 [píng gān yì yáng yào]

wind-extinguishing and spasm-relieving drug [medicinal] 息風止痙藥 [xī fēng zhǐ jīng yào]

aromatic orifice-opening drug [medicinal] 芳香開竅藥 [fāng xiāng kāi qiào yào]

藥 [zhǐ xuè yào]

blood-cooling hemostatic (drug [medicinal]) 涼血止血藥 [liáng xuè zhǐ xuè yào]

astringent hemostatic (drug [medicinal]) 收斂止血藥 [shōu liǎn zhǐ xuè yào]

blood-activating drug [medicinal] 活血藥 [huó xuè yào]

blood-activating and stasis-resolving drug [medicinal] 活血化瘀藥 [huó xuè huà yū yào]

blood-activating analgesic (drug [medicinal]) 活血止痛藥 [huó xuè zhǐ tòng yào]

blood-activating and *qi*-moving drug [medicinal] 活血行氣藥 [huó xuè xíng qì yào]

blood-activating and trauma-curing drug [medicinal] 活血療傷藥 [huó xuè liáo shāng yào]

phlegm-resolving drug [medicinal] 化痰藥 [huà tán yào]

cooling phlegm-resolving drug [medicinal] 清化熱痰藥 [qīng huà rè tán yào]

antasthmatic (drug [medicinal]) 平喘藥 [píng chuǎn yào]

settling tranquilizing drug [medicinal] 重鎮安神藥 [zhòng zhèn ān shén yào]

liver-pacifying and wind-extinguishing drug [medicinal] 平肝息風藥 [píng gān xī fēng yào]

orifice-opening drug [medicinal] 開竅藥 [kāi qiào yào]

stimulant 開竅藥 [kāi qiào yào]

aromatic stimulant 芳香開竅藥 [fāng xiāng kāi qiào yào]

tonifying and nourishing drug [me-

tonifying and replenishing drug [medicinal] 補益藥 [bǔ yì yào]

qi tonic 補氣藥 [bǔ qì yào]

yang-tonifying drug [medicinal] 補陽藥 [bǔ yáng yào]

kidney-yang tonic 補腎陽藥 [bǔ shèn yáng yào]

blood-tonifying drug [medicinal] 補血藥 [bǔ xuè yào]

liver-emolliating drug [medicinal] 柔肝藥 [róu gān yào]

yin tonic 補陰藥 [bǔ yīn yào]

yin-nourishing drug [medicinal] 滋陰藥 [zī yīn yào]

emetic 湧[催]吐藥 [yǒng [cuī] tù yào]

dicinal] 補養藥 [bǔ yǎng yào]

tonic 補益藥 [bǔ yì yào]; 補養藥 [bǔ yǎng yào]

qi-tonifying drug [medicinal] 補氣藥 [bǔ qì yào]

yang tonic 補陽藥 [bǔ yáng yào]

kidney-yang-tonifying drug [medicinal] 補腎陽藥 [bǔ shèn yáng yào]

blood tonic 補血藥 [bǔ xuè yào]

blood-nourishing drug [medicinal] 養血藥 [yǎng xuè yào]

yin-tonifying drug [medicinal] 補陰藥 [bǔ yīn yào]

discharge-arresting drug [medicinal] 收澀藥 [shōu sè yào]

astringent 固澀藥 [gù sè yào]

Discussion

Since the drug classification is in accordance with the therapeutic effects, the terms thus formed are closely related to the treatment principles. The terms in the two categories often match each other. For example, the English equivalent of 補氣 [bǔ qì] is "tonify *qi*" or "*qi* tonification", and so 補氣藥 [bǔ qì yào] is rendered as "*qi*-tonifying drug" or "*qi* tonic". Nevertheless, not all of the terms are treated in this manner. Some terms are expressed by many authors in a simpler but somewhat Westernized way, such as "digestant" (消食藥 [xiāo shí yào]), "antitussive" (止咳藥 [zhǐ ké yào]), and "emetic" (催吐藥 [cuī tù yào]).

ACUPUNCTURE-MOXIBUSTION TERMS

Terms used in acupuncture and moxibustion include the following groups: (1) general terms related to acupuncture and moxibustion, (2) names of meridians, (3) acupuncture points, (4) classification of specific points, (5) terms related to various acupuncture and moxibustion methods. Since the standard names of points have already been approved by the World Health Organization, they will be listed in the annexes with no more discussion.

GENERAL TERMS

Proposed Standard Nomenclature

acupuncture and moxibustion 針灸 [zhēn jiǔ]
acupuncture 針法 [zhēn fǎ]

moxibustion 灸法 [jiǔ fǎ]
acupuncturist 針灸醫生 [zhēn jiǔ yī shēng]

Discussion

The words "acupuncture" and "moxibustion" have been used in the Western world for many years, and are medical subject headings for use in MEDLARS (Medical Literature Analysis and Retrieval System), from which *Index Medicus* is produced. In addition, the term "acupuncture" is also approved by the WHO proposed standard international nomenclature.

The title "acupuncturist", derived from the word "acupuncture", is also widely accepted.

MERIDIANS

Meridian theory is an important component part of traditional Chinese medicine, according to which there exists within the human body a system of conduits through which *qi* and blood circulate, and by which the internal organs are connected with each other and with the superficial organs and tissues. Some of the terms used in the meridian theory are standardized and collected in the WHO Standard Acupuncture Nomenclature. They are listed in the annex, but some of them are repeated here for further discussion.

Proposed Standard Nomenclature

meridian 經 [jīng][1]
meridian and collateral 經絡 [jīng luò][1]

collateral 絡 [luò][1]
three yin meridians of the hand 手三陰經 [shǒu sān yīn jīng][2]

three yang meridians of the hand 手三陽經 [shǒu sān yáng jīng][2]

three yin meridians of the foot 足三陰經 [zú sān yīn jīng][2]

fourteen (main) meridians 十四經 [shí sì jīng][4]

eight extra meridians 奇經八脈 [jì jīng bā mài][5]

large intestine meridian (LI)手陽明大腸經 [shǒu yáng míng dà cháng jīng][6]

heart meridian (HT) 手少陰心經 [shǒu shǎo yīn xīn jīng][6]

bladder meridian (BL) 足太陽膀胱經 [zú tài yáng páng guāng jīng][6]

pericardium meridian (PC) 手厥陰心包經 [shǒu jué yīn xīn bāo jīng][6]

gallbladder meridian (GB) 足少陽膽經 [zú shào yáng dǎn jīng][6]

governor vessel (GV) 督脈 [dū mài][6]

thoroughfare vessel (TV) 衝脈 [chōng mài][6]

belt vessel (BV) 帶脈 [dài mǎi][6]

yang heel vessel (YangHV) 陽蹻脈 [yáng qiāo mài][6]

yang link vessel (YangLV) 陽維脈 [yáng wéi mài][6]

three yang meridians of the foot 足三陽經 [zú sān yáng jīng][2]

regular meridians 正經 [zhèng jīng][3]

twelve (regular) meridians 十二（正）經 [shí èr (zhèng) jīng][3]

lung meridian (LU) 手太陰肺經 [shǒu tài yīn fèi jīng][6]

stomach meridian (ST) 足陽明胃經 [zú yáng míng wèi jīng]

spleen meridian (SP) 足太陰脾經 [zú tài yīn pí jīng][6]

small intestine meridian (SI) 手太陽小腸經 [shǒu tài yáng xiǎo cháng jīng][6]

kidney meridian (KI) 足少陽腎經 [zú shào yáng shènjīng][6]

triple energizer meridian (TE) 手少陽三焦經 [shǒu shào yáng sān jiāo jīng][6]

liver meridian (LR) 足厥陰肝經 [zú jué yīn gān jīng][6]

conception [controller] vessel (CV) 任脈 [rèn mài][4]

yin heel vessel (YinHV) 陰蹻脈 [yīn qiāo mài][6]

yin link vessel (YinLV) 陰維脈 [yīn wéi mài][6]

Discussion

1. The terms "meridian 經 [jīng]", "collateral 絡 [luò]", and "meridian and collateral 經絡 [jīng luò]" were adopted as standard nomenclature by the WHO Working Group on the Standardization of Acupuncture Nomenclature in 1985. At present, some discussion is still necessary for general acceptance of these terms. The Chinese term "經 [jīng]" is an abbreviation of "經脈 [jīng mài]", and "絡 [luò]" is an abbreviation of "絡脈 [luò mài]". There is no doubt that "脈 [mài]" is a body structure equivalent to vessel or blood vessel, including artery and

its pulsation, so that pulse-taking ("診脈 [zhěn mài]") is an important aspect of physical examination in Chinese medicine. The character 經 [jīng] originated from textiles, as shown by its left half 糸 which means silk. The longitudinal line or warp in weaving is called 經 [jīng]. Since the main blood vessels run along the longitudinal axis of the trunk and limbs, these blood vessels were thus called 經脈 [jīng mài]. In the history of acupuncture, needling and blood pricking were closely associated. This is more evidence that the so-called 經絡 [jīng luò] is closely associated with the vascular system. In the later development of acupuncture, the concept of *qi* has become more and more important. Even so, it was believed that either *qi* or blood must circulate in a certain real and concrete structure, and the word "channel" was thus used to express 經脈 [jīng mài].

Modern research, however, has shown that the course of 經脈 [jīng mài] differs greatly from any known structure such as blood vessels and nerves. In addition, no real structure has ever been found to tally with 經脈 [jīng mài]. Therefore, the term "meridian" was initiated and has been adopted at WHO meetings on standard terminology. Now this term is widely used by most authors, although some insist on using the word "channel".

In 1983, Ted Kaptchuk made a comment on this issue. He agreed that "channel" was in fact a better translation than "meridian", but in order to avoid the confusion of using a new term he still used the term meridian*. As the term "meridian" has been recommended as the standard international nomenclature by the WHO since 1991, there is more reason not to change the terminology. For those who prefer "channel", a footnote may be added, like that made by Kaptchuk.

Regarding 絡脈 [luò mài], most authors render it as "collateral", but some call it "network vessel". The latter is closer to the literal meaning of 絡脈 [luò mài], but the former defined as "a small side branch, as of a blood vessel or nerve",** is more concise and can also reflect the meaning of the Chinese term.

2. The disparity in terminology of "three yin [yang] meridians of the hand [foot] 手[足]三陰[陽]經 [shǒu〔zú〕 sān yīn〔yáng〕 jīng]" chiefly

---

*Ted J. Kaptchuk. *The Web That Has No Weaver: Understanding Chinese Medicine.* Congdon & Weed, 1983, p.108.

**Dorland's Illustrated Medical Dictionary*, 29th ed., 2000, p.376.

lies in the word "meridian". (cf. "meridian and collateral")

3. In Chinese medicine 十二經 [shí èr jīng] is also called 十二正經 [shí èr zhèng jīng], or simply 正經 [zhèng jīng]. Most authors translate 正經 [zhèng jīng] as "regular meridians", 十二正經 [shí èr zhèng jīng] as "twelve regular meridians", and 奇經八脈 [jì jīng bā mài] as "extra eight meridians". Other authors prefer "ordinary meridians" for 正經 [zhèng jīng], and extraordinary meridians for 奇經 [jì jīng]. The meridians are so called because each regular meridian has a directly related *zang-fu* organ, while the extra meridians do not. Since the hypothesis of meridians as well as their complicated courses still needs more evidence for their general recognition, it is better not to include the disputable issues as far as possible in the international standard.

The term "twelve (regular) meridians" does not appear in the WHO-proposed standard international acupuncture nomenclature, because "the fourteen main meridians" is taken as a collective term for all the meridians where the acupuncture points are distributed. The term "fourteen meridians" should not be called the "fourteen regular meridians", because it includes governor and conception vessels.

4. The English names and the respective alphabetic codes are listed in the WHO-proposed standard international acupuncture nomenclature. Most authors follow this standard nomenclature without objection. So the WHO nomenclature has really played an important role in the exchange of information. However, the term "conception vessel" is worthy further discussion. Conception means being conceived or becoming pregnant. So it is limited to the females. But it is hard to explain why this vessel also exists in males. In the Chinese language 任 [rèn] and 妊 [rèn] are two different characters, similar in pronunciation but different in meaning. The latter means pregnancy, but the former means the carrying out of duty. Only occasionally, the two characters may be interchangeable, but either in Chinese medical classics or in contemporary textbooks 任脈 [rèn mài] is never written as 妊脈. The translation of 任脈 [rèn mài] into conception vessel is puzzling, particularly when the pair of meridians running along the midline of the body — 督脈 [dū mài] (governor vessel) on the dorsal aspect and 任脈 [rèn mài] on the ventral aspect — are concerned. Because of their important roles in the meridian system, each of them was given a corresponding name, i.e., 督 [dū] and 任 [rèn], which mean governing and controlling, respectively.

These two characters are still in common use, e.g., 總督 [zǒng dū], which means governor, and 主任 [zhǔ rèn] which means director. Nigel Wiseman made a good suggestion about the revision of this translation. In his *Glossary of Chinese Medical Terms* published by Paradigm Publications in 1990, he used "conception vessel CV", but in his *English-Chinese Chinese-English Dictionary of Chinese Medicine* published in 1995, he changed it to "controlling vessel (CV)". The advantage of this revision is that the original alphabetic code CV can still be used. For governor vessel (GV), controller vessel (CV) is proposed here.

5. The "eight extra meridians" (奇經八脈 [jì jīng bā mài]) is a collective term for the main meridians in addition to the twelve regular meridians. They are the governor vessel, conception (or controller) vessel, thoroughfare vessel, belt vessel, yin heel vessel, yang heel vessel, yin link vessel, and yang link vessel (see Annex). These terms are used by most authors, but it is suggested that the term "conception vessel" be replaced by "controller vessel", as discussed above. Another option is the change of "governor vessel (GV)" and "conception vessel (CV)" to "governing vessel (GV)" and "controlling vessel (CV)".

6. All these meridian names are cited from the WHO' Standard Acupuncture Nomenclature.

ACUPUNCTURE POINTS

The World Health Organization has made great efforts to standardize the acupuncture nomenclature. The alphanumeric codes and names of 361 meridian points and 48 extra points are shown in the annex. For acupuncture points, however, there are still some other terms that need standardization.

Proposed Standard Nomenclature

acupuncture point; acupoint; point (針灸) 穴 [zhēn jiǔ xué][1]

meridian point 經穴 [jīng xué][2]

ouch point 阿是穴 [ā shì xué][4]

extra point (經外) 奇穴 [(jīng wài) qí xué][3]

specific points 特定穴 [tè dìng xué][5]

source point 原穴 [yuán xué][6]

eight confluent points (of extra meridians) 八脈交會穴 [bā mài

crossing point 交會穴 [jiāo huì xué][7]

eight influential points 八會穴 [bā

jiāo huì xué][8]

five transport points 五輸穴 [wǔ shù xué][10]

stream point 輸穴 [shù xué][10]

sea point 合穴 [hé xué][10]

back transport points 背俞穴 [bèi shù xué][12]

connecting point 絡穴 [luò xué][14]

ear point 耳穴 [ěr xué][16]

huì xué][9]

well point 井穴 [jǐng xué][10]

spring point 滎穴 [yíng xué][10]

river point 經穴 [jīng xué][10]

lower sea points 下合穴 [xià hé xué][11]

alarm points 募穴 [mó xué][13]

cleft point 郄穴 [xì xué][15]

Discussion

1. In the WHO-proposed standard international acupuncture nomenclature and the WHO Standard Acupuncture Nomenclature, "acupuncture point" 針灸穴 [zhēn jiǔ xué] is taken as the standard term, its abbreviated form "point" is repeatedly used, and the word "acupoint" is also mentioned.

2. The Chinese character "經 [jīng]" is polysemous even when it is used as a medical term. For example, in 經絡 [jīng], 經血 [jīng xuè] and 經方 [jīng fāng], the character 經 [jīng] has entirely different meanings. It means "meridian" in 經絡 (meridian and collateral), "menstrual" in 經血 (menstrual blood), and "classical" in 經方 (classical formula). In acupuncture, even the term 經穴 [jīng xué] has several different meanings: meridian point (one of the 361 points located on the meridians), river point (one of the five transport points), and classical point (one of the points used in ancient times and recorded in classical literature). The former two are technical terms, and so are included in this scheme, while the last one can be regarded as a common expression. The term "meridian point 經穴 [jīng xué]" is adopted in the WHO Standard Acupuncture Nomenclature, and so no more discussion is needed.

3. The term "extra point 奇穴 [qí xué]" is included in the WHO Standard Acupuncture Nomenclature. The points are called "extra" as they are additional points outside the meridians.

4. The ouch point 阿是穴 [ā shì xué] is an acupuncture point with no specific name nor definite location, the site of which is determined by tenderness. The term has been translated in several different ways, such as "Ah Shi (or a-shi, ashi) point", "Oh yes (or Oh-yes-) point", "Ouch (or ouch) point" and "pressure pain point". Of these terms, "ashi point" seems to be most frequently used, while "ouch point" is more English.

5. The specific points 特定穴 [tè dìng xué] are points on the meridians with specific therapeutic effects, and hence specific names. They include the five transport points, source points, connecting points, alarm points, back transport points, the eight influential points, cleft points, crossing points, the eight confluence points, and lower sea points. Most authors prefer the term "specific" points. Others use the term "special" or "specially designated" points. According to the definitions of these points' specific therapeutic effects, the term "specific points" is the best choice.

6. Most authors prefer the term source point as the English equivalent of 原穴 [yuán xué]. Some render it as "primary point", which is not widely accepted. Those who stick to *pinyin* call it "yuan point". Since the *pinyin* name provides no information about the meaning of the term, modifiers are added, for example, "yuan (source) point", and "yuan-primary-point". We cannot see that the term "yuan (source) point" has any advantage over "source point"; on the contrary, it makes the terminology unnecessarily complicated.

7. 交會穴 [jiāo huì xué] is a point where two or more meridians intersect. Its English versions are diversified, including "crossing point", "convergent point", "intersection point", "junction point", "conjunction point", "meeting point" and "influential point". Among these terms, "convergent" is not the correct word because the two meridians do not become identical. Nor is "conjunction", because the two meridians do not join together. "Influential" is even further from the original meaning of 交會 [jiāo huì]. "Meeting" seems to be good, but "crossing", "intersection" and "junction" may be better. The selection can only depend on the frequency of occurrence in recent publications, and hence "crossing point" is chosen.

8. 八脈交會穴 [bā mài jiāo huì xué] are eight specific points where the *qi* of eight extra meridians communicate with that of the twelve main meridians. Most authors use "eight confluent points" to express this term. Some add (of extra meridians) or (connecting extra meridians). The most succinct expression — "eight confluent points" is selected as the standard.

9. The so-called 八會穴 [bā huì xué] are eight specific points where the essential *qi* of *zang* organs, *fu* organs, *qi*, blood, tendons, vessels, bones and marrow flows in and gathers. There have been many arguments regarding the translation of this term. Literally the Chinese character 會 [huì] means "meeting" or "gathering", so some Western

authors use "eight meeting points" or "eight gathering points" as the equivalent of 八會穴 [bā huì xué]. However, in China, some authors have put forward the new term "eight convergent points", although most authors use the term "eight influential points" to indicate the clinical significance of these points. In the present scheme, the latter is selected simply due to its frequency of occurrence.

10. Basically there are two ways to translate the term 五輸穴 [wǔ shù xué]. One is to translate all the three Chinese characters into English, and the other is to use *pinyin* for the character "輸"*. Unlike 陰 [yīn], 陽 [yáng] and 氣 [qì], which have no equivalent in English, 輸 [shū] has a clear meaning without much dispute among different authors. The only dispute is whether it should be translated as "transport" or "transporting". For simplicity, "transport" is selected here.

The five transport points are the well point 井穴 [jǐng xué], spring point 滎穴 [yíng xué], stream point 輸穴 [shù xué], river point 經穴 [jīng xué], and sea point 合穴 [hé xué]. There are also two different ways to designate the five categories of points. One is to render 井 [jǐng], 滎 [yíng], 輸 [shù], 經 [jīng] and 合 [hé] as "well", "spring", "stream", "river" and "sea" respectively. The majority of them are free translations rather than literal translations. The other is to leave the names as they are, and just use *pinyin* to replace the translation. This leads to a lot of confusion. For example, if 五輸穴 is translated as "five shu points", and 輸穴 as "shu point", then we can say that shu point is one of the five shu points. If so, we are speaking nonsense. In addition, the tone symbol is generally not marked when using *pinyin*. If *pinyin* is used to replace translation, 井穴 is "jing point", and 經穴 is also "jing point". Even the *pinyin* enthusiasts have to add some modifiers to make the distinction, e.g., jing-well point for 井穴 and jing-river point for 經穴. In these terms, the *pinyin* "jing" is apparently superfluous, making the terminology chaotic.

11. For the term 下合穴 [xià hé xué], many different expressions have appeared in recent publications, such as lower confluent points, lower He point, xiahe points, lower He-sea point, lower meeting points, lower combination points, lower uniting points, and lower sea points.

---

*In common Chinese language, 輸 is pronounced shū, but in the term 輸穴 it is pronounced shù. — Jian Ming Zhong Yi Zi Dian, *Concise Dictionary of Characters in Chinese Medicine* (in Chinese), Guizhou People's Publishing House, 1985, p.392.

The proper selection chiefly depends on the translation of 合穴. If sea point is good for 合穴 [hé xué], it is natural to use lower sea point for 下合穴 [xià hé xué], as three of the 下合穴 [xià hé xué] are actually 合穴 [hé xué], and they are called 下合穴 [xià hé xué] because they are located in the lower part of the body.

12. The specific points located along the bladder meridian on the back, whither the *qi* of the *zang-fu* organs flows, are called back transport points 背俞穴 [bèi shù xué]. Many authors use *pinyin*, but the three Han characters 俞 [shù], 輸 [shù] and 腧 [shù] are all commonly used in acupuncture. They have exactly the same pronunciation but not always the same meaning, so that *pinyin* will inevitably cause confusion.

13. The difficulty in the English translation of 募穴 [mó xué] lies in the real meaning of the Chinese character 募 [mó]. Certain points on the ventral aspect of the trunk are called 募穴 [mó xué], not only because they are the sites where the *qi* of the corresponding *zang-fu* organ gathers, but particularly because they are the points located close to the corresponding *zang-fu* organs. No appropriate English equivalent has been found, and most authors in China use *pinyin*. Unfortunately they incorrectly pronounce the character 募 as mù and make the transliteration of 募穴 as "mu point". In the common Chinese language, 募 does sound mù, but in the term 募穴 it should be pronounced [mó] (cf. p.15). Other suggestions, such as "collecting point", "accumulation point", and "front point" have been suggested but not widely accepted. Compared with the above-mentioned terms, "alarm point" seems to be more acceptable to a number of authors (e.g., Nigel Wiseman, Chen Jirui, Nissi Wang, Jeremy Ross, and many others use "alarm points" in their publications), though it is not a literal translation.

14. There are basically three different ways to express the term 絡穴 [luò xué]: (1) Some authors regard the Chinese character "絡" as the same as that used in the term 經絡. (2) Another group of authors believe that "絡" in 絡穴 is not exactly the same as is used in the term 經絡. (3) Some prefer to use *pinyin* instead of translation. According to the criteria for the proposed standard nomenclature, the third alternative is definitely not acceptable. The first group of authors translate the term as collateral point which may cause the misunderstanding that the point is on a collateral but not on a meridian. The term "connecting point" used by the second group of authors is more appropriate and acceptable.

15. The Chinese character 郄 [xì] means gap or cleft. The English

term "cleft point" is an appropriate equivalent of 郄穴 [xì xué]. Other translations such as "accumulation point" and "accumulating point" seem to be too general, and "xi point" in *pinyin* is unacceptable. There is no need to put "xi" in front of "cleft", for "xi-cleft point" is confusing in meaning and difficult in pronunciation.

16. Any point on the auricle used in ear acupuncture therapy is called an ear point (耳穴 [ěr xué]). It also has some different names in English, such as "oto-point", "auricular point", and "ear acupoint", but "ear point" is the most common term.

POINT SELECTION

Each acupuncture point has its indication, and proper point selection and combination guarantees the therapeutic effect. Various rules of combination are designated, with specific names.

Proposed Standard Nomenclature

point selection 選穴(法) [xuǎn xué (fǎ)][1]

point combination 配穴(法) [pèi xué (fǎ)][2]

superior-inferior point combination 上下配穴(法) [shàng xià pèi xué (fǎ)][3]

anterior-posterior point combination 前後配穴(法) [qián hòu pèi xué (fǎ)][4]

same-meridian point combination 本經配穴(法) [běn jīng pèi xué (fǎ)][5]

right-left point combination 左右配穴(法) [zuǒ yòu pèi xué (fǎ)][6]

exterior-interior point combination 表裏配穴(法) [biǎo lǐ pèi xué (fǎ)][7]

cleft-influential point combination 郄會配穴(法) [xì huì pèi xué (fǎ)][8]

ventro-dorsal point combination 腹背配穴法[fù bèi pèi xué (fǎ)][10]

source-connecting point combination 原絡配穴(法) [yuán luò pèi xué (fǎ)][9]

Discussion

1. The terms "point selection 選穴（法）[xuǎn xué (fǎ)]" and "point combination 配穴（法）[pèi xué (fǎ)]" are often interchangeable, if more than a single point is used in the treatment. Literally, there is some difference between the two terms. "Point combination" stresses the additive or even synergetic effects of the selected points.

2. For the term "配穴（法）[pèi xué (fǎ)]" a number of expressions have been used: "point prescription", "point compatibility", "point association", "point combining", "point combination", "clinical combination of points", "combination of points", "combining points", and "balance of points". Among these expressions, the verb "combine" or the noun "combination" is most frequently used. Jeremy Ross's *Acupuncture Point Combinations: the Key to Clinical Success* published by Churchill Livingstone, 1995, has become a book of great popularity. Therefore, "point combination" is selected as the proposed standard term.

3. Different expressions have been used for the word "上下" in the term "上下配穴 [shàng xià pèi xué]": "superior and inferior", "upper and lower", "above and below", and "top and bottom". The Chinese textbook defines this term as "the combined use of acupuncture points above the waist and below the waist….e.g., combined use of neiguan (PC6) and zusanli (ST36) for the treatment of stomach diseases."*. According to this definition, "top and bottom" is not an exact equivalent. "Above" and "below" cause difficulty in wording, for they are prepositions or adverbs but not adjectives or nouns. (The originally proposed expression with "above" and "below" is "combining points above with points below".) Both "superior-inferior" and "upper-lower" can be selected as the standard. Their frequencies of use are practically equal.

4. For the word "前後" in "前後配穴（法）[qián hòu pèi xué (fǎ)]", some express it as "front and back", and some others, "anterior and posterior". The latter is much more frequently used, and so selected as the standard. In order to cope with this term, it is better to render "上下配穴 [shàng xià pèi xué]" as "superior-inferior point combination".

5. As for the word "本經" [běn jīng] in 本經配穴（法）[běn jīng pèi xué (fǎ)], some render it as "the same meridian (or channel)", and some others render it as "the diseased meridian (or channel)". Both reflect the original concept of the term. Literally, the word "same-meridian" is closer to the Chinese original.

6. 左右配穴（法）[zuǒ yòu pèi xué (fǎ)] is a method of point combination in which bilateral points of a given meridian are selected and needled. Diversity exists in the word order. In Chinese when "right" and

---

* "將腰部以上腧穴和腰部以下腧穴配合應用的方法。" cited from Sun GJ (chief editor). Zhen Jiu Xue (*Acupuncture and Moxibustion*) (in Chinese), the Textbook Series for Programmed Courses of the TCM Universities and Colleges, Shanghai Science and Technology Press, 1998, p.219.

"left" are put together to denote two sides, the "left" (左 [zuǒ]) always precedes the "right" (右 [yòu]). In English, there is no such rule; on the contrary, "right and left" reads more smoothly than "left and right".

7. If the point combination is based on the exterior-interior relationship of the three yin and three yang meridians (e. g., combined use of zusanli (ST37) and sanyinjiao (SP6) for treating digestive disorders), it is called 表裏(經)配穴（法） [biǎo lǐ pèi xué (fǎ)]. Most authors use exterior and interior to express the concept of 表裏 [biǎo lǐ].

8. 郄會配穴（法） [xì huì pèi xué (fǎ)] refers to the combined use of a cleft point together with an influential point, e.g., kongzui (LU6), the cleft point of the lung meridian with blood influential point geshu (BL17) for arresting hemoptysis. The proposed standard terminology follows the naming of 郄穴 [xì xué] and 會穴 [huì xué], and hence "cleft-influential point combination".

9. 原絡配穴（法） [yuán luò pèi xué (fǎ)] is a method of point combination based on the principle that sources points cure the disorders of the corresponding meridian and connecting points of the interior-exteriorly related meridian relieve the symptoms, e. g., combined use of taiyuan (LI9), source point of the lung meridian, and pianli (LI6), connecting point of large intestine meridian for treating cough and asthma. The proposed standard terminology follows the naming of 原穴 [yuán xué] and 絡穴 [luò xué], and hence "source-connecting point combination".

10. ventro-dorsal point combination 腹背配穴法 [fù bèi pèi xué (fǎ)] is a method of point combination in which both the points on the ventral and dorsal aspects are used for strengthening the therapeutic effects, e.g., combined use of weishu (BL21) on the back and zhongwan (CV12) on the abdomen for treating gastric disorders. For 腹背 [fù bèi], there are two different translations: "abdomen and back", and "ventral and dorsal". The latter is more appropriate, because the Chinese character "腹" [fù] used here is not limited to the abdomen but actually refers to the ventral aspect of the trunk including the part above the abdomen.

POINT LOCATION

The methods of locating acupuncture points are not limited to proportional measurement. Many anatomical landmarks can be taken as the basis for locating points. For example, yintang (EX-HN3) is between the two eyebrows, and shenque (CV8) in the center of the umbilicus. In these cases, no special terms other than anatomical names are used. But the terms related to proportional measurement are specific for acupuncture.

Proposed Standard Nomenclature

point location 腧穴定位 [shù xué dìng wèi]

bone measurement 骨度法 [gǔ dù fǎ][2]

middle finger cun 中指同身寸 [zhōng zhǐ tóng shēn cùn][4]

palm measurement 一夫法 [yī fū fǎ][5]

cun (同身)寸 [(tóng shēn) cùn][1]

bone proportional cun 骨度分寸 [gǔ dù fēn cùn][2]

finger cun 手指同身寸 [shǒu zhǐ tóng shēn cùn][3]

thumb cun 拇指同身寸 [mǔ zhǐ tóng shēn cùn][4]

Discussion

1. At the meeting of the Third Working Group on the Standardization of Acupuncture Nomenclature convened by the WHO Regional Office for the Western Pacific in 1987, the unit for location of points was discussed. Some countries used the term "inch" or other equivalent units in English, but most of the countries used cun or tsun. It was decided to use cun (non-italicized) as the standardized nomenclature for the unit. It was also decided that bone proportional cun (B-cun) and finger cun (F-cun) should be used in each measurement method.

It should be noticed that the full name of cun is body-proportional cun (同身寸 [tóng shēn cùn]), different from an ordinary cun, which equals 1/3 at a decimeter. The body-proportional cun is of no definite length, and varies with the size of the body.

2. In bone measurement (骨度法 [gǔ dù fǎ]), the length of each equally divided portion of a particularly long bone is taken as one cun, also called "bone proportional cun (B-cun)" (骨度分寸 [gǔ dù fēn cùn]) (as decided by the WHO Working Group as the standard nomenclature), a unit of measurement for locating acupuncture points. The full name of this term is "location of point by bone measurement" (骨度折量定位法 [gǔ dù zhé liáng dìng wèi fǎ]). There are other translations, such as "bone standard measurement" and "bone-length measurement". As none of them can avoid misunderstanding without necessary explanation, the

simplest one is selected, for it is most equivalent literally to the original Chinese term.

3. The term "finger cun (F-cun)" (手指同身寸 [shǒu zhǐ tóng shēn cùn]) was suggested by the WHO Working Group on the Standardization of Acupuncture Nomenclature in 1987. In textbooks there are three methods to determine the length of finger cun: middle finger cun, thumb cun, and palm measurement.

4. Middle finger cun (中指同身寸 [zhōng zhǐ tóng shēn cùn]) is the length between the twisted folds at the two ends of the second segment of the patient's middle finger when bent, and a thumb cun (拇指同身寸 [mǔ zhǐ tóng shēn cùn]) is the width of the phalangeal joint of the patient's thumb. Other expressions also exist, such as "middle finger body inch", "middle finger measurement" and "thumb body inch", but they are not widely used.

5. In palm measurement (一夫法 [yī fū fǎ]) the maximal width of the four fingers (namely, the index finger, middle finger, ring finger and little finger) held together with the hand open is taken as a unit of measurement for 3 cun. In fact, the measurement of length by using a part of the human body as a unit also exists in English-speaking countries, for example, foot as a measure of length. Various translations for 一夫法 [yī fū fǎ] have appeared in recent publications in English: "finger breadth measurement", "finger measurement", "hand standard", "*fu* measurement" and "palm measurement". Most authors use the last one, and it is most conformable to the original Chinese and practical measurement.

ACUPUNCTURE NEEDLES

Standard nomenclature for acupuncture needles was adopted or proposed at the WHO meeting of the Third Working Group on the Standardization of Acupuncture Nomenclature in 1987.

Proposed Standard Nomenclature

acupuncture needle 針灸針 [zhēn jiǔ zhēn][1]

handle (of needle) 針柄 [zhēn bǐng][1]

root (of needle) 針根 [zhēn gēn][1]

body (of needle) 針體 [zhēn tǐ][1]

tip (of needle) 針尖 [zhēn jiān][1]

filiform needle 毫針 [háo zhēn][1]

three-edged needle 三棱針 [sān léng zhēn][2]

ringheaded thumbtack needle 撳針 [qìn zhēn][2]

intradermal needle 皮內針 [pí nèi zhēn][2]

dermal needle 皮膚針 [pí fū zhēn][2]

spoon needle 鍉針 [chí zhēn][2]

shear needle 鑱針 [chán zhēn][2]

round-sharp needle 圓利針 [yuán lì zhēn][2]

round-point needle 圓針 [yuán zhēn][2]

lance needle 鋒針 [fēng zhēn][2]

stiletto needle 鈹針 [pī zhēn][2]

long needle 長針 [cháng zhēn][2]

big needle 大針 [dà zhēn][2]

Discussion

1. These terms were adopted as standard nomenclature by the Third Working Group on the Standardization of Acupuncture Nomenclature of the WHO Regional Office for the Western Pacific in 1987. It is by no means an easy task to standardize the nomenclature of Chinese medicine, and it is an even more difficult task to popularize the standard nomenclature. To date, most authors use the term "filiform needle (毫針 [háo zhēn])", but other expressions such as "small needle" and "fine needle" are still in use. Even for such a simple term as "tip of needle (針尖 [zhēn jiān])", another expression "needle end" is recommended in a dictionary of Chinese medicine published in 1994. This expression is apparently not appropriate, for a needle has two ends, and the word end does not necessarily refer to the sharp one.

2. All these terms are listed as Proposed Standard Nomenclature in the pamphlet *Standard Acupuncture Nomenclature Part 2*, published by the WHO Regional Office for the Western Pacific in 1988. Strictly speaking, the exact equivalent of ringheaded thumbtack needle is 圖釘型針 [tú dīng xíng zhēn], but the latter is also called 撳針 [qìn zhēn]. The needles listed from "shear needle 鑱針 [chán zhēn]" below plus "filiform needle (毫針 [háo zhēn])" are collectively called the "nine classical needles" (九針 [jiǔ zhēn]), the majority of which were only used at the ancient times.

FILIFORM NEEDLING

The needles used in acupuncture at present are filiform needles, and the discussion on the methods of needling in recent publications chiefly refer to this kind of needle.

Proposed Standard Nomenclature

filiform needling 毫針刺法 [háo zhēn cì fǎ]

needle insertion 進針 [jìn zhēn][1]

oblique insertion 斜刺 [xié cì][4]

pricking 點刺 [diǎn cì][5]

needle manipulation 行針 [xíng zhēn][7]

needle retention 留針 [liú zhēn][7]

arrival of *qi* 氣至 [qì zhì][10]

reinforcement-reduction manipulation 補瀉手法 [bǔ xiè shǒu fǎ][11]

lifting-thrusting reinforcement and reduction 提插補瀉 [tí chā bǔ xiè][13]

rapid-slow reinforcement-reduction 疾徐補瀉 [jī xú bǔ xiè][15]

reducing method 瀉法 [xiè fǎ][16]

transverse insertion 橫刺 [hén cì][2]

perpendicular insertion 直刺 [zhí cì][3]

joined puncture 透刺 [tòu cì][6]

needle withdrawal 出針 [chū zhēn][8]

needling sensation 針感 [zhēn gǎn][9]

directional reinforcement-reduction 迎隨補瀉 [yíng suí bǔ xiè][12]

twirling reinforcement-reduction 撚轉補瀉 [niǎn zhuǎn bǔ xiè][14]

reinforcing method 補法 [bǔ fǎ][16]

even method 平補平瀉法 [píng bǔ píng xiè fǎ][16]

Discussion

1. Most authors use the word "insertion" to express the penetration of the skin. Either the noun form "needle insertion", or the gerund form "inserting the needle", or the verb form "insert the needle" is used, according to the context.

2. In Chinese 橫刺 [hén cì] is also called 平刺 [píng cì]. The former is often translated as transverse insertion, while the latter, horizontal. The word "horizontal" means "parallel to the horizon", but in 橫刺 [héng cì] or 平刺 [píng cì] the inserted needle is nearly parallel to the skin surface. Therefore, transverse insertion is better than horizontal insertion.

3. For the Chinese character 直 [zhí] in the term 直刺 [zhí cì], most authors use "perpendicular", while some use "vertical". The word "vertical" may be misunderstood as at a right angle to the ground (or the surface of the earth), but its real meaning in this term is at a right angle to the skin surface at the site of puncturing.

4. For the term 斜刺 [xié cì], two expressions are used: "oblique insertion", and "slant (or slanted) insertion". There seems to be no difference between the two, but most authors use the former.

5. 點刺 [diǎn cì] refers to swift insertion and withdrawal of the nee-

needle, chiefly for bloodletting. Most authors render it as "prick" or "pricking". There are other expressions, such as "quick insertion" and "quick puncture", which, reflecting the procedure incompletely, may lead to misunderstanding.

6. Puncture of two or more adjoining points in one insertion of the needle is called 透刺 [tòu cì]. It has several renderings in recent publications: "piercing needling", "point-through-point acupuncture", "point-to-point needling", "joined puncture", "point-joining acupuncture", "point penetration", and "penetration needling". Since it is a special needling technique, and none of the above terms is self-explanatory, the briefest one, "joined puncture" is selected. Terms like "piercing needling" and "point penetration" are also brief, but they may give an impression that the needle should be inserted deep into the tissue. In fact, the needle is often inserted transversely in the superficial tissue to pass through two or more points.

7. Most authors use the noun form "needle manipulation" for 行針 [xíng zhēn] and "needle retention" for 留針 [liú zhēn]. The gerund form "manipulating the needle" and "retaining the needle", and the verb form "manipulate the needle" and "retain the needle" can also be used according to the context.

8. "Needle withdrawal" and "withdrawing the needle" (出針 [chū zhēn]) are very simple terms, but there are several different expressions, such as "removing the needle", "pulling out the needle" and "needle extraction". Comparatively, "withdrawing the needle" or "needle withdrawal" is more frequently used. "Pulling out" and "extraction" usually refer to taking something out with effort or by force.

9. Various expressions for the concept of 針感 [zhēn gǎn] have appeared in recent publications, such as "needling response", "acu-esthesia", "needle sensation", "needling sensation", "needling stimulation", "acupuncture sensation" and "sensation induced by acupuncture". Among these expressions, the word "response" is too general. During needling, local redness may appear as the response, but it is not called 針感. Needling sensation seems to be the most appropriate and simplest one. "Esthesia" means capacity for sensation or feeling, but 針感 refers to the feeling itself. "Needling sensation" is more appropriate than "needle sensation" because the feeling of soreness, numbness, distension or heaviness around the point may exist after withdrawal of the needle.

10. The term 得氣 [dé qì] refers to the patient's feeling of soreness,

numbness, distension or heaviness around the point after insertion of the needle, together with the operator's feeling of tenseness around the needle. From the linguistic perspective, the original Chinese term is such a common expression that it may not be taken as a proper medical term. Grammatically, it is a phrase composed of a transitive verb and a noun as the direct object. English equivalent of this term varies in the following aspects. (1) The translation of 氣 [qì] causes arguments. *Qi* in this phrase is not as mysterious as on other occasions; it can be felt either by the patient or by the practitioner, so many authors use sensation, feeling, needle sensation or acupuncture feeling to represent "*qi*". Many other authors prefer "*qi*" because theoretically *qi* in this phrase refers to meridian *qi*. The latter seems to be more reasonable. (2) The Chinese character 得 [dé] is very easy to understand, but it is very difficult to reach a standard translation. It means to get, to obtain, to achieve, to gain, to acquire, etc. Any of them can be taken as a correct translation, and none is better than the other. Another issue is that, as a medical term, whether the infinitive or the gerund should be used. Different authors also have different opinions: They use "get *qi*", "getting *qi*"; "obtain *qi*", "obtaining *qi*"; "gain *qi*", "gaining *qi*", "gaining of *qi*", and so on. Because of this difficulty, some authors resort to *pinyin*, i.e., *deqi*. This is certainly not the proper way to solve the problem. Among all the translations which have appeared in recent publications, rendering the term as "arrival of *qi*" is an original and appropriate idea. This can be shown with another term 候氣 [hòu qì] which means "waiting for *qi*", or more precisely, "waiting for the arrival of *qi*". Therefore, "arrival of *qi*" may be the best choice for expressing 得氣 [dé qì].

11. In acupuncture, 補 [bǔ] means to activate and restore a decreased function to normal, while 瀉 [xiè] means to expel pathogenic factors and thus to restore the hyperactive function to normal. Different expressions have been used for 補 [bǔ] and 瀉 [xiè]. In herbal medication, "tonification" and "purgation" are often used, closely related to the drugs, as tonics are required for the former and purgatives for the latter. In acupuncture treatment, however, nothing other than needle stimulation is applied. So, other appropriate expressions are required. Among various expressions, "supplementation versus drainage" and "reinforcement versus reduction" are commonly used. The latter pair of expressions seem to be superior to the former, because in the former there should be some material object to be added or flow away, while in the latter the object may

not be material.

12. 迎隨補瀉 [yíng suí bǔ xiè] is a form of needle manipulation in which reinforcement is achieved by selecting the points sequentially along a given meridian and inserting the needle in the direction of the meridian flow, while reduction is achieved by selecting the points counter-sequentially and inserting the needle against the direction of the meridian flow. There are various English equivalents, such as "reinforcement-reduction by puncturing along and against the direction of the meridian (or channel)", "reinforcing-reducing according to needle-direction", "reinforcing and reducing achieved by the direction of the needle tip pointing to", "facing-against reinforcement and reduction", "tonification or purgation with the needle along or against the direction of the channel", "tonifying and draining by directing the needle" and "directional reinforcement-reduction". Since for a technical term the more succinct it is the better, the last one is selected.

13. 提插補瀉 [tí chā bǔ xiè] is a form of needle manipulation in which reinforcement is attained by heavy thrusting and gentle lifting of the needle, and reduction by gentle thrusting and heavy lifting. Most of the authors regard "lifting and thrusting" as the appropriate expression for 提插 [tí chā], and hence "lifting-thrusting reinforcement and reduction" for the whole term.

14. In the manipulation 撚轉補瀉 [niǎn zhuǎn bǔ xiè], the differentiation of reinforcement and reduction is based on the degree of twirling: reinforcement by twirling the needle with a heavy force at a high frequency for a long period for reducing, and reinforcement by twirling the needle with a mild force at a low frequency for a short period. For the word 撚轉 [niǎn zhuǎn], the majority of the authors use "twirling", while some prefer "rotating".

15. 疾徐補瀉 [jí xú bǔ xiè] is a form of needle manipulation in which reinforcement or reduction is achieved by insertion and withdrawal of the needle at different speeds, namely, slow insertion and rapid withdrawal for reinforcement, and swift insertion and slow withdrawal for reduction. Most authors prefer "rapid-slow" for expressing 疾徐 [jí xú], and only a few authors use "quick-slow".

16. 平補平瀉 [píng bǔ píng xiè] is most commonly used in practice but least described in textbooks. For example, in two Chinese national textbooks of acupuncture, one edited by Qiu Mao-liang and published in 1985, and the other edited by Sun Guo-jie and published in 1997, this

technique is similarly described in one simple sentence: "lifting, thrusting and twirling the needle evenly after the arrival of *qi*". Indeed, one of the literal meanings of the Han character 平 [píng] is "equal" or "at the same level". Thus the following words are considered by different authors as its equivalent: "uniform", "even", "neutral", and "balanced". Among them, the word "uniform" is most frequently used. However, the crucial question is what the whole term 平補平瀉 [píng bǔ píng xiè] means. In ancient texts, 平補 [píng bǔ] and 平瀉 [píng xiè] are two independent terms. In both the character 平 [píng] certainly does not mean "equal" or "at the same level". It means "mild" or "moderate", and is synonymous with 和 [hé] and 緩 [huǎn], both meaning "gentle". Therefore, 平補 [píng bǔ] and 平瀉 [píng xiè] refer to "moderate reinforcement" and "moderate reduction", respectively. At present, in some Chinese authoritative books it is also emphasized that the key point of 平補平瀉 [píng bǔ píng xiè] is to twirl, thrust and lift the needle with moderate force.* Based on the above discussion, this technique can be defined as a form of needle manipulation in which the needle is lifted, thrust and twirled evenly with a proper amplitude and moderate angle, indicated in cases of combined excess and deficiency or no distinct excess or deficiency.

General Comments on Nomenclaure of Needling Manipulations

Although Chinese medicine describes a series of effective manipulations which are still useful at present, the terminology regarding the manipulations needs careful consideration. In fact, in modern publications on acupuncture a detailed description of manipulative procedure is much more useful than simply mentioning the name of the reinforcement-reduction method. As the standard nomenclature it may be better to put forward a series of basic elements of the manipulation rather than the traditional names of reinforcement-reduction manipulations. First of all, the terms 補 [bǔ] and 瀉 [xiè] can hardly be well defined. This is unlike herbal medication, in which each medicinal or drug has its own ingredients with certain effects. For example, ginseng is a tonic, and. rhubarb is a purgative. Their effects can be confirmed both pharmaco-

---

*Qiu PR and Chen HP. Xin Bian Zhong Guo Zhen Jiu Xue, *Newly Compiled Chinese Acupuncture and Moxibustion* (in Chinese), Shanghai Science and Technology Press, 1992, p. 341, and Li JW, Yu YA et al. Zhong Yi Da Ci Dian, *Grand Dictionary of Traditional Chinese Medicine* (in Chinese), People's Health Publishing House, 1995, p. 396

logically and clinically. In acupuncture, the situation is different; no confirming evidence has been achieved to show the effect of reinforcing or reducing merely due to the change of the manipulation. In fact, besides the manipulation, the patient's condition and the point selection also determine the effect of acupuncture. It is not infrequently encountered that in different patients the same manipulation may lead to different reactions. Therefore, it is better to describe in detail all the elements of manipulation, including the form (whirling, thrusting, lifting, vibrating or handle rubbing), force, speed, amplitude of thrusting and lifting, degree and frequency of twirling, number of needle manipulations, duration of needle retention, and so forth, rather than labeling the manipulation as a certain kind of reinforcement or reduction. MacPherson and Kaptchuk edited *Acupuncture in Practice — Case History Insights from the West* (published by Churchill Livingstone, 1997) in this way successfully. It is a collection of forty papers contributed by authors from Australia, Canada, France, Germany, Israel, Italy, Norway, the UK, and the USA. The needling method or technique is described in detail, and only in exceptional cases are the terms "reinforcing method", "reducing method" and "even method" used. In this scheme of proposed standard nomenclature, these terms are recommended, particularly if they are used together with detailed descriptions of the manipulation.

ACUPUNCTURE ACCIDENTS

Accidents that are sometimes encountered in acupuncture are fainting of the patient, and sticking, bending or breaking of the needle. All these terms are better expressed by using common words rather than special ones.

Proposed Standard Nomenclature

fainting during acupuncture 晕針 [yūn zhēn][1]

sticking of needle 滯針 [zhì zhēn][2]

bending of needle 彎針 [wān zhēn][3]

breaking of needle 折針 [shé zhēn][4]

Discussion

1. For the Chinese character 晕 [yūn], most authors translate it as

"fainting" or "faint", while others use "syncope" or "sickness". "Syncope" is too serious, and a patient suffering from 暈針 [yūn zhēn] is not necessarily in a state of syncope. Sickness is a word with a vague and broad sense. It refers to 暈 [yūn] only in some special terms, such as sea sickness, and car sickness.

2. There are basically two forms of wording to express 滯針 [zhì zhēn]: "sticking of needle" and "stuck needle". The former seems to be better, and is used by most authors; the latter describes the needle in a certain condition rather than the condition that happens to the needle. Other expressions such as "difficult withdrawal of the needle", and "sticking of the inserted needle" are explanatory, exceeding the scope of the original term. As a technical term, "sticking of needle" is clear enough. It goes without saying that the needle refers to the inserted one.

3. The basic wordings to express 彎針 [wān zhēn] are "bent needle", "bending needle" and "bending of needle". Both "bent needle" and "bending of needle" are commonly used terms in acupuncture, but the former is often used to describe the condition of the needle, particularly in the preparatory examination of the instruments before performing the manipulation, while the latter refers to what happens during the manipulative procedure.

4. In recent publications, quite a few expressions are used for 折針 [shé zhēn]: "broken needle", "breaking needle", "breaking of needle", "breaking of the inserted needle", and "needle breakage". "Broken needle" is a common expression, not necessarily related to an acupuncture accident. "Breaking of needle" and "needle breakage" are suitable expressions for the accident, and it is self-evident that the needle referred to is the inserted needle.

MOXIBUSTION

Moxibustion is a kind of thermotherapy. The character 灸 [jiǔ] means "burn", and 灸法 [jiǔ fǎ] refers to therapy involving applying heat from some burning substance to a certain site on the body surface. In the original Chinese terminology, the burning substance is not confined to moxa or mugwort. Practically, moxa is the substance most frequently used, because of its easy ignition and gentle heat-production

Proposed Standard Nomenclature

moxibustion (therapy) 灸(法) [jiǔ (fǎ)][1]

moxa 艾 [ài][2]

moxa roll 艾卷 [ài juǎn][3]

moxa cone 艾炷 [ài zhù][4]

moxa-roll moxibustion 艾卷灸 [ài juǎn jiǔ][5]

mild moxibustion 溫和灸 [wēn hé jiǔ][6]

pecking moxibustion 雀啄灸 [què zhuó jiǔ][7]

circling moxibustion 迴旋灸 [huí xuán jiǔ][8]

moxa-cone moxibustion 艾炷灸 [ài zhù jiǔ][9]

scarring moxibustion 瘢痕灸 [bān hén jiǔ][10]

direct moxibustion 直接灸 [zhí jiē jiǔ][11]

indirect moxibustion 間接灸 [jiàn jiē jiǔ][11]

ginger moxibustion 隔薑灸 [gé jiāng jiǔ][12]

garlic moxibustion 隔蒜灸 [gé suàn jiǔ][12]

salt moxibustion 隔鹽灸 [gé yán jiǔ][12]

Discussion

1. As mentioned above, the word "moxibustion" is already taken as a medical subject heading for use in MEDLARS (Medical Literature Analysis and Retrieval System).

2. The word "moxa" has already been included in *Dorland's Illustrated Medical Dictionary* (29th edition, 2000) with the following definition: "a tuft of soft, combustible substance to be burned upon the skin, popularly used in the Orient as a cautery and counterirritant."

3. There are different names both in Chinese and in English for the round long roll made of moxa wool: "艾卷 [ài juǎn]", "艾條 [ài tiáo]", "moxa roll", "moxa stick", "moxa cigar", and "moxa pole". Among these terms "moxa roll (艾卷 [ài juǎn])" is the best, because it precisely describes the reality — a roll of moxa wool enclosed in thin paper for ignition. A cigar is tight roll of tobacco leaves for smoking, and most cigars have a shape different from a moxa roll. A pole usually refers to a long thin rounded piece of wood or metal, e.g., flag pole, telegraph pole and tent pole.

4. Most authors use the term "moxa cone" for 艾炷 [ài zhù], but some prefer "mugwort cone". If we agree to adopt moxa as the standard name for the combustible substance used in moxibustion, moxa cone is the most appropriate term.

5. The term "moxa-roll moxibustion 艾卷灸 [ài juǎn jiǔ]" comes

from moxa roll. The three common procedures for performing moxa-roll moxibustion are mild moxibustion 溫和灸 [wēn hé jiǔ], pecking moxibustion 雀啄灸 [què zhuó jiǔ] and revolving moxibustion 迴旋灸 [huí xuán jiǔ].

6. For the term "mild moxibustion 溫和灸 [wēn hé jiǔ]", there are many other expressions:, "gentle moxibustion", "warming moxibustion", "warm moxibustion", "lukewarm moxibustion" and "mild-warm moxibustion". It should be noted that 溫和 [wēn hé] does not mean warm or lukewarm. The present Chinese national textbook of acupuncture and moxibustion describes this form of moxibustion as follows: "It makes the patient feel local hotness but no burning pain… and is to be applied until a red halo appears."[*] "Mild moxibustion" and "gentle moxibustion" are equally suitable for designating this treatment, but most authors use the former.

7. The English names corresponding to 雀啄灸 [què zhuó jiǔ] include "bird-peck moxibustion", "sparrow-pecking moxibustion", "pecking moxibustion with moxa stick" and "pecking moxibustion". The last one is simple and explicit.

8. There are several different expressions for 迴旋灸 [huí xuán jiǔ]: "moving moxibustion", "waving moxibustion", "revolving moxibustion", "circling moxibustion" and "circle moxibustion". Most authors prefer "circling moxibustion".

9. The English equivalents of 艾炷灸 [ài zhù jiǔ] include "moxibustion with moxa cone", "moxibustion with a mugwort cone", "moxa cone moxibustion" and "cone moxibustion". If moxa-roll moxibustion is appropriate for 艾卷灸 [ài juǎn jiǔ], then it is rational to select moxa-cone moxibustion for 艾炷灸 [ài zhù jiǔ].

10. Three wordings — "scar-producing moxibustion", "scar-forming moxibustion" and "scarring moxibustion" — have often appeared in recent publications expressing 瘢痕灸 [bān hén jiǔ]. Most authors adopt the last one.

11 Basically, there are two ways to translate the terms 直接灸 [zhí jiē jiǔ]: "direct contact moxibustion" and "direct moxibustion"; and similarly two ways to translate 間接灸 [jiàn jiē jiǔ]: "indirect contact moxibus-

---

[*] "使患者局部有溫熱感而無灼痛，…至皮膚紅暈爲度。" – cited from Sun GJ. (chief editor) Zhen Jiu Xue, *Acupuncture and Moxibustion* (in Chinese), the Textbook Series for Programmed Courses of the TCM Universities and Colleges, Shanghai Science and Technology Press, 1998, p.178.

tion" and "indirect moxibustion". Comparatively speaking, the addition of the word "contact" gives more information about the type of moxibustion, but after all it is additional and explanatory. In fact, more explanatory words can be added, such as "moxa-cone direct (or indirect) contact moxibustion". In order to make the term simple, clear and concise, most authors prefer "direct moxibustion" and "indirect moxibustion".

12. The English terms for 隔薑灸 [gé jiāng jiǔ] include "ginger moxibustion", "ginger interposed moxibustion", "ginger-partition moxibustion", "ginger-partitioned moxibustion", "moxibustion with ginger", "indirect moxibustion with ginger", etc. Among these terms, "ginger moxibustion" is the simplest and most frequently used. It seems unlikely to cause misunderstanding due to deletion of the word "interposed", "partition" or "partitioned". The same reasoning applies to "garlic moxibustion 隔蒜灸 [gé suàn jiǔ]" and "salt moxibustion 隔鹽灸 [gé yán jiǔ]".

OTHER ACUPUNCTURE-RELATED THERAPIES

A variety of therapies have been developed on the basis of meridian theory and point stimulation. These therapies are named in two ways: according to the local site where the specific points are distributed, and according to the stimulus applied to the point. Ear acupuncture, scalp acupuncture, hand acupuncture, etc., belong to the first system of naming, and they are collectively called "microsystem acupuncture". Electroacupuncture, point injection, etc. belong to the second system of naming. The two systems of naming can be used in combination, in such expressions as ear electroacupuncture.

Proposed Standard Nomenclature

microsystem acupuncture 微針系統 [wēi zhēn xì tǒng][1]

ear acupuncture (therapy) 耳針(療法) [ěr zhēn (liáo fǎ)][3]

electroacupuncture (therapy) 電針(療法) [diàn zhēn (liáo fǎ)][5]

electric stimulator 電針儀 [diàn zhēn yí][5]

scalp acupuncture (therapy) 頭(皮)針(療法) [tóu (pí) zhēn (liáo fǎ)][2]

hand acupuncture (therapy) 手針(療法) [shǒu zhēn (liáo fǎ)][4]

(acu)point injection (therapy) 穴位注射(療法) [xué wèi zhù shè (liáo fǎ)][6]

Discussion

1. Microsystem acupuncture 微針系統 [wēi zhēn xì tǒng] is a newly developed collective term for various types of acupuncture in a specific local area, including scalp acupuncture, ear acupuncture, nose acupuncture, hand acupuncture, foot acupuncture, etc.

2. 頭(皮)針(療法) [tóu (pí) zhēn (liáo fǎ)] is a special form of acupuncture developed on the combined basis of traditional medical understanding and modern knowledge of the cerebral cortical function. Its equivalent, "scalp acupuncture", has already been stipulated in the WHO- proposed standard international nomenclature, and widely used by various authors.

3. 耳針(療法) [ěr zhēn (liáo fǎ)] is one of the microsystem acupuncture therapies, in which points located on the auricle are needled for therapeutic purpose. Different authors have used various English names, including "oto-acupuncture", "auriculo-acupuncture", "auricular acupuncture" and "ear acupuncture". The last one is selected because of its simplicity and popularity.

4. 手針(療法) [shǒu zhēn (liáo fǎ)] is one of the microsystem acupuncture therapies, in which given points of the hand are needled for treating disorders elsewhere in the body. It is called "hand acupuncture" in English, and there seems to be no dispute about the naming. It should be noted that "manual acupuncture" is an entirely different term, which some authors use to indicate that the stimulation in acupuncture is performed by the physician's hand (not by electricity).

5. There has not been much argument about the term "electroacupuncture". Some authors use electric acupuncture instead of electroacupuncture, and some prefer electro-acupuncture with the insertion of a hyphen. The word "electroacupuncture" has already been included in *Dorland's Illustrated Medical Dictionary* (29th edition, 2000) with the following definition: "acupuncture in which the needles are stimulated electrically." The instrument that applies pulses of current to stimulate the acupuncture site is called an "electric stimulator".

6. 穴位注射（療法） [xué wèi zhù shè (liáo fǎ)] is a therapy by which liquid medicine is injected into the acupuncture point to cure diseases. Several different names have been given to this therapy: "point injection", "acupoint injection", "acupuncture point injection therapy", and "hydro-acupuncture". Acupoint injection or point injection seem to be explicit enough.

SELECTED CLASSICAL WORKS

The ancient classics form an important part of traditional Chinese medicine. To date, they are often cited in the writings. Theoretically, whether the titles of medical books should be regarded as medical terms and whether they should be transliterated or translated according to the meanings or contents are all questionable, but practically there is an urgent need for standardizing the titles of the classical TCM works, as they have already been rendered into English, but in disparate ways by different authors. In addition, the original Chinese title may also vary. Some authors prefer the full title, while others prefer the abbreviated title. For example, 普濟本事方 [pǔ jì běn shì fāng] is often abbreviated as 本事方 [běn shì fāng], but 普濟方 [pǔ jì fāng] is another classical formulary. Indication of the author's name may still cause confusion, as Chinese authors often had three names: formal name, alternative name, and style. For example, 李時珍 [lǐ shí zhēn], the author of 本草綱目 [běn cǎo gāng mù], is also called 李東璧 [lǐ dōng bì], and styled 瀕湖 [bīn hú], and hence his book on the pulse is titled *Binhu's Sphygmology* (瀕湖脈學 [bīn hú mài xué]).

Another problem is how to select the classics. Some of the TCM classics are generally recognized, such as 內經 [nèi jīng] (*Canon of Medicine*) and 本草綱目 [běn cǎo gāng mù] (*Compendium of Materia Medica*), but some others are not public knowledge. Unlike the clinical terms, no official standard terminology in Chinese can be taken as reference. In the present scheme, a provisional criterion is used for deciding the selection, i.e., a classic that has been cited by at least three recent publications.

Some of the TCM classics have already been totally or partly rendered into English. Such a title of the English translation, of course, should be accepted as a *fait accompli*, and the citation should be strictly in accordance with the English book title. The same classic may have two or more translated editions, each with a different English title. In this case, the reference should be written in complete conformity with the title of the translated edition from which the citation is made.

More frequently the citation is made from the original classic in Chinese. The correct reference is the original Chinese title in Chinese characters, in Romanized Chinese (derived from pinyin) or in both, preferably with an English translation of the title attached. For example, the reference of a citation from the Chinese edition of 內經 [nèi jīng] is written as "Nei Jing (*Canon of Medicine*)" or "內經 (Nei Jing, *Canon of Medicine*)". What we are going to discuss is the attachment.

CANON OF MEDICINE AND RELATED WORKS

Proposed Standard Annotations

The Yellow Emperor's Canon of Medicine 黃帝內經 [huáng dì nèi jīng][1]
The Yellow Emperor's Internal Classic 黃帝內經 [huáng dì nèi jīng][1]
Canon of Medicine 內經 [nèi jīng][1]
Internal Classic 內經 [nèi jīng][1]
Plain Questions 素問 [sù wèn][2]
Spiritual Pivot 靈樞 [líng shū][2]
Canon of Acupuncture 針經 [zhēn jīng][2]
Essentials of the Canon of Medicine 內經知要 [nèi jīng zhī yào][3]
Essentials of the Internal Classic 內經知要 [nèi jīng zhī yào][3]
The Yellow Emperor's Canon of Medicine: Great Simplicity 黃帝內經太素 [huáng dì nèi jīng tài sù][4]
The Yellow Emperor's Internal Classic: Great Simplicity 黃帝內經太素 [huáng dì nèi jīng tài sù][4]
Classified Canon 類經 [lèi jīng][5]
Classic of Difficult Issues 難經 [nàn jīng][6]
Genuine Meaning of the Classic of Difficult Issues 難經本義 [nàn jīng běn yì][7]
Variorum of the Classic of Difficult Issues 難經集注 [nàn jīng jí zhù][7]

Discussion

1. Although this famous TCM classic has been repeatedly mentioned in many TCM publications in English, the rendering of the book title varies greatly. First of all, 黃帝 [huáng dì] is rendered in two ways: "the Yellow Emperor" and "Huangdi". Most Westerners prefer the for-

mer, for its long existence and easy remembrance, while some Chinese translators insist on the latter, believing that a proper name should only be rendered into English by transliteration. Indeed, 黄帝 [huáng dì] is a proper noun that refers to a legendary monarch in ancient China, but it is not the real name of the person. His surname was 姬 [jì], belonging to the clan of 軒轅 [xuān yuán]. 黄帝 [huáng dì] was actually a title for the chief of a tribe living in the central area. In fact, most of the titles of Chinese emperors' reigns are transliterated. However, rendering 黄帝 [huáng dì] as "the Yellow Emperor" gives no cause for criticism because the character 黄 [huáng] does mean "yellow", indicating the central area.*

In one of the English editions, "Yellow Emperor" is changed to "Yellow Empero". This is apparently not a printing mistake, for "Empero" repeatedly appears on the front cover, the title page, and the color plate. The translators did not give any explanation. Perhaps, they might not totally agree with the word "Emperor" because the Chinese empire started with the Qin Dynasty (221–206 B.C.), thousands of years after the legendary monarch.

Since the term "Yellow Emperor" has been used by many authors and translators for a long period of time (at least for more than half a century since Ilza Veith published *The Yellow Emperor's Classic of Internal Medicine* in 1949), it should be considered as widely accepted. In addition, it does not misrepresent the original meaning, and so it is selected as the proposed standard.

As for the term 内經 [nèi jīng], it is rendered as "Inner Classic", "Internal Classic", "Canon of Medicine", "Inner Canon", "Canon of Internal Medicine", "Classic of Internal Medicine", "Internal Classic of Medicine" "Canon of Internal Medicine", and "Classic of Medicine". Among these renderings, "Internal Classic" and "Canon of Medicine" are the two most frequently used.

2. The Canon of Medicine is composed of two parts: 素問 [sù wèn] and 靈樞 [líng shū], each of which contains 81 chapters. For the first part, "Simple Questions", "Plain Questions", "Elementary Questions" and "Basic Questions" are the common equivalents. According to the frequency of practical use, "Plain Questions" takes the first place, and

---

*In ancient Chinese culture, the colors corresponded to directions, namely, blue to the east, red to the south, yellow to the center, white to the west and black to the north.

"Simple Questions" the second. Comparatively speaking, "Plain Questions" is more appropriate, because the questions discussed in the classic are not simple, but they are put forward in a frank and direct manner.

Regarding the rendering of 靈樞 [líng shū], four words are used for 靈 [líng]: "spiritual", "divine", "miraculous", and "magic", of which "spiritual" is recommended for the majority of authors use this word. Two words are used for 樞 [shū]: "axis" and "pivot". Of these two words, "pivot" is recommended because (1) more authors use this word, and (2) besides the meaning of the shaft on which something turns, it also means the central or most important thing. In conclusion, "spiritual pivot" is recommended as the standard annotation of 靈樞 [líng shū], and this English expression is also in conformity with the only translated edition at present.

靈樞 [líng shū] is also called 針經 [zhēn jīng], which is rendered as "Canon of Acupuncture" by most authors.

3. 內經知要 [nèi jīng zhī yào] (1642) is a rearrangement of excerpts from 內經 [nèi jīng], compiled by 李中梓 [lǐ zhōng zǐ] (called also 李士材 [lǐ shì cái] and 李念莪 [lǐ niàn é]). The title of the book has many different renderings. Most authors render 知要 [nèi jīng zhī yào] as "Essentials", but some render it as "Abstracts". Judged from the contents of the book, "Essentials" is better than "Abstracts". As for 內經 [nèi jīng], most authors represent it as "Canon of Medicine" or "Internal Classic".

4. 黃帝內經太素 [huáng dì nèi jīng tài sù] is an early version of the Yellow Emperor's Internal Classic. Among several renderings of 太素 [tài sù], "Great Simplicity" is better than such expressions as "Comprehensive Notes to ……" and "Elements Written in ……"

5. 類經 [lèi jīng] was compiled by 張介賓 [zhāng jiè bīn] (also called 張景嶽 [zhāng jǐng yuè]), who rearranged the contents of the Internal Classic in a new and systematic way. Some authors render the book title as "Systematic Compilation of the Internal Classic". This reflects the real contents, but is not consistent with the original title. Other authors render it as "Classic of Categories", which is literally accurate but difficult to understand. So, most authors render it as "Classified Canon".

6. 難經 [nàn jīng] is rendered as "Classic of Difficulties", "Classic on Medical Problems", "Difficult Classic", "Classic of Difficult Issues", and "The Classics on Difficulty", with only minor differences. "Classic of Difficult Issues" is selected, for it is clear, causing no misunderstanding.

In addition, it is same as the title of the translation edition.

7. 難經本義 [nàn jīng běn yì] (1361) is a re-edited version of the Classic of Difficult Issues with notes and commentaries by 滑壽 [huá shòu] (also called 滑伯仁 [huá bó rén]). 本義 [běn yì] is rendered as "Meaning", "Genuine Meaning", and "Proper Sense". The majority opinion is in favor of "Genuine meaning".

難經集注 [nàn jīng jí zhù] is an edition of the Classic of Difficult Issues containing various notes and commentaries. 集注 [jí zhù] in this book title is rendered as "Collected Commentaries", "Notes" and "Variorum". The last one seems most appropriate.

ZHANG ZHONG-JING'S WORKS AND THEIR COMMETARIES

Zhang Ji (called also Zhang Zhong-jing) was one of the most influential physicians in the history of Chinese medicine. He created the system of traditional Chinese diagnosis and treatment, and his 傷寒雜病論 [shāng hán zá bìng lùn] is believed to be the most authoritative classic of clinical medicine. It was later rearranged as two books — 傷寒論 [shāng hán lùn] and 金匱要略方論 [jīn guì yào lüè fāng lùn]

Proposed Standard Annotations

Treatise on Cold-induced and Miscellaneous Diseases 傷寒雜病論 [shāng hán zá bìng lùn][1]

Treatise on Cold-induced Diseases 傷寒論 [shāng hán lùn][1]

General Treatise on Cold-induced Diseases 傷寒總病論 [shāng hán zǒng bìng lùn][2]

Annotated Treatise on Cold-induced Diseases 注解傷寒論 [zhù jiě shāng hán lùn][3]

Rationale of the Treatise on Cold-induced Diseases 傷寒明理論 [shāng hán míng lǐ lùn][4]

Renewal Variorum of Cold-induced Diseases 傷寒來蘇集 [shāng hán lái sū jí][5]

String-of-Pearls Variorum of Cold-induced Diseases 傷寒貫珠集 [shāng hán guàn zhū jí][5]

Synopsis of Prescriptions of the Golden Chamber 金匱要略方論 [jīn guì yào lüè fāng lùn][6]

Synopsis of the Golden Chamber 金匱要略 [jīn guì yào lüè][6]

Discussion

1. Great disparity exists in English translations of 傷寒論 [shāng hán lùn]. The book actually deals with exogenous febrile diseases but they are called "cold damage". This is based on the following statement in the *Canon of Medicine*: "Now, febrile diseases are all of the cold damage kind."* (*Plain Questions* · Chapter 31). To render the book title into English, there are two opposite ways: one is direct and literal translation as "On Cold Damage", the other is a reflection of the contents as "Treatise on Exogenous Febrile Diseases" or "Treatise on Febrile Diseases". The intermediate and compromise way is a combination of the two expressions as "Treatise on Febrile Diseases Caused by Cold".

To date, there are three English editions with three different titles: (1) Shang Han Lun (1981), (2) Treatise on Febrile Diseases Caused by Cold (1993) and (3) On Cold Damage (1999). In addition, certain paragraphs of the contents were rendered into English, with the book title translated as "Discussion of Cold-induced Disorders" (1996). Comparatively speaking, most authors prefer the wording "cold-induced diseases" for 傷寒 [shāng hán], probably because "febrile diseases caused by cold" does not match the Chinese original, and "cold damage" is likely to be misunderstood as frostbite. Therefore, in this scheme "Treatise on Cold-induced and Miscellaneous Diseases" is proposed for 傷寒雜病論 [shāng hán zá bìng lùn], and "Treatise on Cold-induced Diseases" for 傷寒論 [shāng hán lùn].

2. It is generally agreed to render 總病論 [zǒng bìng lùn] as "General Treatise". If the equivalent of 傷寒 [shāng hán] is "Cold-induced Diseases, the whole title then becomes "General Treatise on Cold-induced Diseases".

3. There are three expressions for the phrase 注解 [zhù jiě] in the book title 注解傷寒論 [zhù jiě shāng hán lùn]: "Annotated", "Commentary on", and "with Notes". The first one seems the most suitable, and hence the whole title is "Annotated Treatise on Cold-induced Diseases".

4. Expressions for 明理論 [míng lǐ lùn] include "clear rationale", "concise expositions", "expoundings", etc. According to the preface to

---

*"今夫熱病者，皆傷寒之類也。"（素問·熱論）

the book, this phrase is explained as "let the readers know the reasons"[*]
So, "rationale" suits the Chinese original best.

5. 集 [jí] means collection. 傷寒來蘇集 [shāng hán lái sū jí] and 傷寒貫珠集 [shāng hán guàn zhū jí] are two books containing various notes and comments, and so the word "variorum" is more appropriate. Other selections are made between "Renewal" and "Revival" for 來蘇 [lái sū], and between "String-of-Pearls" and "String of Beads" for 貫珠 [guàn zhū].

6. 金匱 [jīn guì] is not a technical term, and Zhang Zhong-jing is not the person who first used this phrase in medical writings. This can be illustrated by the Canon of Medicine, in which the fourth chapter of the Plain Questions is entitled 金匱真言論 [jīn guì zhēn yán lùn]. The character 匱 [guì] means a big box, chest or cabinet, and 金匱 [jīn guì] is an abbreviation of 金滕之匱 [jīn téng zhī guì], referring to a container for storing literature written on bamboo slips bound with wires. Translators render the character 匱 [guì] in various ways, such as "bookcase", "cabinet", "chest", "coffer" and "chamber", but all of them use the word "golden" for 金 [jīn]. It is interesting to note that, except for the word "chamber", all the words used to express 匱 [guì] is literally correct, but most translators prefer the word "chamber". As for the rendering of 金 [jīn], none of the translators use any word other than "golden", but it does not strictly reflect the original meaning literally. So, it can be concluded that ancient Chinese idioms usually cannot be translated literally into English. Acceptance through common practice is probably the best way to solve the problem. In this scheme, "Synopsis of Prescriptions of the Golden Chamber" is selected not only because most authors prefer this title in English, but also because an English edition is so titled.

ETIOLOGY AND PATHOGENESIS

Proposed Standard Annotations

Treatise on Causes and Symptoms of Diseases 諸病源候論 [zhū bìng yuán hòu lùn][1]
Treatise on Three Causes of Diseases with Syndromes and Remedies 三因

---

[*]"使習醫者流，讀其論而知其理。"（傷寒明理論·嚴器之序）

極一病證方論 [sān yīn jí yī bìng zhèng fāng lùn][2]
Three Causes of Diseases with Remedies 三因方 [sān yīn fāng][2]

Discussion

1. The major disparity in the translation of the book title 諸病源候論 [zhū bìng yuán hòu lùn] lies in the grammatical understanding of the two characters 源 [yuán] (origin) and 候 [hòu] (symptoms). Some authors take 源候 [yuán hòu] as a noun phrase with the second character in the genitive case, and so render it as "Origins of Symptoms". This goes against the grammar of the Chinese language. In Chinese, if a phrase consists of a noun as principal part and another noun in the genitive case as the subordinate part, the subordinate should always precede the principal, and not follow the principal. Therefore, for "origins of symptoms" the corresponding Chinese is 證候之源 [zhèng hòu zhī yuán], or 候源 [hòu yuán] for short. In fact, this book deals with etiology and symptomatology as two main parts, and 源候 [yuán hòu] is a coordinative word group composed of 源 [yuán] (abbreviation of 病源 [bìng yuán], i.e., cause of disease) and 候 [hòu] (abbreviation of 證候 [zhèng hòu], i.e., symptoms) in parallel.

2. 三因極一病證方論 [sān yīn jí yī bìng zhèng fāng lùn] is also called 三因方 [sān yīn fāng] for short. In order to avoid a lengthy book title, some authors translate the full title as an abbreviated one, e.g., "A Treatise on the Three Categories of Causes of Disease", "Prescriptions Assigned to the Three Categories of Pathogenic Factors", "Discussion of Pathology Based on the Triple-Etiology Doctrine", "Treatise on the Three Categories of Pathogenic Factors and Prescriptions" and "Three Causes Formulary". The full title is rendered as "Discussion of Illnesses, Patterns, and Prescriptions Related to the Unification of the Three Etiologies", and "Unified Treatise on Diseases, Patterns, and Remedies According to the Three Causes". Based on the above renderings, the following title is suggested: "Treatise on Three Causes of Diseases with Syndromes and Remedies" and "Three Causes of Diseases with Remedies". The reasons are: (1) 三因極一 [sān yīn jí yī] means "under the unified top heading of three causes". This book mainly discusses the causes of disease, classifying them into three categories in the company of syndromes and remedies. (2) 病證 [bìng zhèng] does not necessarily mean 病 [bìng] and 證 [zhèng]. In order to avoid monosyllabic words, 證 [zhèng] is seldom

used singly. In addition, "cause of disease" already involves disease.

STUDIES OF THE PULSE AND OTHER EXAMINATIONS

Proposed Standard Annotations

Pulse Classic 脈經 [mài jīng][1]
Binhu's Studies on the Pulse 瀕湖脈學 [bīn hú mài xué][2]
Tongue Differentiation with Cold-induced Diseases 傷寒舌鑒 [shāng hán shé jiàn][3]
The Essential Four Diagnostic Examinations 四診抉微 [sì zhěn jué wēi][4]

Discussion

1. 脈經 [mài jīng] is rendered by different authors as "Classic of the Pulse", "Classic on Pulse", "Pulse Classic", "Pulse Canon", "Classic of Sphygmology". They are practically the same, with minor differences.

2. 李時珍 [lǐ shí zhēn], the author of Compendium of Materia Medica, styled himself 瀕湖 [bīn hú], and titled his writing on pulse studies with his styled name. Some authors render 瀕湖脈學 [bīn hú mài xué] as "Pulse Studies of the Lakeside Master", and some other authors render it as "The Pulse Studies of Li Shi-zhen", but most authors prefer the simple and direct expression "Binhu's Studies on the Pulse".

3. Among the renderings of 傷寒舌鑒 [shāng hán shé jiàn], "Tongue Differentiation with Febrile Diseases" seems most succinct, but the term "Febrile Diseases" should be changed to "Cold-induced Diseases" as discussed in Zhang Zhong-Jing's works.

4. 四診抉微 [sì zhěn jué wēi] (1723) is a compilation of the essentials chosen from contemporary and old works on diagnostic examinations. In the title, 四診 [sì zhěn] means "four diagnostic examinations", 抉 [jué] means "pick out" or "choose", and 微 [wēi] is an abbreviation of 精微 [jīng wēi], i.e., "essence" or "essentials". There are two trends in translation of the book title: Some authors emphasize accurate reflection of the Chinese book title, such as "The Four Examinations Pared Down to Their Essence", and "The Essential Four Diagnostic Examinations". Some others stress that the book is a compilation of other authors' works, and hence "Compilation of the Four Examination Methods".

MATERIA MEDICA

Proposed Standard Annotations

Shen Nong's Classic of Materia Medica 神農本草經 [shén nóng běn cǎo jīng][1]

Shen Nong's Herbal 神農本草經 [shén nóng běn cǎo jīng][1]

Classic of Materia Medica 本草經 [běn cǎo jīng][1]

The Herbal 本草經 [běn cǎo jīng][1]

Variorum of the Classic of Materia Medica 本草經集注 [běn cǎo jīng jí zhù][2]

Variorum of the Herbal 本草經集注 [běn cǎo jīng jí zhù][2]

Lei's Treatise on Medicinal Processing 雷公炮炙論 [léi gōng páo zhì lùn][3]

Newly Revised Materia Medica 新修本草 [xīn xiū běn cǎo][4]

Tang Materia Medica 唐本草 [táng běn cǎo][3]

Supplement to Materia Medica 本草拾遺 [běn cǎo shí yí][5]

Classified Materia Medica for Emergencies 經史證類備急本草 [jīng shǐ zhèng lèi bèi jí běn cǎo][6]

Classified Materia Medica 證類本草 [zhèng lèi běn cǎo][6]

Drug Nature of the Pearl Bag in Songs 珍珠囊藥性賦 [zhēn zhū náng yào xìng fù][7]

The Pearl Bag 珍珠囊 [zhēn zhū náng][7]

Materia Medical for Decoctions 湯液本草 [tāng yè běn cǎo][8]

Compendium of Materia Medica 本草綱目 [běn cǎo gāng mù][9]

Essential of Materia Medica 本草備要 [běn cǎo bèi yào][10]

Supplement to Compendium of Materia Medica 本草綱目拾遺 [běn cǎo gāng mù shí yí][11]

Discussion

1. According to legends, China had three monarchs in three ancient historical periods. 伏羲 [fú xī] introduced livestock raising, and was said to be the inventor of acupuncture (with stone needles). 神農 [shén nóng] started farming, and was said to be the inventor of herbal medication. 黃帝 [huáng dì] invented sericulture, boats and carts, music, writing, arithmetic, and medicine. Since "Yellow Emperor" is generally regarded as the equivalent of 黃帝 [huáng dì], 神農 [shén nóng] is rendered as

"Divine Husbandman" or "Divine Farmer" by some authors. However, these translations are not so impressive as the "Yellow Emperor", and so many authors would rather use the transliteration Shen Nong.

As for the term 本草經 [běn cǎo jīng], among various renderings "Classic of Materia Medica" and "(The) Herbal" are commonly used either as a part of the book title 神農本草經 [shén nóng běn cǎo jīng] or as the abbreviation of that title.

2. Among the words used by different authors for expressing the term 集注 [jí zhù], "Variorum" is better than "Collective Notes" or "Collection of Commentaries", for the book also contains other versions of materia medica.

3. Disparity lies in the rendering of 炮炙 [páo zhì]: "Preparation of Drugs", "Preparing Materia Medica" and "Processing of Medicinals".

4. Most authors render 新修本草 [xīn xiū běn cǎo] as "Newly Revised Materia Medica". The book is also titled 唐本草 [táng běn cǎo] for it was sponsored by the Tang court as the earliest pharmacopoeia published officially. Some authors render the book title as "The Materia Medica of the Tang Dynasty", which is explanatory and somewhat lengthy. Most authors prefer "Tang Materia Medica".

5. 拾遺 [shí yí] means "to make good the omissions". Since this is too lengthy to put in a book title, some authors render 本草拾遺 [běn cǎo shí yí] as "Omissions from the Materia Medica", but more authors prefer "Supplement to Materia Medica".

6. 經史證類備急本草 [jīng shǐ zhèng lèi bèi jí běn cǎo] compiled by Tang Shen-wei in 1082～1098, is a lengthy title, often abbreviated as 證類本草 [zhèng lèi běn cǎo]. Before making the proposed standard annotation, two key questions must be answered first. 經史 [jīng shǐ] are two of the main traditional categories of Chinese writings, namely classics and history. The reason why the book title contains the term 經史 [jīng shǐ] is because "Tang Shen-wei (the compiler) recorded every medicinal name and every discussion of formulae he found in all the classics and historical books, and then compiled this book."* Does 證類 [zhèng lèi] mean "Arranged According to Pattern Group" or "Arranged According To Pattern"? Here, we are not discussing whether 證 should be rendered as "pattern" or "syndrome". It has nothing to do with disease and symptoms. It is an abbreviation of 考證 [kǎo zhèng], which

---

*"唐慎微……每于經史諸書得一藥名，一方論，遂集爲此書。"（宇文虛中氏跋）

means "textual research". Textual research is an important work for compiling materia medica, because in different areas of China the same medicinal may have different names and different medicinals may have the same name. 證類 [zhèng lèi] is classification according to the results of such research. In fact, the medicinals in this book are classified as minerals, herbs, woody plants, fruits, cereals, vegetables, animals, birds, insects, etc., and described with illustrations. Therefore, many English renderings of this book title are incorrect. The only selection is "Classified Materia Medica for Emergencies" as the full title, and "Classified Materia Medica" as the abbreviation.

7. In the book title 珍珠囊 [zhēn zhū náng], 珍珠 [zhēn zhū] ("pearl") actually refers to very precious things. Two words are used for expressing 囊 [náng]: "bag" and "pouch" and two collocations for 珍珠囊 [zhēn zhū náng]: "bag [pouch] of pearls" and "pearl bag [pouch]". Based on the various renderings, "The Pearl Bag" is proposed for 珍珠囊 [zhēn zhū náng] and "Drug Nature of the Pearl Bag in Songs" for 珍珠囊藥性賦 [zhēn zhū náng yào xìng fù]

8. There are three different expressions for 湯液本草 [tāng yè běn cǎo] (1289): "Materia Medica for Decoctions" "Decoction and Materia Medica", and "Materia Medica of Decoctions". The first one seems the most appropriate.

9. There are several different renderings of 本草纲目 [běn cǎo gāng mù] (1590), among which most authors use the title "Compendium of Materia Medica".

10. Most authors use the word "Essential" to represent 備要 [bèi yào].

11. Most authors express 拾遺 [shí yí] in 本草纲目拾遺 [běn cǎo gāng mù shí yí] (1765) as "Supplement".

FORMULARIES

Proposed Standard Annotations

Handbook of Prescriptions for Emergencies 肘後備急方 [zhǒu hòu bèi jí fāng][1]
Thousand Ducat Prescriptions 千金方 [qiān jīn fāng][2]
Thousand Ducat Essential Prescriptions 千金要方 [qiān jīn yào fāng][2]
Supplement to the Thousand Ducat Prescriptions 千金翼方 [qiān jīn yì

fāng]²

Imperial Benevolence Formulary of the Taiping Era 太平聖惠方 [tài píng shèng huì fāng]³

Formulary of the Taiping Welfare Dispensary Bureau 太平惠民和劑局方 [tài píng huì mín hé jì jú fāng]⁴

General Collection of Imperial Remedies 聖濟總錄 [shèng jì zǒng lù]⁵

Universal Aid Formulary with Basic Facts 普濟本事方 [pǔ jì běn shì fāng]⁶

Formulary for Succoring the Sick 濟生方 [jì shēng fāng]⁷

Effective Formulae Tested by Physicians for Generations 世醫得效方 [shì yī dé xiào fāng]⁸

Elaboration of the Bureau Formulary 局方發揮 [jú fāng fā huī]⁹

Universal Aid Formulary 普濟方 [pǔ jì fāng]¹⁰

Non-Classical Formulae in Rhyme 時方歌括 [shí fāng gē kuò]¹¹

Discussion

1. 肘後 [zhǒu hòu] literally means "behind the elbow". A book so labeled usually refers to a guidebook close at hand while practicing. So many authors render it as handbook, and the whole book title as "Handbook of Prescriptions for Emergencies".

2. 千金方 [qiān jīn fāng] is a collective title of 千金要方 [qiān jīn yào fāng] and 千金翼方 [qiān jīn yì fāng]. Literally 千金 [qiān jīn] means a thousand pieces of gold, a figure of speech to express great value. Among various renderings, many authors, particularly Europeans, prefer "thousand ducat", as a ducat was a gold coin formerly current in Europe.

3. Many authors translate 太平 [tài píng] as "Peaceful" or "Great Peace". This is certainly not acceptable because 太平 [tài píng] is the abbreviated title of the second emperor of the Song Dynasty's reign. (The full title is 太平興國 [tài píng xīng guó].) For 聖惠方 [shèng huì fāng], "Holy Benevolent Prescriptions", "Sages' Benevolent Prescriptions", "Sage-like Prescriptions", "Sacred Remedies", and "Sagacious Benevolence Formulary" are roughly the same, but none of them exactly reflect the original sense. The compilation of this formulary was organized by the imperial government of the early Song Dynasty. 聖 [shèng] refers to the emperor, and 聖上 [shèng shàng] is an equivalent of "His Majesty". So, 聖惠 [shèng huì] means "benevolence bestowed by the emperor", and the whole book

title can be rendered as "Imperial Benevolence Formulary of the Taiping Era".

4. The crux of rendering 聖濟總錄 [shèng jì zǒng lù] into English is also the character 聖 [shèng]. The 8th emperor of the Song Dynasty paid much attention to medicine. He himself wrote a book on medical theories, and titled it 聖濟經 [shèng jì jīng]. Afterwards, he issued an edict to collect medical formulae used in the Imperial Court and from other sources, and organized medical officials to compile a voluminous formulary titled 聖濟總錄 [shèng jì zǒng lù]. As discussed in the above passage, 聖 [shèng] signifies the ruler of the Chinese empire. Based on the present translations of "General Record of Sagelike Benefit", "General Collection for Holy Relief", "Sages' Aid Records" and "Complete Record of Holy Benevolence", a new one is suggested: "General Collection of Imperial Remedies".

5. In the 11th ― 14th centuries the Chinese government set up such organizations as 惠民局 [huì mín jú] (Bureau of People's Welfare) for the administration of drug preparation and sale, and 和劑局 [hé jì jú] (Dispensary House) for dispensing prescriptions and manufacturing prepared drugs. The names of these organizations were changed several times, such as 太平惠民局 [tài píng huì mín jú] (Taiping Welfare Bureau) and 醫藥和劑局 [yī yào hé jì jú] (Medical Dispensary Bureau). For 太平惠民和劑局方 [tài píng huì mín hé jì jú fāng], there are various translations, from which the following one is selected: "Formulary of the Taiping Welfare Dispensary Bureau".

6. 普濟本事方 [pǔ jì běn shì fāng] (1132) was compiled by Xu Shu-wei. The key question is why it is called 本事方 [běn shì fāng], or what 本事方 [běn shì fāng] is. Xu lived in an era when poetry was in vogue. There came into being a well-known book titled 本事詩 [běn shì shī], which literally means "poems with the original facts". It is a collection of poems together with basic facts or events upon which the poems were written. Following the layout of 本事詩 [běn shì shī], Xu compiled the book with detailed descriptions of the basic data under each formula, and named it 本事方 [běn shì fāng] or 普濟本事方 [pǔ jì běn shì fāng] in full. According to the above discussion, none of the available translations found in recent publications can express the real meaning of Chinese book title, nor reflect the distinguishing feature of the book. Therefore, a new suggestion is necessary: "Universal Aid Formulary with Basic Facts" as the full name, and "Formulary with Ba-

sic Facts" for short.

7. Rendering 濟生 [jì shēng] as "life-saving" or "saving life" is excessive. Many of the formulae listed in 濟生方 [jì shēng fāng] are not used for this purpose. Some authors express it as "beneficial to life" or "succoring the sick", which are more appropriate.

8. The renderings of 世醫得效方 [shì yī dé xiào fāng] include "Effective Formulae [Formulas] Tested by Physicians for Generations", "Effective [Efficacious] Prescriptions for Generations", "Tested Prescriptions of Veteran Physicians", etc. They are generally the same, with minor differences.

9. In the book 局方發揮 [jú fāng fā huī], 局方 [jú fāng] "Formulary of the Bureau" is an abbreviation of "Formulary of the Taiping Welfare Dispensary Bureau". 發揮 [fā huī] is rendered as "Elaboration", "Elucidation", "Exposition" and "Expounding" by different authors.

10. Among the available renderings of 普濟方 [pǔ jì fāng], "Universal Aid Formulary" is the most succinct and exact to the Chinese original.

11. Many authors render 時方 [shí fāng] as "Contemporary Formulae" or "Popular Prescriptions" in 時方歌括 [shí fāng gē kuò]. In traditional Chinese medicine, 時方 [shí fāng] is specially defined as the opposite of 經方 [jīng fāng] (classical formulae). The latter refers to the formulae initiated by Zhang Zhong-jing in the second century and recorded in his famous book *Treatise on Cold-induced and Miscellaneous Diseases*. All the formulae developed by later generations are called 時方 [shí fāng], which is better called "non-classical formulae" in English. The book 時方歌括 [shí fāng gē kuò] was compiled and published in 1801, but the formulae recorded were widely used in the previous millennium and more. It is unreasonable to describe such a long period as "contemporary". The word "popular" is even more unacceptable, because the classical formulae excluded from this book are also popular or even more popular.

ACUPUNCTURE AND MOXIBUSTION

Proposed Standard Annotations

Systematic Classic of Acupuncture and Moxibustion 針灸甲乙經 [zhēn jiǔ jiǎ yǐ jīng][1]

Illustrated Manual of Acupoints on the Bronze Figure 銅人俞穴針灸圖經

[tóng rén shù xué zhēn jiǔ tú jīng][2]

Nourishing Life with Acupuncture and Moxibustion 針灸資生經 [zhēn jiǔ zī shēng jīng][3]

Elaboration of the Fourteen Meridians 十四經發揮 [shí sì jīng fā huī][4]

Gatherings from Eminent Acupuncturists 針灸聚英 [zhēn jiǔ jù yīng][5]

Great Compendium of Acupuncture and Moxibustion 針灸大成 [zhēn jiǔ dà chéng][6]

Discussion

1. In Chinese, 甲 [jiǎ] and 乙 [yǐ] are so-called heavenly stems used as serial numbers, like A, B, C in English. But as a book title, ABC refers to the simplest and most basic facts about a subject, while 甲乙 [jiǎ yǐ] means that the contents are arranged in serial order. Some authors express 針灸甲乙經 [zhēn jiǔ jiǎ yǐ jīng] as "ABC of Acupuncture" or "The ABC Classic of Acupuncture and Moxibustion". But these might belittle the importance of this book. In fact, it is a book with substantial content and systematic exposition, reflecting ancient China's great achievements in acupuncture. Therefore, "Systematic Classic of Acupuncture and Moxibustion" or "The Systematized Canon of Acupuncture and Moxibustion" suggested by some authors is recommended.

2. Translation of the character 經 [jīng] in book titles may cause difficulty. It has three meanings. (1) a work recognized as being of high quality and lasting value, and generally regarded as sacred or standard, e.g., 內經 [nèi jīng] (*Canon of Medicine*) and 针經 [zhēn jīng] (*Canon of Acupuncture*); (2) the Confucian classics, e.g., 詩經 [shī jīng] (*The Book of Songs*), 書經 [shū jīng] (*The Book of History*) and 易經 [yì jīng] (*The Book of Changes*); (3) a detailed scholarly study of one subject or systematic exposition of one technique, roughly equivalent to a monograph. The character 經 [jīng] in 銅人俞穴針灸圖經 [tóng rén shù xué zhēn jiǔ tú jīng] belongs to the third category. Some authors render the book title as "The Illustrated Classic of Acupuncture Points as Found on the Bronze Model", but more authors render it as "(An) Illustrated Manual of Acupuncture Points [Acupoints] (as shown [as found]) on the Bronze Man [Figure]".

3. 針灸資生經 [zhēn jiǔ zī shēng jīng] (1220) is a monograph written by 王執中 [wáng zh zhōng], chiefly discussing his own experience of acupuncture and moxibustion. The title has been rendered in

two different ways: "Classic of Nourishing Life with Acupuncture and Moxibustion" and "Experience in Acupuncture and Moxibustion Therapy". The latter conforms to the contents but departs from the original title. Thus, the first one is selected with omission of the word "Classic".

4. To reflect 發揮 [fā huī] in the book title 十四經發揮 [shí sì jīng fā huī] (1341), the following expressions have appeared in recent publications: "Elaboration", "Elucidation", "Expounding", "Exposition" and "Enlargement". Most authors prefer the first one.

5. Among various renderings that have appeared in recent publications, "Gatherings from Eminent Acupuncturists" most succinctly represents the original book title 針灸聚英 [zhēn jiǔ jù yīng], though the word moxibustion is omitted.

6. Almost all authors render 針灸大成 [zhēn jiǔ dà chéng] (1601) as "Compendium of Acupuncture and Moxibustion"; the only difference is that the majority of them add "Great" at the beginning of the title.

GENERAL MEDICINE AND INTERNAL MEDICINE

Proposed Standard Annotations

Essential Secrets from the Imperial Library 外臺秘要 [wài tái mì yào][1]

Confucians' Duties to Their Parents 儒門事親 [rú mén shì qīn][2]

Treatise on Differentiation of Endogenous and Exogenous Injuries 內外傷辨惑論 [nèi wài shāng biàn huò lùn][3]

Differentiation of Endogenous and Exogenous Injuries 內外傷辨 [nèi wài shāng biàn][3]

Treatise on the Spleen and Stomach 脾胃論 [pí wèi lùn][4]

Supplementary Treatise on Knowledge from Practice 格致餘論 [gé zhì yú lùn][5]

Dan-Xi's Experiential Therapy 丹溪心法 [dān xī xīn fǎ][6]

Prolonging Life and Preserving Vitality 壽世保元 [shòu shì bǎo yuán][7]

Key Link of Medicine 醫貫 [yī guàn][8]

Jing-Yue's Complete Works 景嶽全書 [jǐng yuè quán shū][9]

Supplement to the Synopsis of the Golden Chamber 金匱翼 [jīn guì yì][10]

Orthodox Tradition of Medicine 醫學正傳 [yī xué zhèng zhuàn][11]

Correction of Errors in Medicine 醫林改錯 [yī lín gǎi cuò][12]

Treatment Planning According to Syndrome Categories 類證治裁 [lèi zhèng zhì cái][13]
Treatise on Blood Syndromes 血證論 [xuè zhèng lùn][14]

Discussion

1. 外臺 [wài tái] is another name for the imperial library, and 秘要 [mì yào] means something secret and important. The author of the book, Wang Tao (670—755), was the chief of the Imperial Library for 20 years. He sorted out secret and important data from the books in the library, and compiled this book, which is praised by historians as a "treasure of the era". The following translations are found in recent publications: "Medical Secrets of an Official", "Medical Secrets Held by an Official", "Necessities of a Frontier Official", and "Essential Secrets from Outside the Metropolis". None of them well reflects the real meaning of the original book title. The key problem lies in the rendering of 外臺 [wài tái]. 臺 [tái] is a high and flat building. Since the official mansions in ancient China were built in such a form, the character 臺 [tái] was often used as a term of respect, especially for high-ranking officials. That is why many translators use the word "official", and the author of the book, chief of the Imperial Library, was really an official. However, "official" is not the real meaning of 外臺 [wài tái] in the book title. Even if the word "official" could be reluctantly agreed upon, "Frontier Official" is definitely unacceptable. A new suggestion is thus made: "Essential Secrets from the Imperial Library".

2. 儒門事親 [rú mén shì qīn] is rendered in various ways. Among them "Confucians' Duties to Their Parents" is accepted by most authors.

3. The key words in the book 內外傷辨惑論 [nèi wài shāng biàn huò lùn] are 內傷 [nèi shāng] and 外傷 [wài shāng]. The existing expressions are "External and Internal Injuries", "Endogenous and Exogenous Injuries" and "Endogenous and Exogenous Diseases". Comparatively speaking, "injuries" is more appropriate than "diseases", and "endogenous-exogenous" than "internal-external". "External diseases" refers to diseases visible from the outside, mainly including subcutaneous and cutaneous lesions. "External injury" is equivalent to trauma. These are not what this book discusses.

4. 脾胃論 [pí wèi lùn] is rendered by most authors as "Treatise on the Spleen and Stomach", and its English edition (1993) is also called

this.

5. 格致 [gé zhì] is an abbreviation of 格物致知 [gé wù zhì zhī], a proposition of ancient Chinese philosophy, interpreting the process of cognition.* Among the various translations of 格致餘論 [gé zhì yú lùn], some are close to the Chinese original, but others are miles apart from the Chinese original. "Supplementary Treatise on Knowledge from Practice" may be the best choice.

6. The English edition of 丹溪心法 [dān xī xīn fǎ] is titled "The Heart and Essence of Dan Xi's Methods of Treatment", but many other authors use different names such as "Essential Methods of Dan Xi", "Teachings of Dan-Xi", "Dan-Xi's Experiential Methods", "Experiential Therapy of Dan Xi", "Therapy in Danxi's Mind", and "Secrets of the Cinnabar Creek Master". Among these expressions, most authors prefer "Dan-Xi's Experiential Therapy".

7. 壽世保元 [shòu shì bǎo yuán] literally means "Prolonging Life and Preserving the Origin". Here, "the Origin" is the abbreviation of original *qi*, the source of all kinds of life activities. So, other authors prefer "Life-prolonging and Vitality-preserving" or "Longevity and Life Preservation".

8. The author of 醫貫 [yī guàn] advocated the theory of the life fire, and stressed that taking good care of the life fire could connect all kinds of treatment and prevention as the key link. Among the expressions "Medical Connection", "Thorough Knowledge of Medicine", and "Key Link of Medicine", the last one may be the best.

9. There are several expressions for 全書 [quán shū]: "Complete Book", "Complete Works", "Collected Treatises", and "Complete Compendium". 景嶽全書 [jǐng yuè quán shū] is better rendered as "Complete Book" or "Complete Works".

10. In the book title 金匱翼 [jīn guì yì], 金匱 [jīn guì] refers to 金匱要略 [jīn guì yào lüè] (Synopsis of the Golden Chamber).

11. Translations of 醫學正傳 [yī xué zhèng zhuàn] include "Orthodox Medical Record(s)", "Orthodox Medical Problems", and "Orthodox Tradition of Medicine". The last one is a close translation.

12. There is not much disparity in translating 醫林改錯 [yī lín gǎi

---

* "致知在格物，物格而後知至"（《礼记》）"If you want to get knowledge, you have to go deeply into the matter. From thorough study of the matter, knowledge emerges." (*The Book of Rites*)

cuò]. The only difference lies in the character 林 [lín]. Some authors omit it in their translation, and some others render it as "Works" or "Literature". The precise meaning of 醫林 [yī lín] is "medical circles". So, the simple and clear expression "Medicine" is recommended.

13. The main problem with rendering 類證治裁 [lèi zhèng zhì cái] into English is the character 裁 [cái]. Some authors render 治裁 [zhì cái] as "Clear-Cut Treatments". 裁 [cái] does mean "cut" in dress-making, but in this case it means "judge" or "decide". So, among the various translations "Treatment Planning according to Syndrome Categories" is close to the Chinese original.

14. Various renderings of 血證論 [xuè zhèng lùn] occur in recent publications, such as "Discussion on Blood", "Discussion of Blood Patterns", "Treatise on Blood Troubles", "Treatise on Blood Syndromes", "Discussion of Blood Syndromes", and "Treatise on Hemorrhagic Diseases". The first and the last ones are inaccurate. The disadvantage of rendering 證 [zhèng] as "pattern" is apparent in this case.

EXTERNAL MEDICINE AND TRAUMATOLOGY

Many authors translate 外科 [wài kē] as "surgery", simply because the word "surgery" is translated into Chinese as 外科 [wài kē]. In modern medicine, these two terms are equivalent, but in traditional Chinese medicine 外科 [wài kē] was defined in a different way: a branch of medicine concerned with diseases and conditions that are visible from without.* So, it dealt not only with surgical diseases involving the body surface, but also with skin diseases. Since many external diseases are not treated with operative or manual procedures, it is better to avoid using the word "surgery", particularly where the ancient works are concerned.

Proposed Standard Annotations

Liu Juanzi's Remedies Bequeathed by a Ghost 劉涓子鬼遺方 [liú quān

---

*"外科者，以其癰疽瘡瘍皆見於外，故以外科名之。" (汪机·外科理例) "It is called external medicine because the diseases such as carbuncles, sores, wounds and ulcers are all visible from the outside." (Wang Ji. *Theory and Examples of External Medicine*, 1519)

zǐ guǐ yí fāng][1]

Essence of External Medicine 外科精要 [wài kē jīng yào][2]

Essentials of External Medicine 外科精義 [wài kē jīng yì][2]

Pivot of External Medicine 外科樞要 [wài kē shū yào][2]

Orthodox External Medicine 外科正宗 [wài kē zhèng zōng][3]

Great Compendium of External Medicine 外科大成 [wài kē dà chéng][4]

Life-for-all Manual of External Medicine: Diagnosis and Treatment 外科
證治全生集 [wài kē zhèng zhì quán shēng jí][5]

Secret Methods of Treating Traumas and Fractures 理傷續斷秘方 [lǐ
shāng xù duàn mì fāng][6]

A Complete Book on Surgery 瘍醫大全 [yáng yī dà quán][7]

Discussion

1. 劉涓子鬼遺方 [liú quān zǐ guǐ yí fāng] was drafted by 劉涓子
[liú quān zǐ] in the fifth century. He made the draft in the name of the
ghost of Huang's father (黃父鬼 [huáng fù guǐ]), and so the book was
thus called when it was later edited by 龔慶宣 [gōng qìng xuān]. Among
the available translations, "Liu Juanzi's Remedies Left by a Ghost" is the
closest to the Chinese original, and the word "bequeathed" used by others
may be better than "left".

2. 精要 [jīng yào], 精義 [jīng yì] and 樞要 [shū yào] all mean
the necessary, indispensable and most important thing. The most common word used to express this meaning in the book titles is "Essentials",
but it will cause confusion if all the three books are designated the same
way. According to the frequency of the word used by different translators, "Essence" is selected for 精要 [jīng yào], "Essentials" for 精義
[jīng yì], and "Pivot" for 樞要 [shū yào]. In addition, it is suggested
that the author's name and the year of the first publication of the book be
added, namely, Wai Ke Jing Yao (*Essence of External Medicine* by Chen
Zi-Ming, 1263), Wai Ke Jing Yi (*Essentials of External Medicine* by Qi
De-Zhi, 1335), and Wai Ke Shu Yao (*Pivot of External Medicine* by Xue
Ji, 1571).

3. 正宗 [wài kē zhèng zōng] is most frequently translated as "orthodox". Many authors render 外科正宗 [wài kē zhèng zōng] as "Orthodox
Manual of External Diseases" or "Orthodox Manual of External Medicine". Since it is a voluminous book with substantial contents and detailed
discussions, the title "Orthodox External Medicine" is recommended.

4. "Complete Book", "Comprehensive Summary" and "Great Compendium" are used to express 大成 [dà chéng] in this book title. In order to match other books so titled, "Great Compendium" is selected.

5. The renderings of the book title 外科證治全生集 [wài kē zhèng zhì quán shēng jí] are multifarious and can be hardly unified. A practical way to solve the problem is to divide the book title into several parts, and select the proper expression for each part from the various renderings: (1) For the rendering of 外科 [wài kē], "External Medicine" is preferable. (2) "Diagnosis and Treatment" is a simple and clear way to express 證治 [zhèng zhì]. (3) For expressing 全生 [quán shēng], "Life-for-All" is a choice phrase. (4) 集 [jí] literally means "collection", but no translator uses this word in translating this book title, while many translators use the word "Manual", for the book gives practical instructions. (5) The whole title is often abbreviated as 外科全生集 [wài kē quán shēng jí], and so the desirable word order is to place "Diagnosis and Treatment" at the end, as suggested by some translators. In conclusion, the proposed translation is "Life-for-all Manual of External Medicine: Diagnosis and Treatment" or "Life-for-all Manual of External Medicine" for short.

6. Translation of 理傷續斷秘方 [lǐ shāng xù duàn mì fāng] word by word may cause difficulty. 理 [lǐ], being an abbreviation of 治理 [zhì lǐ], means "treat", and 續斷 [xù duàn] ("rejoin the fracture") is a treatment. Despite the various complicated renderings, "Secret Methods of Treating Traumas and Fractures" probably suits the book best.

7. In traditional Chinese medicine, 瘍醫 [yáng yī] or 瘍科 [yáng kē] is equivalent to surgery.

OBSTETRICS AND GYNECOLOGY

Proposed Standard Annotations

Tested Treasure in Obstetrics 經效産寶 [jīng xiào chǎn bǒo][1]
The Complete Book of Efficacious Prescriptions for Women 婦人大全良方 [fù rén dà quán liáng fāng][2]
Fu Qing-zhu's Obstetrics and Gynecology 傅青主女科 [fù qīng zhǔ nǚ kē][3]
Principles of Obstetrics and Gynecology 女科經綸 [nǚ kē jīng lún][4]

Discussion

1. Among various expressions, "Tested Treasure in Obstetrics" reflects the original title best.

2. Most authors render 婦人大全良方 [fù rén dà quán liáng fāng] as "The Complete Book of Effective Prescriptions for Women". There are modifications, such as replacing "Efficacious Prescriptions" with "Effective Prescriptions", "Good Prescriptions" or "Useful Prescriptions", changing "Women" into "Women's Diseases", etc.

3. 傅青主女科 [fù qīng zhǔ nǚ kē] is generally rendered as Fu Qing-zhu's Obstetrics and Gynecology. Some authors delete "Obstetrics" from the title. This is not recommended, because obstetrics is a very important part of the book.

4. Most authors render 女科經綸 [nǚ kē jīng lún] as "Principles of Obstetrics and Gynecology". Other renderings include "Discussion of Women's Disorders", "Classified Treatise on Obstetrics and Gynecology", etc.

PEDIATRICS

Proposed Standard Annotations

Key to Differentiation and Treatment of Children's Diseases 小兒藥證直訣 [xiǎo ér yào zhèng zhí jué][1]

A New Book of Pediatrics 幼幼新書 [yòu yòu xīng shū][2]

Children's Diseases: Sources and Remedies 小兒病源方論 [xiǎo ér bìng yuán fāng lùn][3]

Elaboration of Pediatrics 幼科發揮 [yòu kē fā huī][4]

A Complete Work on Pediatrics 幼幼集成 [yòu yòu jí chéng][5]

Discussion

1. Most authors use the word "key" to express 直訣 [zhí jué].

2. For the book title 幼幼新書 [yòu yòu xīng shū] in English, most authors prefer "A New Book of Pediatrics", while some others render it as "New Pediatrics" or "New Book for Infants".

3. "Children's Diseases: Remedies and Sources" is a recommended translation of 小兒病源方論 [xiǎo ér bìng yuán fāng lùn], but it is

better to transpose the two words "Remedies" and "Sources".

4. 發揮 [fā huī] may be rendered as "Elaboration", "Elucidation", "Expounding", "Exposition" or "Enlargement". For 幼科發揮 [yòu kē fā huī], "Elaboration of Pediatrics" is selected.

5. Most authors express 幼幼 [yòu yòu] as pediatrics, but some other authors render it as "young child". A brief discussion on this phrase is necessary. Grammatically, 幼幼 [yòu yòu] is a verb-object word group, in which the first character is a verb with the meaning of "care for", and the second character is a noun with the meaning of "children". Primarily, 幼 [yòu] is an adjective signifying "young". It can be used as a noun, i.e., the young, and can also be used as a verb meaning to care for a child. A famous remark from *Mencius* showing universal fraternity reads as follows: 幼吾幼，以及人之幼 [yòu wú yòu, yǐ jí rén zhī yòu]. (Love my own children, and love others' children alike.) Therefore, 幼幼 [yòu yòu] means "caring for children" but not "young child", and pediatrics is a branch of medicine dealing with the care of children.

OPHTHALMOLOGY

Proposed Standard Annotations

A Precious Book of Ophthalmology 審視瑤函 [shěn shì yáo hán][1]
Essentials of Ophthalmology 銀海精微 [yín hǎi jīng wēi][2]

Discussion

1. 審視瑤函 [shěn shì yáo hán] is also called 眼科大全 [yǎn kē dà quán] (Great Compendium of Ophthalmology) and 眼科審視瑤函 [yǎn kē shěn shì yáo hán], but in Chinese medical circles the first one is the best known. The renderings of 審視瑤函 [shěn shì yáo hán] are practically identical, with minor differences. Among "A Precious Book of Ophthalmology", "A Valuable Manual of Ophthalmology" and "A Precious Work on Ophthalmology" the first is regarded as the most suitable.

2. 銀海 [yín hǎi] is a euphemistic term referring to the eye in Chinese. Its directly literal translation as "silver(y) sea" is probably unintelligible. Among other renderings, "Essentials of Ophthalmology" is recommended.

DISEASES OF THE MOUTH AND THROAT

Proposed Standard Annotations

Analysis of Diphtheria 白喉條辨 [bái hóu tiáo biàn][1]
Jade Key to the Secluded Chamber 重樓玉鑰 [chóng lóu yù yào][2]
Essentials of Diseases of the Mouth and Teeth 口齒類要 [kǒu chǐ lèi yào][3]

Discussion

1. 條辨 [tiáo biàn] means study of something by differentiating and examining its parts, equivalent to "analysis". Among the available translations, "Detailed Analysis of Diphtheria" is a close one, though the word "Detailed" may not be necessary.

2. 重樓玉鑰 [chóng lóu yù yào] reads like the title of a novel. It is difficult to find a generally recognized English equivalent. Such titles as "Precious Works on Throat Diseases" and "Treatment of Laryngological Diseases" are far from the Chinese original. Most authors render it literally as "Jade Key to the Secluded Chamber".

3. For 口齒類要 [kǒu chǐ lèi yào], "Essentials of the Mouth and Teeth" is a close translation, but addition of "Diseases" seems necessary.

WARM DISEASES

Proposed Standard Annotations

Treatise on Pestilence 溫疫論 [wēn yì lùn][1]
Treatise on Warm Diseases 溫熱論 [wēn rè lùn][2]
Analysis of Warm Diseases 溫病條辨 [wēn bìng tiáo biàn][3]
Compendium of Epidemic Febrile Diseases 溫熱經緯 [wēn rè jīng wěi][4]
Treatise on Seasonal Diseases 時病論 [shí bìng lùn][5]

Discussion

1. 溫疫論 [wēn yì lùn] was written by Wu You-xing, and published in 1642. There are different renderings of 溫疫 [wēn yì]: "Acute Epidemic Febrile Diseases", "Warm Epidemics", and "Pestilence". This term

is confusing, because 溫 [wēn] (warm diseases) and 疫 [yì] (pestilential diseases) are not the same. In 1864, Zheng Chong-guang made supplementary notes to the book, and changed the book title to 瘟疫論 [wēn yì lùn] (Treatise on Pestilence). He named his own book 瘟疫論補注 [wēn yì lùn bǔ zhù] (Supplementary Notes to the Treatise on Pestilence). This certainly makes the term 溫疫 [wēn yì] clear, but the original book title could not be changed, because it had already been published. To date, most translators prefer "Treatise on Pestilence" as the equivalent of 溫疫論 [wēn yì lùn].

2. The term 溫熱 [wēn rè] is also a problematic one. It has been vaguely defined either as a synonym for warm diseases (溫病 [wēn bìng]) or as one category of warm diseases. In the latter case, it is translated as "warm-heat" to be juxtaposed with "wind-warm", "damp-warm" etc. Later, the term 溫熱 [wēn rè], used in its broad sense, was changed to 溫病 [wēn bìng], but the original book title should be kept. As for the English title of this book, many authors prefer "Treatise on Warm Diseases". This causes no confusion, for no book known to-day is titled as 溫病論 [wēn bìng lùn].

3. Divergent opinions exist in translating the terms 溫病 [wēn bìng] and 條辨 [tiáo biàn]. Some authors render 溫病 [wēn bìng] as "Epidemic Febrile Diseases", while others prefer "Warm Diseases" to keep the unique flavor of traditional Chinese medicine. For the book title, the latter is selected. 條辨 [tiáo biàn] is rendered in various ways, such as "Differentiation", "Treatise on Differentiation and Treatment", "Systematized Idenitification", "Detailed Analysis" and "Analysis". The last one is close to the Chinese original, as discussed in 白喉條辨 [bái hóu tiáo biàn].

4. 經緯 [jīng wěi] (warp and weft) has a similar meaning to 綱目 [gāng mù] (head rope and mesh wire), and can be translated as "compendium" or "outline". For the phrase 經緯 [jīng wěi] in the book title 溫熱經緯 [wēn rè jīng wěi] most translators prefer "Compendium" to "Outline", and for 溫熱 [wēn rè], "Epidemic Febrile Diseases".

5. 時病論 [shí bìng lùn] is rendered as "Treatise on Seasonal Diseases" or "Treatise on Seasonal Febrile Diseases" by different authors. The former is more appropriate, because diarrhea without fever is also dealt with in this book.

COMPREHENSIVE OR SERIAL MEDICALBOOKS

Proposed Standard Annotations

Secret Collection of the Orchid Chamber 蘭室秘藏 [lán shì mì cáng][1]
Precious Warnings for Health Service 衛生寶鑒 [wèi shēng bǎo jiàn][2]
Outline of Medicine 醫學綱目 [yī xué gāng mù][3]
Complete Compendium of Medical Tradition, Ancient and Contemporary 古今醫統大全 [gǔ jīn yī tǒng dà quán][4]
Medical Tradition, Ancient and Contemporary 古今醫統 [gǔ jīn yī tǒng][4]
Introduction to Medicine 醫學入門 [yī xué rù mén][5]
Standards of Diagnosis and Treatment in Six Branches of Medicine 六科證治準繩 [liù kē zhèng zhì zhǔn shéng][6]
Standards of Diagnosis and Treatment 證治準繩 [zhèng zhì zhǔn shéng][6]
Essential Readings in Medicine 醫宗必讀 [yī zōng bì dú][7]
Principles and Prohibitions of Medical Practice 醫門法律 [yī mén fǎ lǜ][8]
Zhang's General Medicine 張氏醫通 [zhāng shì yī tōng][9]
Medicine Comprehended 醫學心悟 [yī xué xīn wù][10]
Golden Mirror of Medicine 醫宗金鑒 [yī zōng jīn jiàn][11]
Orthodox Medicine 醫學正宗 [yī xué zhèng zōng][12]

Discussion

1. Most authors translate 蘭室 [lán shì] as "Orchid Chamber". For 秘藏 [mì cáng], the available translations include "Secret Record", "Secret Book Kept", "Secret Treasure", and "Secret Collection", which are roughly the same.

2. In modern Chinese, 衛生 [wèi shēng] is equivalent to hygiene, which refers to conditions or practices (as of cleanliness) conductive to health. In this book, 衛生 [wèi shēng] (protection of health or life) refers to the proper treatment of disease. In addition, the first part of the book is 藥誤永鑒 [yào wù yǒng jiàn], i.e., "Perpetual Warning from Improper Medication". This explains why the book is titled 寶鑒 [bǎo jiàn], and is also evidence that "Hygiene" is not the proper translation. Some authors use "Health Service", which is more acceptable.

3. 綱目 [gāng mù] is equivalent to "compendium" or "outline". Most authors translate it in the title 本草綱目 [běn cǎo gāng mù] as "Compendium", but in 醫學綱目 [yī xué gāng mù] as "Outline". This

is related to the respective contents of the books.

4. The available translations of 古今醫統大全 [gǔ jīn yī tǒng dà quán] include "Complete Compendium of Medical Works, Ancient and Modern", "A Complete Work of Ancient and Modern Medicine", "Ancient and Modern Medicine Encyclopedia", and "The General Medicine of the Past and Present". The first one is recommended for its word order, but it does not reflect the Chinese original 醫統 [yī tǒng], nor do the other translations. 統 [tǒng] means "interconnected system", and in the present title it may be translated as "Tradition".

5. Among the available English translations of 入門 [rù mén], "Introduction" is the exact word, because almost all books titled "Introduction" are rendered into Chinese as 入門 [rù mén].

6. Although 證治 [zhèng zhì] is an abbreviation of 辨證 [biàn zhèng] (syndrome differentiation or pattern identification) and 治療 [zhì liáo] (treatment), most authors prefer to skirt round the problematic character 證 [zhèng]. There is no dispute when 證治 [zhèng zhì] is rendered as "diagnosis and treatment". Thus, 證治準繩 [zhèng zhì zhǔn shéng] is "Standards of [for] Diagnosis and Treatment", and the full title 六科證治準繩 [liù kē zhèng zhì zhǔn shéng] is "Standards of [for] Diagnosis and Treatment in Six Branches of Medicine"

7. In order to express the book title 醫宗必讀 [yī zōng bì dú] precisely, the translation is often complicated, e.g., "Essential Readings for Those in the Medical Lineage", "Required Reading(s) for Medical Professionals". However, if these are compared with "Essential Readings in Medicine" or "Indispensable Medical Reading", the direct literal translation of the character 宗 [zōng] seems unnecessary. In addition, there are many Chinese medical books containing the phrase 醫宗 [yī zōng], e.g., 醫宗金鑒 [yī zōng jīn jiàn], in which the character 宗 [zōng] is usually omitted in translation.

8. In modern Chinese, the term 法律 [fǎ lǜ] is equivalent to law. But the 醫門法律 [yī mén fǎ lǜ] was a book published in 1658. At that time, this term was not used in the modern sense. 法 [fǎ] and 律 [lǜ] refer to 法則 [fǎ zé] (principle) and 禁律 [jìn lǜ] (prohibition). In fact, most authors render the title of this book as "Principles and Prohibitions of Medical Practice [Profession]".

9. 張氏醫通 [zhāng shì yī tōng] is a comprehensive book covering almost all branches of medicine from the ancient to the contemporary, including the author's own experience. The character 通 [tōng] in the book

title has the following meanings: (1) general, and (2) having a thorough knowledge from the ancient to the contemporary. Among various translations, "Zhang's Treatise on General Medicine" is most frequently encountered. Since the book deals with more than one subject, it is better to omit the words "Treatise on".

10. 醫學心悟 [yī xué xīn wù] is rendered in various ways by different authors. The candidates for selection include "Medical Revelations", "Medicine Comprehended", "Medical Insights" and "Insightful Medicine". Most authors prefer "Medicine Comprehended".

11. Almost all authors render 醫宗金鑒 [yī zōng jīn jiàn] as "Golden Mirror of Medicine".

12. 正宗 [zhèng zōng] and "Orthodox" are generally recognized equivalents.

OTHERS

Proposed Standard Annotations

Classified Case Records of Famous Physicians 名醫類案 [míng yī lèi àn][1]
Clinical Guide with Case Histories 臨證指南醫案 [lín zhèng zhǐ nán yī àn][2]
Collected Records of Medical Jurisprudence 洗冤集錄 [xǐ yuān jí lù][3]
Collected Records of Medical Jurisprudence 洗冤錄 [xǐ yuān lù][3]
Herbal Dietotherapy 食療本草 [shí liáo běn cǎo][4]
Dietary Herbal 食物本草 [shí wù běn cǎo][4]
Principles of Correct Diet 飲膳正要 [yǐn shàn zhèng yào][5]
Medical Talks in a Deserted House 冷廬醫話 [lěng lú yī huà][6]

Discussion

1. Although 名醫類案 [míng yī lèi àn] is composed of only four commonly used characters in two phrases, and no disagreement exists in the translations, this book title is rendered in multifarious ways. The available renderings of 名醫 [míng yī] include "Famous Physicians", "Well- known Physicians" and "Distinguished Physicians", and those of 類案 [lèi àn] include "Ordered Case Histories", "Classified Case Records", 'Classified Medical Records" and "Classified Medical Case Records". Then, there are various combinations, and it is hard to say which

combination definitely has more advocates.

2. In translating English into Chinese, "Guidebook" is equivalent to 指南 [zhǐ nán]. So, it is natural to render 指南 [zhǐ nán] as "Guidebook" or "Guide". Among various renderings of 臨證指南醫案 [lín zhèng zhǐ nán yī àn], "Clinical Guide with Case Histories" is the most succinct.

3. 洗冤集錄 [xǐ yuān jí lù], also called 洗冤錄 [xǐ yuān lù] for short, has the following renderings: "Instruction to Coroners", "Manual of Forensic Medicine" and "Collected Records of Medical Jurisprudence". The last seems the most appropriate, as it accords with the Chinese original and can be abbreviated by omitting the word "Collected".

4. 食療本草 [shí liáo běn cǎo] is not only a book of materia medica, but also a book of dietotherapy. All the medicinals listed in the book are foodstuffs. There are various renderings of the book title: "A Dietetic Materia Medica", "Dietary Herbal", "Dietotherapy of Materia Medica", "Materia Medica of Diet Therapy", and "Materia Medica as Dietetic Therapy". The first two are suitable translations for another book, titled 食物本草 [shí wù běn cǎo].

5. All authors translate 飲膳正要 [yǐn shàn zhèng yào] as "Principles of Correct Diet".

6. In ancient China, many distinguished physicians were also *literati*. They often gave their houses or studies elegant names. Their writings often contained such house or study names in the title. 冷廬 [lěng lú] is such a name. Some authors leave it in pinyin, while others render it as "Cold Shack" or "Deserted House".

APPENDIX: ENGLISH EDITIONS OF CLASSICAL CHINESE MEDICAL WORKS PUBLISHED IN RECENT DECADES

黃帝內經 [huáng dì nèi jīng]

The Yellow Emperor's Classic of Internal Medicine [Huang Di Nei Jing — Su Wen], translated by Ilza Veith, Williams & Wilkins, 1949

The Yellow Emperor's Classic of Internal Medicine [Huang Di Nei Jing — Su Wen] translated by Ilza Veith, University of California Press, Berkeley and Los Angeles, 1966

Ling Shu or The Spiritual Pivot. Asia Spirituality, translated by Wu J.N., Taoist Studies Series, the Taoist Center, Washington, D.C., 1993.

The Yellow Emperor's Classic of Medicine translated by Maoshing Ni,

Shambhala, Boston and London, 1995.

Yellow Empero's Canon Internal Medicine translated by Nelson Lian-sheng Wu and Andrew Qi Wu, China Science & Technology Press, Bei-jing, 1999.

難經 [nàn jīng]

The Classic of Difficult Issues [Nan Jing] translated by Paul Unschuld, University of California Press, Berkeley, Los Angeles, London, 1986.

傷寒論 [shāng hán lùn]

Treatise on Febrile Diseases Caused by Cold with 500 Cases: A Clas-sic of Traditional Chinese Medicine with Ancient and Contemporary Case Studies [Shang han lun] translated by Luo Xiwen, New World Press, Bei-jing, 1993.

On Cold Damage [Shang han Lun] translated by Craig Mitchell, Feng Ye and Nigel Wiseman, Paradigm Publications, Brookline, Massachusetts, 1999.

金匱要略 [jīn guì yào lüè]

Synopsis of Prescriptions of the Golden Chamber [Jin Gui Yao Lue Fang Lun] translated by Luo Xiwen, New World Press, Beijing, 1987.

Synopsis of Prescriptions of the Golden Chamber with 300 Cases: A Classic of Traditional Chinese Medicine with Ancient and Contemporary Case Studies [Jin Kui Yao Lue] translated by Luo Xiwen, New World Press, Beijing, 1995

神農本草經 [shén nóng běn cǎo jīng]

The Divine Farmer's Materia Medica: a Translation of the Shen Nong Ben Cao Jing, translated by Yang Shou-zhong, Blue Poppy Press, Boulder, 1998.

脈經 [mài jīng]

The Pulse Classic: a Translation of the Mai-jing by Wang Shu-he, translated by Yang Shou-zhong, Blue Poppy Press, Boulder, 1997.

脾胃論 [pí wèi lùn]

Li Dong-yuan's Treatise on the Spleen & Stomach: a Translation of the Pi Wei Lun, translated by Yang Shou-zhong, Blue Poppy Press, Boulder, 1993.

丹溪心法 [dān xī xīn fǎ]
The Heart and Essence of Dan-xi's Methods of Treatment [Dan Xi Xin Fa], translated by Yang Shou-zhong, Blue Poppy Press, Boulder, 1993.

BIBLIOGRAPHY

Advanced Textbook on Traditional Chinese Medicine and Pharmacology. Vol. I, II, III and IV New World Press, Beijing, 1995 to 1997.

Bensky D and Gamble A (comp. and transl.) *Materia Medica*, revised ed. Eastland Press, Seattle, 1993.

Chen JR, Wang N. *Acupuncture Case Histories from China*. Eastland Press, Seattle, 1988.

Chen P, ed. *Acupuncture and Moxibustion* in Advanced TCM Series vol. 6. Science Press, Beijing, and IOS Press, Amsterdam, Ohmsha, Tokyo, 2000.

Chen P. et al, (ed.) *Chinese Herbs and Compatibility* in Advanced TCM Series vol. 4. Science Press, Beijing, and IOS Press, Amsterdam, Ohmsha, Tokyo, 1997.

Chen ZL and Chen MF. *A Comprehensive Guide to Chinese Herbal medicine*. Castle Books, 1992.

Editorial Committee of the Chinese-English Medical Dictionary: *Chinese-English Medical Dictionary*. People's Medical Publishing House, China, 1987

Ehling D. *The Chinese Herbalist's Handbook*. Inword Press, 1994.

Ergil M and Yi SM, (transl.) *Practical Diagnosis in Traditional Chinese Medicine* written by Deng TT. Churchill Livingstone, 1999.

Fan WJ. *A Manual of Chinese Herbal Medicine. Principles and Practice for Easy Reference*. Shambhala, Boston and London, 1996.

Flaws B. *The Secret of Chinese Pulse Diagnosis*. Blue Poppy Press, Colorado, USA, 1995.

Fung (transl.) *The Basis of Traditional Chinese Medicine* written by Shen ZY. The Commercial Press (Hong Kong) Ltd. 1994

Guillaume G, Chieu M. *Rheumatology in Chinese Medicine*. Eastland Press, Seattle, 1996.

Hammer L. *Dragon rise, red bird flies: Psychology of Chinese Medicine*. Station Hill Press, 1990.

Hopwood V, Lovesey M and Mokone S. *Acupuncture & Related Techniques in Physical Therapy*. Churchill Livingstone, New York, Edinburgh, London, Madrid, Melbourne, San Francisco and Tokyo, 1997.

Hou JL, Chen G, eds. *Treatment of Paediatric Diseases in Traditional Chinese Medicine*. Academy Press [Xue Yuan], Beijing, 1995.

Hsu HY (ed.) *Natural Healing with Chinese Herbs* written by Keisetsu Otsuka. Oriental healing Arts Institute, Los Angeles, California, USA,

Hsu HY and Hsu CS. *Commonly Used Chinese Herb Formulas with Illustrations*. Oriental Healing Arts Institute, Long Beach, CA, 1980.

Hsu HY and Peacher WG, (transl. and eds.) *Wellspring of Chinese Medicine*. Keats Publishing, Inc., 1981.

Hsu HY. *Chinese Herb Medicine and Therapy*. Oriental Healing Arts Institute, USA, 1982

Hsu HY. *Oriental Materia Medica – a concise guide*. Oriental Healing Arts Institute, USA, 1986

Institute of History of Natural Sciences, Chinese Academy of Sciences. *Ancient China's Technology and Science*. Foreign Languages Press, Beijing, 1983.

Jin HD (transl.) *Essentials of Traditional Chinese Pediatrics*. Foreign Language Press, Beijing, 1990.

Kaptchuk TJ. *The Web That Has No Weaver.* Congdon & Weed, Inc., Chicago, 1983.

Larre C. *Rooted in Spirit: The Heart of Chinese Medicine*. Station Hill Press, 1995.

Li ZG, ed. *A Comprehensive Chinese-English Dictionary of Traditional Chinese Medicine*. World Book Publications, 1997.

Luo XW, (comp. and transl.) *Treatise on Febrile Diseases Caused by Cold* [Shang Han Lun] *with 500 Cases*. New World Press, 1993.

Luo XW (transl.) *Synopsis of Prescriptions of the Golden Chamber* [Jin Gui Yao Lue Fang Lun]. New World Press, Beijing, 1987.

Maciocia G. *Obstetrics and Gynecology in Chinese Medicine*. Churchill Livingstone, New York, Edinburgh, London, Madrid, Melbourne, San Francisco and Tokyo, 1998.

Maciocia G. *The Foundations of Chinese Medicine – A Comprehensive Text for Acupuncturists and Herbaslists*. Churchill Livingstone, Edinburgh, Londong, Melbourne and New York, 1989.

Maciocia G. *The Practice of Practice of Chinese Medicine – The Treatment of Diseases with Acupuncture and Chinese Herbs*. Churchill Livingstone,

New York, Edinburgh, London, Madrid, Melbourne, San Francisco and Tokyo, 1994.

Maciocia G. *Tongue Diagnosis in Chinese Medicine*. Eastland Press, Seattle, 1987.

MacPherson H and Kaptchuk TJ. *Acupuncture in Practice – Case History Insights from the West*. Churchil Livingstone, 1997.

McNamara S. *Traditional Chinese Medicine*. Hamish Hamilton, London, 1995.

Mitchell C, Ye F, Wiseman N (transl.). *Shang han Lun: On Cold Damage*. Paradigm Publications, Brookline, Massachusetts, 1999.

Ni MS (transl.) *The Yellow Emperor's Classic of Medicine*. Shambhala, Boston and London, 1995.

O'Connor J and Bensky D. *Acupuncture – A Comprehensive Text*. Eastland Press, Chicago, 1981.

Ou M (ed.) *Chinese-English Dictionary of Traditional Chinese Medicine*. Guangdong Science & Technology Press, 1986.

Pharmacopoeia of the People's Republic of China (English Edition). Chemical Industry Press, Beijing, China, 1997.

Porkert M. *Chinese Medicine*. William Morrow & Co., Inc. New York and Seattle, 1988.

Ross J. *Acupuncture Point Combinations – The Key to Clinical Success*. Churchill Livingstone, Edinburgh, Hong Kong, London, Madrid, Melbourne, New York and Tokyo, 1995.

Shen DH, Wu XF and Wang N. *Manual of Dermatology in Chinese Medicine*. Eastland Press, Seattle, 1995.

Shuai XZ (transl.) *Fundamentals of Traditional Chinese Medicine* written by Yin HH et al. Foreign Language Press, Beijing, 1992.

Shuai XZ, ed. *Chinese-English Terminology of TCM*. Hunan Science and Technology Press, 1983.

Sivin N. *Traditional Medicine in Contemporary China*. Center for Chinese Study, the University of Michigan, 1987.

Unschuld PU (ed.) *Approaches to Traditional Chinese Medical Literature*. Kluwer Academic Publishers, 1989.

Unschuld PU (transl.) *The Classic of Difficult Issues* [Nan Jing]. University of California Press, Berkeley, Los Angeles, London, 1986.

Unschuld PU. *Introductory Readings in Classical Chinese Medicine*. Kluwer Academic Publishers, Dordrecht/Boston/London, 1988.

Veith I (transl.) *The Yellow Emperor's Classic of Internal Medicine* [Huang

Di Nei Jing – Su Wen]. The Williams & Wilkins Company, 1949.

Veith I (transl.) *The Yellow Emperor's Classic of Internal Medicine* [Huang Di Nei Jing – Su Wen]. University of California Press, Berkeley and Los Angeles, 1966.

Wang BX and Dong XM (eds.) *Chinese-English Glossary of Traditional Chinese Medicine*. Science Press, Beijing, 1993.

Williams T. *Chinese Medicine*. Element Books Ltd., 1997.

Williams T. *The Complete Illustrated Guide to Chinese Medicine*. Element Books, 1996.

Wiseman N (ed.) *English-Chinese Chinese-English Dictionary of Chinese Medicine*. Hunan Science and Technology Press, 1996.

Wiseman N. *Fundamentals of Chinese Medicine,* Paradigm Publications, Brookline, Massachusetts, 1995.

World Health Organization Regional Office for the Western Pacific (WPRO). *Standard Acupuncture Nomenclature*. WPRO, Manila, Philippines, 1991.

World Health Organization (WHO). *A propose standard international acupuncture nomenclature*. WHO, Geneva, 1991.

Wu JN (transl.) *Ling Shu or The Spiritual Pivot.* Asia Spirituality, Taoist Studies Series, the Taoist Center, Washington, D.C., 1993.

Wu LC et al. (eds.) *Chinese Traditional medicine and Materia Medica Subject Headings*. China Ancient Book Publications, 1996.

Wu NL and Wu AQ, (transl.) *Yellow Empero's Canon Internal Medicine.* China Science & Technology Press, Beijing, 1999.

Wu Y and Fisher W. *Practical Therapeutics of Traditional Chinese Medicine*. Paradigm Publications, Brookline, Massachusetts, 1997.

Xie ZF et al., (transl.) *Chinese Acupuncture and Moxibustion.* 1st and revised eds. Foreign Language Press, Beijing, 1987 and 1999.

Xie ZF and Huang XK (eds.) *Common Terms of Traditional Chinese Medicine in English*. Beijing Medical College, 1981 and *Dictionary of Traditional Chinese Medicine*, Commercial Press, Hong Kong, 1984.

Xie ZF, Lou ZQ and Huang XK (eds.) *Classified Dictionary of Traditional Chinese Medicine*. New World Press, Beijing, 1994.

Yan MH and Zhang F (transl.) *Tuina Therapy* written by Wang DQ. Shandong Science and Technology Press, 1996.

Yuan YX et al. (eds.) *Chinese-English Dictionary of Traditional Chinese Medicine*. People's Medical Publishing House, China, 1997.

Zhang RF et al. (eds.) *Illustrated TCM Dictionary of Chinese Acupuncture.* Sheep's Publications (HK) and People's Medical Publishing House, China,

1985.

Zhao JY and Li XM. *Patterns & Practice in Chinese Medicine*. Eastland Press, Seattle, WA, USA, 1998.

Zheng FQ (eds.) *Traditinal Chinese Medicine Dictionary in Chinese-English and English-Chinese*. Tianjin University Press, 1994

Zhou ZY and Jin HD. *Clinical manual of Chinese Herbal medicine and Acupuncture*. Churchill Livingstone, New York, Edinburgh, London, Madrid, Melbourne, San Francisco and Tokyo, 1997.

ANNEX

LIST OF ACUPUNTURE POINTS ACCORDING TO WHO'S STANDARD INTERNATIONAL ACUPUNCTURE NOMENCLATURE

The 361 classical acupuncture points

LU 1	zhōngfǔ	中府	LU 2	yúnmén	雲門
LU 3	tiānfǔ	天府	LU 4	xiábái	俠白
LU 5	chǐzé	尺澤	LU 6	kǒngzuì	孔最
LU 7	lièquē	列缺	LU 8	jīngqú	經渠
LU 9	tàiyuān	太淵	LU 10	yújì	魚際
LU 11	shàoshāng	少商			
LI 1	shāngyáng	商陽	LI 2	èrjiān	二間
LI 3	sānjiān	三間	LI 4	hégǔ	合谷
LI 5	yángxī	陽谿	LI 6	piānlì	偏歷
LI 7	wēnliū	溫溜	LI 8	xiàlián	下廉
LI 9	shànglián	上廉	LI 10	shǒusānlǐ	手三里
LI 11	qūchí	曲池	LI 12	zhǒuliáo	肘髎
LI 13	shǒuwǔlǐ	手五里	LI 14	bìnào	臂臑
LI 15	jiānyú	肩髃	LI 16	jùgǔ	巨骨
LI 17	tiāndǐng	天鼎	LI 18	fútū	扶突
LI 19	kǒuhéliáo	禾髎	LI 20	yíngxiāng	迎香
ST 1	chéngqì	承泣	ST 2	sìbái	四白
ST 3	jùliáo	巨髎	ST 4	dìcāng	地倉
ST 5	dàyíng	大迎	ST 6	jiáchē	頰車
ST 7	xiàguān	下關	ST 8	tóuwéi	頭維
ST 9	rényíng	人迎	ST 10	shuǐtū	水突
ST 11	qìshè	氣舍	ST 12	quēpén	缺盆
ST 13	qìhù	氣戶	ST 14	kùfáng	庫房
ST 15	wūyì	屋翳	ST 16	yīngchuāng	膺窗
ST 17	rǔzhōng	乳中	ST 18	rǔgēn	乳根
ST 19	bùróng	不容	ST 20	chéngmǎn	承滿
ST 21	liángmén	梁門	ST 22	guānmén	關門

ST 23	tàiyǐ	太乙		ST 24	huáròumén	滑肉門
ST 25	tiānshū	天樞		ST 26	wàilíng	外陵
ST 27	dàjù	大巨		ST 28	shuǐdào	水道
ST 29	guīlái	歸來		ST 30	qìchōng	氣衝
ST 31	bìguān	髀關		ST 32	fútù	伏兔
ST 33	yīnshì	陰市		ST 34	liángqiū	梁丘
ST 35	dúbí	犢鼻		ST 36	zúsānlǐ	足三里
ST 37	shàngjùxū	上巨虛		ST 38	tiáokǒu	條口
ST 39	xiàjùxū	下巨虛		ST 40	fēnglóng	豐隆
ST 41	jiěxī	解谿		ST 42	chōngyáng	衝陽
ST 43	xiàngǔ	陷谷		ST 44	nèitíng	內庭
ST 45	lìduì	厲兌				
SP 1	yǐnbái	隱白		SP 2	dàdū	大都
SP 3	tàibái	太白		SP 4	gōngsūn	公孫
SP 5	shāngqiū	商丘		SP 6	sānyīnjiāo	三陰交
SP 7	lòugǔ	漏谷		SP 8	dìjī	地機
SP 9	yīnlíngquán	陰陵泉		SP 10	xuèhǎi	血海
SP 11	jīmén	箕門		SP 12	chōngmén	衝門
SP 13	fǔshè	府舍		SP 14	fùjié	腹結
SP 15	dàhéng	大橫		SP 16	fùāi	腹哀
SP 17	shídòu	食竇		SP 18	tiānxī	天谿
SP 19	xiōngxiāng	胸鄉		SP 20	zhōuróng	周榮
SP 21	dàbāo	大包				
HT 1	jíquán	極泉		HT 2	qīnglíng	青靈
HT 3	shàohǎi	少海		HT 4	língdào	靈道
HT 5	tōnglǐ	通里		HT 6	yīnxì	陰郄
HT 7	shénmén	神門		HT 8	shàofǔ	少府
HT 9	shàochōng	少衝				
SI 1	shàozé	少澤		SI 2	qiángǔ	前谷
SI 3	hòuxī	後谿		SI 4	wàngǔ	腕骨
SI 5	yánggǔ	陽谷		SI 6	yǎnglǎo	養老
SI 7	zhīzhèng	支正		SI 8	xiǎohǎi	小海
SI 9	jiānzhēn	肩貞		SI 10	nàoshù	臑俞
SI 11	tiānzōng	天宗		SI 12	bǐngfēng	秉風
SI 13	qūyuán	曲垣		SI 14	jiānwàishù	肩外俞
SI 15	jiānzhōngshù	肩中俞		SI 16	tiānchuāng	天窗
SI 17	tiānróng	天容		SI 18	quánliáo	顴髎
SI 19	tīnggōng	聽宮				
BL 1	jīngmíng	睛明		BL 2	cuánzhú	攢竹
BL 3	méichōng	眉衝		BL 4	qūchā(qūchāi)	曲差
BL 5	wǔchù	五處		BL 6	chéngguāng	承光
BL 7	tōngtiān	通天		BL 8	luòquè	絡卻
BL 9	yùzhěn	玉枕		BL 10	tiānzhù	天柱
BL 11	dàzhù	大杼		BL 12	fēngmén	風門
BL 13	fèishù	肺俞		BL 14	juéyīnshù	厥陰俞
BL 15	xīnshù	心俞		BL 16	dūshù	督俞

BL 17	géshù	膈俞	BL 18	gānshù	肝俞
BL 19	dǎnshù	膽俞	BL 20	píshù	脾俞
BL 21	wèishù	胃俞	BL 22	sānjiāoshù	三焦俞
BL 23	shènshù	腎俞	BL 24	qìhǎishù	氣海俞
BL 25	dàchángshù	大腸俞	BL 26	guānyuánshù	關元俞
BL 27	xiǎochángshù	小腸俞	BL 28	pángguāngshù	膀胱俞
BL 29	zhōnglǚshù	中膂俞	BL 30	báihuánshù	白環俞
BL 31	shàngliáo	上髎	BL 32	cìliáo	次髎
BL 33	zhōngliáo	中髎	BL 34	xiàliáo	下髎
BL 35	huìyáng	會陽	BL 36	chéngfú	承扶
BL 37	yínmén	殷門	BL 38	fúxì	浮郄
BL 39	wěiyáng	委陽	BL 40	wěizhōng	委中
BL 41	fùfēn	附分	BL 42	pòhù	魄戶
BL 43	gāohuāng	膏肓	BL 44	shéntáng	神堂
BL 45	yìxǐ	譩譆	BL 46	géguān	隔關
BL 47	húnmén	魂門	BL 48	yánggāng	陽綱
BL 49	yìshè	意舍	BL 50	wèicāng	胃倉
BL 51	huāngmén	肓門	BL 52	zhìshì	志室
BL 53	bāohuāng	胞肓	BL 54	zhìbiān	秩邊
BL 55	héyáng	合陽	BL 56	chéngjīn	承筋
BL 57	chéngshān	承山	BL 58	fēiyáng	飛揚
BL 59	fūyáng	跗陽	BL 60	kūnlún	崑崙
BL 61	púcān	僕參	BL 62	shēnmài	申脈
BL 63	jīnmén	金門	BL 64	jīnggǔ	京骨
BL 65	shùgǔ	束骨	BL 66	zútōnggǔ	足通谷
BL 67	zhìyīn	至陰			
KI 1	yǒngquán	湧泉	KI 2	rángǔ	然谷
KI 3	tàixī	太谿	KI 4	dàzhōng	大鍾
KI 5	shuǐquán	水泉	KI 6	zhàohǎi	照海
KI 7	fùliū	復溜	KI 8	jiāoxìn	交信
KI 9	zhùbīn	築賓	KI 10	yīngǔ	陰谷
KI 11	hénggǔ	橫骨	KI 12	dàhè	大赫
KI 13	qìxué	氣穴	KI 14	sìmǎn	四滿
KI 15	zhōngzhù	中注	KI 16	huāngshù	肓俞
KI 17	shāngqū	商曲	KI 18	shíguān	石關
KI 19	yīndū	陰都	KI 20	fùtōnggǔ	腹通谷
KI 21	yōumén	幽門	KI 22	bùláng	步廊
KI 23	shénfēng	神封	KI 24	língxū	靈墟
KI 25	shēncáng	神藏	KI 26	yùzhōng	彧中
KI 27	shùfǔ	俞府			
PC 1	tiānchí	天池	PC 2	tiānquán	天泉
PC 3	qūzé	曲澤	PC 4	xìmén	郄門
PC 5	jiānshǐ	間使	PC 6	nèiguān	內關
PC 7	dàlíng	大陵	PC 8	láogōng	勞宮
PC 9	zhōngchōng	中衝			
TE 1	guānchōng	關衝	TE 2	yèmén	液門

TE 3	zhōngzhǔ	中渚	TE 4	yángchí	陽池
TE 5	wàiguān	外關	TE 6	zhīgōu	支溝
TE 7	huìzōng	會宗	TE 8	sānyángluò	三陽絡
TE 9	sìdú	四瀆	TE 10	tiānjǐng	天井
TE 11	qīnglěngyuān	清冷淵	TE 12	xiāoluò	消濼
TE 13	nàohuì	臑會	TE 14	jiānliáo	肩髎
TE 15	tiānliáo	天髎	TE 16	tiānyǒu	天牖
TE 17	yìfēng	翳風	TE 18	chìmài	瘈脈
TE 19	lúxī	顱息	TE 20	jiǎosūn	角孫
TE 21	ěrmén	耳門	TE 22	ěrhéliáo	和髎
TE 23	sīzhúkōng	絲竹空			
GB 1	tóngzǐliáo	瞳子髎	GB 2	tīnghuì	聽會
GB 3	shàngguān	上關	GB 4	hànyàn	頷厭
GB 5	xuánlú	懸顱	GB 6	xuánlí	懸釐
GB 7	qūbìn	曲鬢	GB 8	shuàigǔ	率谷
GB 9	tiānchōng	天衝	GB 10	fúbái	浮白
GB 11	tóuqiàoyīn	頭竅陰	GB 12	wángǔ	完骨
GB 13	běnshén	本神	GB 14	yángbái	陽白
GB 15	tóulínqì	頭臨泣	GB 16	mùchuāng	目窗
GB 17	zhèngyíng	正營	GB 18	chénglíng	承靈
GB 19	nǎokōng	腦空	GB 20	fēngchí	風池
GB 21	jiānjǐng	肩井	GB 22	yuānyè	淵腋
GB 23	zhéjīn	輒筋	GB 24	rìyuè	日月
GB 25	jīngmén	京門	GB 26	dàimài	帶脈
GB 27	wǔshū	五樞	GB 28	wéidào	維道
GB 29	jūliáo	居髎	GB 30	huántiào	環跳
GB 31	fēngshì	風市	GB 32	zhōngdú	中瀆
GB 33	xīyángguān	膝陽關	GB 34	yánglíngquán	陽陵泉
GB 35	yángjiāo	陽交	GB 36	wàiqiū	外丘
GB 37	guāngmíng	光明	GB 38	yángfǔ	陽輔
GB 39	xuánzhōng	懸鍾	GB 40	qiūxū	丘墟
GB 41	zúlínqì	足臨泣	GB 42	dìwǔhuì	地五會
GB 43	xiáxī	俠谿	GB 44	zúqiàoyīn	足竅陰
LR 1	dàdūn	大敦	LR 2	xíngjiān	行間
LR 3	tàichōng	太衝	LR 4	zhōngfēng	中封
LR 5	lígōu	蠡溝	LR 6	zhōngdū	中都
LR 7	xīguān	膝關	LR 8	qūquán	曲泉
LR 9	yīnbāo	陰包	LR 10	zúwǔlǐ	足五里
LR 11	yīnlián	陰廉	LR 12	jímài	急脈
LR 13	zhāngmén	章門	LR 14	qīmén	期門
GV1	chángqiáng	長強	GV2	yāoshù	腰俞
GV3	yāoyángguān	腰陽關	GV4	mìngmén	命門
GV5	xuánshū	懸樞	GV6	jǐzhōng	脊中
GV7	zhōngshū	中樞	GV8	jīnsuō	筋縮
GV9	zhìyáng	至陽	GV10	língtái	靈臺
GV11	shéndào	神道	GV12	shēnzhù	身柱

GV13	táodào	陶道	GV14	dàzhuī	大椎
GV15	yǎmén	瘂門	GV16	fēngfǔ	風府
GV17	nǎohù	腦戶	GV18	qiángjiān	強間
GV19	hòudǐng	後頂	GV20	bǎihuì	百會
GV21	qiándǐng	前頂	GV22	xìnhuì	顖會
GV23	shàngxīng	上星	GV24	shéntíng	神庭
GV25	sùliáo	素髎	GV26	shuǐgōu	水溝
GV27	duìduān	兌端	GV28	yínjiāo	齦交
CV1	huìyīn	會陰	CV2	qūgǔ	曲骨
CV3	zhōngjí	中極	CV4	guānyuán	關元
CV5	shímén	石門	CV6	qìhǎi	氣海
CV7	yīnjiāo	陰交	CV8	shénquè	神闕
CV9	shuǐfēn	水分	CV10	xiàwǎn	下脘
CV11	jiànlǐ	建里	CV12	zhōngwǎn	中脘
CV13	shàngwǎn	上脘	CV14	jùquè	巨闕
CV15	jiūwěi	鳩尾	CV16	zhōngtíng	中庭
CV17	dànzhōng	膻中	CV18	yùtáng	玉堂
CV19	zǐgōng	紫宮	CV20	huágài	華蓋
CV21	xuánjī	璇璣	CV22	tiāntū	天突
CV23	liánquán	廉泉	CV24	chéngjiāng	承漿

The 48 extra points

EX-HN1	sìshéncōng	四神聰	EX-HN2	dāngyáng	當陽
EX-HN3	yìntáng	印堂	EX-HN4	yùyāo	魚腰
EX-HN5	tàiyáng	太陽	EX-HN6	ěrjiān	耳尖
EX-HN7	qiúhòu	球後	EX-HN8	shàngyíngxiāng	上迎香
EX-HN9	nèiyíngxiāng	內迎香	EX-HN10	jùquán	聚泉
EX-HN11	hǎiquán	海泉	EX-HN12	jīnjīn	金津
EX-HN13	yùyè	玉液	EX-HN14	yìmíng	翳明
EX-HN15	jǐngbǎiláo	頸百勞			
EX-CA1	zǐgōng	子宮			
EX-B1	dìngchuǎn	定喘	EX-B2	jiájǐ	夾脊
EX-B3	wèiwǎnxiàshù	胃脘下俞	EX-B4	pǐgēn	痞根
EX-B5	xiàzhìshì	下志室	EX-B6	yāoyí	腰宜
EX-B7	yāoyǎn	腰眼	EX-B8	shíqīzhuī	十七椎
EX-B9	yāoqí	腰奇			
EX-UE1	zhǒujiān	肘尖	EX-UE2	èrbái	二白
EX-UE3	zhōngquán	中泉	EX-UE4	zhōngkuí	中魁
EX-UE5	dàgǔkōng	大骨空	EX-UE6	xiǎogǔkōng	小骨空
EX-UE7	yāotòngdiǎn	腰痛點	EX-UE8	wàiláogōng	外勞宮
EX-UE9	bāxié	八邪	EX-UE10	sìfèng	四縫
EX-Uē	shíxuān	十宣			
EX-LE1	kuāngǔ	髖骨	EX-LE2	hèdǐng	鶴頂
EX-LE3	xīnèi	膝內	EX-LE4	nèixīyǎn	內膝眼
EX-LE5	xīyǎn	膝眼	EX-LE6	dǎnnáng	膽囊

EX-LE7	lánwěi	闌尾	EX-LE8	nèihuáijiān	內踝尖
EX-LE9	wàihuáijiān	外踝尖	EX-LE10	bāfēng	八風
EX-Lē	dúyīn	獨陰	EX-LE12	qìduān	氣端

INDEX

ACKNOWLEDGEMENT

I am indebted to Dr. Zhang Xue-zhi, deputy director, and Ms Li Ning, senior technician, department of integrated Chinese and Western medicine, the First College of Clinical Medicine, Peking University, for their great help with collecting the source materials.

ABOUT THE AUTHOR

Dr. Xie Zhufan is a professor of both Western and Chinese medicine and honorary director of the Institute of Integrative Chinese-Western Medicine of the First Clinical Medical College, Peking University. He has been appointed three times as a consultant on traditional medicine by the World Health Organization, and has been invited on many occasions to give lectures on Chinese medicine at overseas medical schools. He has great experience in expressing Chinese medical concepts and knowledge in English. He and his associates compiled the *Common Terms of Traditional Chinese Medicine* in English. It was published by the Beijing Medical College Press in 1980, as the first Chinese-English dictionary of traditional Chinese medicine in China. Since it was widely welcomed, the Commercial Press, Hong Kong, published a revised edition titled *Beijing Medical College Dictionary of Traditional Chinese Medicine* (1984). Prof. Xie was then asked to help with the compilation of the traditional Chinese medicine part of the *Chinese-English Medical Dictionary* by the Ministry of Health, People's Republic of China (1987). He won a special award from the Ministry of Health for his outstanding contributions to that work. Together with his colleagues, he compiled the *Classified Dictionary of Traditional Chinese Medicine* (1994). In 2000, he was assigned by the State Administration of Traditional Chinese Medicine to pursue a research project on the standardization of the English translation of Chinese medical terminology. In this research he collected a large amount of source materials for the new edition of the *Classified Dictionary of Traditional Chinese Medicine* (2002). In the same year, he drafted a technical document relating to "International Standard Acupuncture Terminology for Basic Training" for the World Health Organization. The present book provides the groundwork for the standard nomenclature of commonly used traditional Chinese medical terms, including those that are necessary for the training of acupuncturists.

Dr. Xie graduated from the Medical College of Peking University (also called Beijing Medical College or Beijing Medical University at different periods) in 1946. He then practiced Western internal medicine for more than 20 years at the First Hospital of the College. Because of his achievements in cardiology and nephrology, he was promoted to deputy director of the department of internal medicine. In 1955, he was trained as an acupuncture teacher at a special course organized by the Ministry of Health. He then set up the department of acupuncture in the First Hospital of the College, practicing Western medicine at the same time. In the late 1960s he took a refresher course in traditional Chinese medicine, and in 1970 he became the director of the department of traditional Chinese medicine at the First Hospital of the College, and in 1987 the director of the Institute of Integrative Chinese-Western Medicine. He won the State Administration of Traditional Chinese Medicine Award for Scientific and Technological Advancement in 1992 for his systematic studies of basic traditional medical theory.

His educational and professional experience has provided him with extensive knowledge, which he has used to compile the present book. In recent years, he has published the following books on traditional Chinese medicine in English, besides dictionaries:

Chinese Acupuncture and Moxibustion, translated by Xie et al., Foreign Languages Press, 1987.

Traditional Chinese Internal Medicine, written by Xie and Liao, Foreign Languages Press, 1993.

Best of Traditional Chinese Medicine, New World Press, 1995.

Practical Traditional Chinese Medicine, Foreign Languages Press, 2000.

Prof. Xie was one of the editors of the *Pharmacopoeia of the People's Republic of China* (English Edition) Vol. I, 1997. In addition, he has contributed two special papers to the publications of the World Health Organization:

``The Harmonization of Traditional and Modern Medicine,'' *Traditional Medicine in Asia*, edited by Ranjit Roy Chaudhury and Uton Muchtar Rafei, World Health Organization Regional Office for South-East Asia, 2002, pp. 115-134.

The draft of *Acupuncture: Review and Analysis of Reports on Controlled Clinical Trials*, World Health Organization, Geneva, 2002.

图书在版编目（CIP）数据

英文中医名词术语标准化 / 谢竹藩 著.
－北京：外文出版社，2003.10
ISBN 7－119－03339－5

I. 英… II. 谢… III. 中国医药学－名词术语－英文
IV. R2－61

中国版本图书馆 CIP 数据核字（2003）第 048555 号

责任编辑　胡开敏
英文编辑　郁　苓
封面设计　蔡　荣
印刷监制　冯　浩

英文中医名词术语标准化

谢竹藩　著

*

©外文出版社
外文出版社出版
（中国北京百万庄大街 24 号）
邮政编码　100037
外文出版社网址: http://www.flp.com.cn
外文出版社电子信箱: info@flp.com.cn
sales@flp.com.cn

三河市汇鑫印务有限公司印刷
中国国际图书贸易总公司发行
（中国北京车公庄西路 35 号）
北京邮政信箱第 399 号　邮政编码　100044
2003 年 (小 16 开) 第 1 版
2003 年 10 月第 1 版第 1 次印刷
（英）
ISBN 7－119－03339－5 / R·189 (外)
07200(平)
14－E－3554 P